ISGE Series

Series Editor

Andrea R. Genazzani, International Society of Gynecological Endocrinology, Pisa, Italy

The ISGE Book Series is the expression of the partnership between the International Society of Gynecological Endocrinology and Springer. The book series includes single monographs devoted to gynecological endocrinology relevant topics as well as the contents stemming from educational activities run by ISGRE, the educational branch of the society. This series is meant to be an important tool for physicians who want to advance their understanding of gynecological endocrinology and master this difficult clinical area. The International Society of Gynecological ad Reproductive Endocrinology (ISGRE) School fosters education and clinical application of modern gynecological endocrinology throughout the world by organizing high-level, highly focused residential courses twice a year, the Winter and the Summer Schools. World renowned experts are invited to provide their clinical experience and their scientific update to the scholars, creating a unique environment where science and clinical applications melt to provide the definitive update in this continuously evolving field. Key review papers are published in the Series, thus providing a broad overview over time on the major areas of gynecological endocrinology.

More information about this series at http://www.springer.com/series/11871

Andrea R. Genazzani • Lourdes Ibáñez
Andrzej Milewicz • Duru Shah
Editors

Impact of Polycystic Ovary, Metabolic Syndrome and Obesity on Women Health

Volume 8: Frontiers in Gynecological Endocrinology

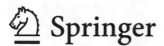

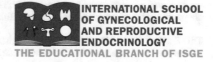

INTERNATIONAL SCHOOL
OF GYNECOLOGICAL
AND REPRODUCTIVE
ENDOCRINOLOGY
THE EDUCATIONAL BRANCH OF ISGE

Editors
Andrea R. Genazzani
International Society of Gynecological
Endocrinology
Pisa
Italy

Lourdes Ibáñez
Endocrinology Department
Hospital Sant Joan de Déu Barcelona
Barcelona
Spain

Andrzej Milewicz
Department of Endocrinology, Diabetology
Wrocław Medical University
Wroclaw
Poland

Duru Shah
Obstetrics and Gynecology
Gynaecworld
Mumbai
India

ISSN 2197-8735 ISSN 2197-8743 (electronic)
ISGE Series
ISBN 978-3-030-63652-4 ISBN 978-3-030-63650-0 (eBook)
https://doi.org/10.1007/978-3-030-63650-0

This Springer imprint is published by the registered company Springer Nature Switzerland AG
The registered company address is: Gewerbestrasse 11, 6330 Cham, Switzerland

Preface

This volume analyzes the impact of polycystic ovary syndrome (PCOS), metabolic syndrome (MS), and obesity on women's reproductive function and health from adolescence to elderly.

Starting from the description and importance of Brain Phenotype in PCOS, the volume analyzes the impact of adolescence as a high-risk period for PCOS development and the strategies to be used toward adolescent PCOS to prevent adult anovulation.

The possible responsibility of environmental factors in developing obesity and insulin resistance as well as the metabolic and neuroendocrine aspects of PCOS pathogenesis are presented considering their implications on the future therapeutic strategies.

The impact of PCOS, MS, and obesity on follicular growth arrest in women's health and the role of PCOS on women's quality of life and sexual health are extensively discussed as well as the impact on female infertility and treatment and on the management of PCOS women preparing pregnancy and pregnancy outcome.

Specific chapters are also dedicated to the role of insulin resistance in benign breast diseases and the impact of PCOS on inflammation, metabolic changes, and menopause, on cardiovascular function, and, last but not least, on how to prevent, diagnose, and treat gynecological cancers in PCOS patients.

This volume represent a very comprehensive effort to clarify how to better understand, recognize, and treat PCOS patients with personalized therapies according to the goals to be reached for their health, reproductive needs, and quality of life.

Pisa, Italy   Andrea R. Genazzani
Barcelona, Spain   Lourdes Ibáñez
Wroclaw, Poland   Andrzej Milewicz
Mumbai, India   Duru Shah

Contents

The Brain Phenotype in Polycystic Ovary Syndrome (PCOS): Androgens, Anovulation, and Gender

Sarah L. Berga

1.1 Introduction

Polycystic ovary syndrome (PCOS) is a common condition with reproductive and metabolic features. Recent studies confirmed that women with PCOS have multiple genetic allelic variants that are independently associated with hyperandrogenism, gonadotropin regulation, timing of menopause, depression, and metabolic disturbances, including insulin resistance [1]. Of note, the data cited above showed that not all women with PCOS possess the full complement of the 14 genetic variants identified. Genetic heterogeneity results in clinical heterogeneity. We have long recognized that there is a spectrum of clinical presentation, with some women having a more pronounced reproductive phenotype and others presenting primarily with metabolic features. Despite variation related to PCOS genotype and phenotype, however, two long-recognized pathogenic themes remain the same: excess androgen exposure and insulin resistance. Since androgens and insulin modulate of brain architecture and function, it is not surprising that PCOS is associated with a brain phenotype, but also one that presents variably. Building on the notion that the brain is a target of hormones of all classes, in this chapter we characterize the brain phenotype in PCOS and explore the evidence that the brain phenotype is the result of androgen exposure that not only predisposes to anovulation and obesity but also has the potential to skew gender identity and sexual orientation.

S. L. Berga (✉)
Department of Obstetrics and Gynecology, Jacobs School of Medicine and Biomedical Sciences, University at Buffalo SUNY, Buffalo, NY, USA
e-mail: slberga@buffalo.edu

© International Society of Gynecological Endocrinology 2021
A. R. Genazzani et al. (eds.), *Impact of Polycystic Ovary, Metabolic Syndrome and Obesity on Women Health*, ISGE Series,
https://doi.org/10.1007/978-3-030-63650-0_1

1.2   Anovulation Reflects the PCOS Brain Phenotype

A key paradox in the presentation of PCOS is chronic anovulation despite an abundance of oocytes (polycystic ovaries). This paradox was one of the first clues to the unique brain phenotype in PCOS associated with reproductive dysfunction. Subsequent studies found that the primary cause of anovulation in PCOS was not resistance to FSH but an insufficient rise in FSH to initiate folliculogenesis. It is now widely appreciated that exogenous FSH administration readily initiates folliculogenesis in women with PCOS and that follicle development is often so exuberant that ovarian hyperstimulation results. Not only are FSH levels insufficient, paradoxically, LH levels are tonically high. The elevated LH/FSH ratio characteristic of women with PCOS catalyzed an investigative search for an explanation. As shown in Fig. 1.1, one likely contributor to increased LH and reduced FSH levels is increased GnRH-LH drive [2, 3]. As shown in Fig. 1.2, GnRH-LH pulse frequency in women with PCOS approaches that of men, namely, one LH pulse per hour, rather than one pulse every 90 minutes observed in eumenorrheic, ovulatory women [2]. Studies in men with idiopathic hypothalamic hypogonadism revealed that the more rapid the pulse frequency of exogenously administered GnRH, the higher the

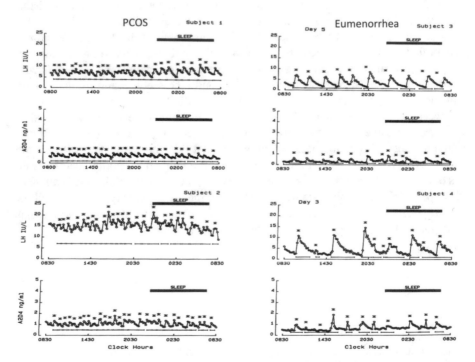

Fig. 1.1 GnRH-LH and alpha-subunit pulse patterns in 9 women with polycystic ovary syndrome (PCOS) (left) and 9 eumenorrheic, ovulatory women (right). Blood samples were obtained at 10-min intervals fro 24 h from an indwelling intravenous catheter and pulse patterns were analyzed using a computer-based algorithm. Berga et al. [2]

Fig. 1.2 24-h LH and alpha-subunit number in eumenorrheic, ovulatory women eumenorrhea and women with polycystic ovary syndrome (PCOS). EW mean 17.1 ± 1.7 (SEM) vs PCOS 23.0 ± 0.7, p < 0.01. The mean interpulse interval was 84 min for EW and 63 min for PCOS. Original graph. Berga et al. [2]

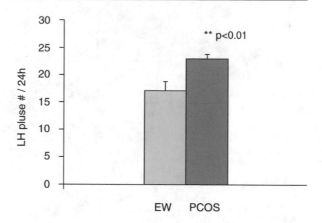

LH and the lower the FSH levels [4]. Subsequent studies showed that low dose testosterone increased GnRH-LH pulse frequency in eumenorrheic women and that high dose testosterone increased GnRH-LH pulse frequency in women with PCOS. Further, we and others also showed that the increased GnRH-LH drive in PCOS was resistant to suppression by sex steroids [5, 6] and that sensitivity to sex steroid suppression was restored by the androgen receptor blocker flutamide [7], but not by metformin [8]. The above evidence suggests that androgen exposure causes the rapid GnRH pulse frequency and explains the skewed LH/FSH ratio observed in women with PCOS.

1.3 Neuroregulation of GnRH and the Brain Phenotype in PCOS

An explosion in knowledge regarding the regulation of GnRH over the last 30 years has afforded us the opportunity to identify factors that mediate the development of the brain phenotype in women with PCOS. We now understand that neurodevelopment and neuroregulation is much more than sex steroid exposure, although clearly androgens, estrogens, and progesterone are major modifiers of both. However, other hormones, including peptides, growth, and immune factors also influence neurodevelopment and neuroactivity.

The discovery that the kisspeptin peptide system serves as a key proximate regulator of GnRH pulsatility revolutionized our understanding of the neuroregulation of reproductive function. Within the arcuate nucleus, kisspeptin/neurokinin B/dynorphin (KNDy) neurons release the prohormone kisspeptin, a 145 amino acid protein that is enzymatically cleaved to a 54 amino acid peptide known as kisspeption-54. The kisspeptin receptor, abbreviated GPR54 for G protein-coupled receptor 54, is expressed on GnRH neurons, allowing kisspeptin to activate GnRH neurons [9]. Exogenously administered kisspeptin exerts a profound stimulatory effect on gonadotropin secretion in animal and human models. Both testosterone and

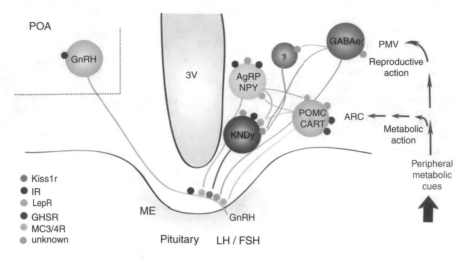

Fig. 1.3 Schematic representation of neural interactions between metabolic and reproductive functions depicting likely sites of action of leptin, insulin, and ghrelin to control GnRH release. 3 V, third ventricle; ARC, arcuate nucleus; ME, median eminence; PMV, ventral pre-mammillary nucleus; POA, preoptic area. Navarro and Kaiser [11]

estradiol regulate *Kiss1* gene expression. In addition to activating GnRH neurons, kisspeptin neurons also form synapses with GnRH neuron terminals in the median eminence, where GnRH release (exocytosis) is stimulated by kisspeptin [10]. Figure 1.3 shows the central cascade that regulates GnRH and highlights the role of KNDy neurons [11].

As shown in Fig. 1.3, GABA (gamma-aminobutyric acid) neuronal input modulates the entire cascade, including kisspeptin neurons, and directly and indirectly regulates GnRH drive. Importantly, the GABAergic network integrates external environmental and internal host signals to align reproductive function with individual circumstance. Thus, stress, sex steroids, and metabolic signals regulate GABAergic tone and the entire cascade by direct and indirect mechanisms. For example, in a monkey model, the administration of the CRH antagonist, astressin B, reversed the impact of the chronic social stress of subordination on GABA-A receptor binding in the prefrontal cortex, a site implicated in the regulation of the limbic-hypothalamic-pituitary-adrenal, −gonadal, and -thyroidal axes [12]. A recent study found that chronic administration of letrozole to female mice induced polycystic ovaries, anovulation, elevated testosterone, increased LH pulsatility, and elevated kisspeptin and neurokinin B gene expression in the arcuate nucleus [13]. In a murine model, leptin-responsive GABAergic neurons regulated fertility through pathways that reduced kisspeptinergic tone [14].

Androgens play a fundamental role in the organization and activation of the hypothalamic circuitry shown in Fig. 1.3. The mechanisms by which androgens act are many. Androgens increase GABAergic innervation of KNDy neurons and alter sex steroid feedback sensitivity [15]. Administration of dihydrotestosterone (DHT), a non-aromatizable androgen, to mice increased GnRH firing activity [16]. In a sheep model of PCOS, prenatal testosterone exposure increased GABAergic synaptic inputs to and stimulation of GnRH and KNDy neurons [17]. Androgen exposure acting via an androgen receptor mechanism also impaired progesterone receptor transcription, impaired negative feedback, and resulted in GnRH neuronal hyperactivity [18]. Absence of progesterone signaling in kisspeptin neurons disrupted the LH surge and impaired fertility in female mice [19]. In a mouse model of DHT-induced PCOS, selective deletion of the androgen receptor (AR) in neurons, but not granulosa cells, reversed the impact of DHT, leading the investigators to conclude that neuroendocrine genomic AR signaling is an important extra-ovarian mediator of the PCOS phenocopy in mice [20]. The above preclinical studies likely explain why GnRH drive in women with PCOS was resistant to suppression by progestin and progesterone feedback [5–7]. Thus, as shown in Fig. 1.3, KNDy neurons and kisspeptin-GPR54 receptors form the final common pathway in the hypothalamic circuitry that regulates GnRH drive [9]; GABAergic tone modulates the function of the kisspeptinergic pathway and confers feedback sensitivity to sex steroids and metabolic signals.

The term hyperandrogenic anovulation parsimoniously conceptualizes PCOS and conveys the notion that androgens of ovarian origin initiate and maintain the brain phenotype responsible for anovulation, namely, increased GnRH-LH drive and chronic insufficiency of FSH. To investigate the role of androgens and GABA in human PCOS, we compared cerebrospinal fluid (CSF) levels of GABA, testosterone, and estradiol in eumenorrheic, ovulatory women and those with PCOS [21]. Figure 1.4 shows that women with PCOS not only have higher CSF levels of

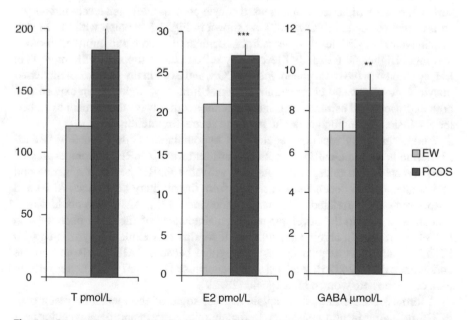

Fig. 1.4 Increased cerebrospinal fluid levels of GABA, testosterone (T), and estradiol (E2) in 12 women with polycystic ovary syndrome as compared to 15 eumenorrheic, ovulatory women (EW). Original graph. Kawwass et al. [21]

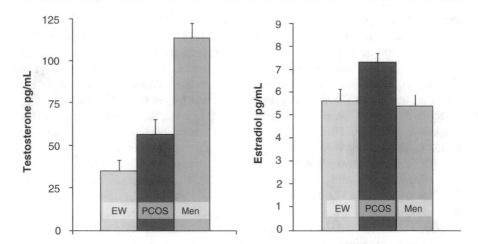

Fig. 1.5 Cerebrospinal fluid levels of testosterone and estradiol in 15 eumenorrheic, ovulatory women, 14 women with PCOS, and 6 men. Unpublished data from Berga lab

testosterone and GABA but also higher CSF levels of estradiol. While the CSF levels of testosterone in PCOS were not as high as the levels in men (Fig. 1.5), they were clearly higher than the levels in eumenorrheic, ovulatory women. Thus, the brain phenotype in PCOS that predisposes to chronic anovulation despite increased oocyte endowment most likely results from chronically increased androgen exposure, which, in turn, reflects an increased oocyte pool, as androgen levels and oocyte endowment correlate in PCOS [22]. As shown in Fig. 1.5, women with PCOS also displayed higher CSF levels of estradiol as compared to both eumenorrheic women and men. Higher CSF estradiol levels may differentially suppress FSH more than LH, contribute to the brain phenotype in PCOS, and explain the paradox of increased oocyte endowment and chronic anovulation. Ultimately, higher brain exposure to both androgens and estradiol imprints the brain in other ways that remain to be better elucidated, including gender identity and sexual orientation.

Another recently reported regulator of hypothalamic GnRH function is anti-Müllerian hormone (AMH). In both humans and mice, GnRH neurons expressed AMH receptors. In mice, AMH potently activated GnRH neuron firing rate and accentuated GnRH-dependent LH release from the pituitary [23]. Since AMH and testosterone are correlated with oocyte endowment [22], AMH also could play a fundamental role in the development and maintenance of the brain phenotype in PCOS that results in chronic anovulation. If so, this may explain why women with PCOS display more regular cycles as they age because AMH levels and oocyte endowment drop [24, 25]; a later age at menopause [1, 26, 27]; and better fertility than eumenorrheic women after age 40 [28, 29].

Androgen excess may also explain at least some of the metabolic features of PCOS including insulin resistance. In female mice, excess androgen receptor activation in neurons caused peripheral insulin resistance and pancreatic beta cell dysfunction [30]. In contrast, selectively knocking out the androgen receptor in neurons of female mice decreased glucose and insulin levels in fasted and fed states as compared to wild-type female mice [31]. Ultimately, the most parsimonious explanation for PCOS, including the reproductive brain phenotype, is androgen excess in an XX genotype.

1.4   Gender Identity and Sexual Orientation

The brain orchestrates many functions in addition to reproductive function. What are the possible consequences of brain androgenization in women with PCOS other than increased GnRH pulsatility? Both insulin resistance and a tendency to weight gain likely reflect brain androgenization. Other behavioral variables that could be attributable at least in part to brain androgenization include stress sensitivity, mood, gender identity, and sexual orientation. While sex refers to genetic sex, which is readily determined because it is a biological attribute, gender refers to a set of behavioral expectations assigned according to genetic sex. However, gender is a cultural construct; the attributes considered male and female varies somewhat across cultures. Some cultures define gender as male, female, and other, while other cultures have a strictly binary view. Currently, cultures around the world are grappling with a more expanded perspective on gender.

At least two key important questions deserve increased clinical attention to better care for women with PCOS. First, do women with PCOS differ in terms of gender identity from eumenorrheic, ovulatory women? Second, do women with PCOS differ in terms of sexual orientation from eumenorrheic, ovulatory women? Given that our understanding of the role of prenatal and postnatal hormone exposures as contributors to brain organization and activation is limited, it should not be surprising that our understating of the impact of hormones on gender identity and sexual orientation is also constrained. However, current evidence based on neuroimaging and clinical studies suggests that women with PCOS differ from eumenorrheic women in terms of the proportion that report nonconforming gender identity and lesbianism.

To delve into the topic of gender identify and sexual orientation requires an appreciation of the notion that sex steroid exposures in utero organize the brain. At the time of puberty and during the ensuring reproductive years, gonadal hormones activate the already sexually dimorphic brain, which results in gender asymmetries and sex-specific attributes [32, 33]. There are many clinical studies showing that sex hormone exposures modulate attention, comprehension, reaction time, and memory. One of the critical behavioral consequences of gonadal hormonal exposures is altered information processing [34]. In a recent review, McCarthy and Arnold suggested that estradiol is a masculinizing hormone and exerts multiple region-specific effects via distinct cellular mechanisms [35]. During the perinatal sensitive period, estradiol promotes cell survival, cell death, and cell proliferation in separate brain regions and promotes the formation of new dendritic spine synapses in some brain regions while suppressing them in others. Essentially, hormonal exposures "sculpt" the brain. The enduring organizational effects of exposure to estradiol are mediated in part via epigenetic changes to the DNA and chromatin in processes that are region-specific. Given the organizational complexity of the brain and the spectrum of hormonal exposures, the potential for neurocomplexity is enormous. Unfortunately, neither our lexicon nor our cultural and medical constructs adequately capture the neurocomplexity of gender identity and sexual orientation. Certainly, it is unlikely that gender is dichotomous. At this time, it might be best to assume that the actual range of neurodiversity is not "visible" due to the dissonance between biological complexity and cultural stereotypes that constrain individual expression.

Our study of CSF levels of estradiol and testosterone in women with PCOS revealed increased brain exposure to both estradiol and testosterone as compared to eumenorrheic women [21]. For women with PCOS, altered sex steroid exposure likely began in utero, resumed at puberty, and continued at least until menopause. The altered steroid milieu differentially organizes the brain architecture and then differentially activates brain function. As McCarthy and Arnold [35] suggest, altered sex steroid hormone exposures likely result in a spectrum, mosaic or hybrid of brain masculinization versus feminization that might be best termed gender neurodiversity.

Few investigations have directly determined the gender identity and sexual orientation of women with PCOS. Agrawal et al. [36] found that 80% of lesbian women versus 32% of heterosexual women had polycystic ovarian morphology (PCOM) on ultrasound. Nearly all transmen (female to male transgender) had PCOM [37]. Women with congenital adrenal hyperplasia showed increased rates of bisexual and homosexual orientation that correlated with prenatal androgenization. Bisexual and homosexual orientation also correlated with global measures of masculinization of non-sexual behavior and was predicted by childhood behavior [38, 39].

Neuroimaging of women with PCOS and congenital adrenal hyperplasia has revealed additional neurocomplexity that likely reflects the interaction of hyperandrogenism in an XX genotype, including sex-specific hormone action. The findings do not easily fit into the conventional mindset that gender identity and sexual orientation exist on a spectrum of maleness to femaleness. Rather the data suggest that gender nonconforming is a unique brain state. Lentini et al. [40] analyzed the contributions of genetic sex and androgen exposure and found that cerebellar and precentral gray matter volume was related to X-chromosome escapee genes in the amygdala, parahippocampus, and occipital cortex and that gray matter volume correlated with testosterone levels regardless of sex. They concluded that brain asymmetries are attributable to sex hormones and X-chromosome genes in a regionally differentiated manner [41]. Using PET scanning with ^{15}O-H$_2$O, Savic et al. [42] showed that sex-specific pheromones elicited sex-differentiated hypothalamic activation in heterosexual women and men; however, homosexual men and women responded to pheromone exposure according to sexual orientation rather than biological sex [43, 44]. Two parameters previously shown to be sexually dimorphic are hemispheric asymmetry and functional connectivity. Extending earlier studies, Savic and Lindström [45] found that PET and MRI revealed differences in cerebral asymmetry and functional connectivity between homo- and heterosexual subjects.

Heterosexual men and homosexual women showed rightward cerebral asymmetry while all homosexuals showed sex-atypical amygdala connections. They concluded that these results were not due to learning. Other investigators found that white matter microstructure was altered and cognitive function was compromised in young adults with PCOS independent of education and BMI [46]. Further, women with PCOS who displayed insulin resistance had greater regional activation during an emotion task than controls, and this difference resolved with metformin therapy [47]. The best synopsis of the few neuroimaging findings currently available is that brain function in women with PCOS is neither strictly male nor female and reflects a hybrid or mosaic of features.

The brain is complex. There are more than 86 billion neurons in the mammalian brain, which exceeds the number of stars in the Milky Way. In the cortex, each neuron forms about 10,000 synapses with target cells. Astonishingly, a cubic millimeter of brain contains as many as 90,000 neurons. The human brain is also an energy hog; rodents require about 5% of daily energy intake to fuel their brains while monkeys require 10%, human adults 20%, and human infants 60%. In contrast the brain is only 2% of the human body by weight, requires only 16% of cardiac output, and 25% of oxygen consumption. No wonder our brains drive us to eat. Indeed, insulin resistance may well be an adaptive response to constrain energy utilization that until recently would have represented a survival advantage as it would have rendered insulin-resistant humans "fuel independent" relative to other humans. It is important to consider PCOS in the context of human evolution and recognize that genes that conferred "energy parsimony" may have provided reproductive and survival advantages in fuel-deficient environments, which until recently have been normative. Humans generally now have fuel abundance as even nutrient poor foods fuel the brain. One has to consider that hyperandrogenism in women may have increased rather than decreased reproductive opportunity by allowing survival and conferring prolonged fertility [29]. Thus, while women with PCOS display chronic anovulation and obesity in fuel replete settings, they also display neurodiversity with regard to cognition, behavior, gender identity, and sexual orientation. Clinically it is best to acknowledge and recognize that women with PCOS may not conform to cultural expectations with regard to gender identity and sexual orientation and that they may initiate care for a variety of reasons including gender-affirming hormone therapy.

1.5   Summary

PCOS is generally understood to be a reproductive condition characterized by chronic anovulation, hyperandrogenism, obesity, and metabolic dysfunction. In PCOS, chronic anovulation reflects increased GnRH drive resulting in chronically suppressed FSH. The most likely explanation for increased GnRH drive is prenatal and sustained postnatal brain androgenization. Recent studies suggest both genotypic and phenotypic variability. Given the complexities of brain development, brain androgenization not only manifests as altered reproductive function but also gender neurodiversity. Thus, gender identity in women with PCOS may be culturally nonconforming. Gender diversity carries psychological consequences for individuals, families, and society and must be recognized and managed for better overall health. Clinical decision trees need to incorporate the variation in, and complexity of, the clinical presentation of PCOS. The medical profession must be able to offer more than ovarian suppression with oral contraceptives, ovulation induction for infertility, and metformin for metabolic dysfunction. Women with PCOS will undoubtedly benefit from holistic diagnostic and treatment algorithms that incorporate recognition of gender identity and sexual orientation and screening for mood disorders [48]. A deeper appreciation of the nuances of PCOS affords an opportunity for individualized and improved care.

References

1. Day F, Karaderi T, Jones MR, Meun C, He C, Drong A, et al. Large-scale genome-wide meta-analysis of polycystic ovary syndrome suggests shared genetic architecture for different diagnosis criteria. PLoS Genet. 2018;14(12):e1007813. https://doi.org/10.1371/journal.pgen.1007813.
2. Berga SL, Guzick DS, Winters SJ. Increased luteinizing hormone and alpha-subunit secretion in women with hyperandrogenic anovulation. J Clin Endocrinol Metab. 1993;77:895–901.
3. Kalro BN, Loucks TL, Berga SL. Neuromodulation in polycystic ovary syndrome. Obstet Gynecol Clin N Am. 2001;28:35–62.
4. Gross KM, Matsumoto AM, Berger RE, Bremner WJ. Increased frequency of pulsatile luteinizing hormone-releasing hormone administration selectively decreases follicle-stimulating hormone levels in men with idiopathic azoospermia. Fertil Steril. 1986;45:392–6.
5. Daniels TL, Berga SL. Resistance of gonadotropin releasing hormone drive to sex steroid-induced suppression in hyperandrogenic anovulation. J Clin Endocrinol Metab. 1997;82:4179–83.
6. Pastor CL, Griffin-Korf ML, Aloi JA, Evans WS, Marshall JC. Polycystic ovary syndrome: evidence for reduced sensitivity of the gonadotropin-releasing hormone pulse generator to inhibition by estradiol and progesterone. J Clin Endocrinol Metab. 1998;83:582–90.
7. Eagleson CA, Gingrich MB, Pastor CL, Arora TK, Burt CM, Evans WS, Marshall JC. Polycystic ovarian syndrome: evidence that flutamide restores sensitivity of the gonadotropin-releasing hormone pulse generator to inhibition by estradiol and progesterone. J Clin Endocrinol Metab. 2000;85:4047–52.
8. Eagleson CA, Bellows AB, Hu K, Gingrich MB, Marshall JC. Obese patients with polycystic ovary syndrome: evidence that metformin does not restore sensitivity of the gonadotropin-releasing hormone pulse generator to inhibition by ovarian steroids. J Clin Endocrinol Metab. 2003;88:5158–62.
9. Dungan HM, Clifton DK, Steiner RA. Minireview: kisspeptin neurons as central processors in the regulation of gonadotropin-releasing hormone secretion. Endocrinology. 2006;147:1154–8.
10. Ramaswamy S, Guerriero KA, Gibbs RB, Plant TM. Structural interactions between kisspeptin and GnRH neurons in the mediobasal hypothalamus of the male rhesus monkey (Macaca mulatta) as revealed by double immunofluorescence and confocal microscopy. Endocrinology. 2008;149:4387–95.
11. Navarro VM, Kaiser UB. Metabolic influences on neuroendocrine regulation of reproduction. Curr Opin Endocrinol Diabetes Obes. 2013;20:335–41.
12. Michopoulos V, Embree M, Reding K, Sanchez MM, Toufexis D, Votaw JR, Voll RJ, Goodman MM, Rivier J, Wilson ME, Berga SL. CRH receptor antagonism reverses the effect of social

subordination upon Central GABAA receptor binding in estradiol-treated ovariectomized female rhesus monkeys. Neuroscience. 2013;250:300–8.

13. Esparza LA, Schafer D, Ho BS, Thackray VG, Kauffman AS. Hyperactive LH pulses and elevated kisspeptin and neurokinin B gene expression in the arcuate nucleus of a PCOS mouse model. Endocrinology 161(4). Pii: bqaa018. 2020; https://doi.org/10.1210/endocr/bqaa018.

14. Martin C, Navarro VM, Simavli S, Vong L, Carroll RS, Lowell BB, Kaiser UB. Leptin-responsive GABAergic neurons regulate fertility through pathways that result in reduced kisspeptinergic tone. J Neurosci. 2014;34:6047–56.

15. Moore AM, Prescott M, Marshall CJ, Yip SH, Campbell RE. Enhancement of a robust arcuate GABAergic input to gonadotropin-releasing hormone neurons in a model of polycystic ovarian syndrome. Proc Natl Acad Sci U S A. 2015;112:596–601.

16. Pielecka J, Quaynor SD, Moenter SM. Androgens increase gonadotropin-releasing hormone neuron firing activity in females and interfere with progesterone negative feedback. Endocrinology. 2006;147:1474–9.

17. Porter DT, Moore AM, Cobern JA, Padmanabhan V, Goodman RL, Coolen LM, Lehman MN. Prenatal testosterone exposure alters GABAergic synaptic inputs to GnRH and KNDy neurons in a sheep model of polycystic ovarian syndrome. Endocrinology. 2019; 160:2529–42.

18. Ruddenklau A, Campbell RE. Neuroendocrine impairments of polycystic ovary syndrome. Endocrinology. 2019;160:2230–42.

19. Stephens SB, Tolson KP, Rouse ML Jr, Poling MC, Hashimoto-Partyka MK, Mellon PL, Kauffman AS. Absent progesterone signaling in kisspeptin neurons disrupts the LH surge and impairs fertility in female mice. Endocrinology. 2015;156:3091–7.

20. Caldwell ASL, Edwards MC, Desai R, Jimenez M, Gilchrist RB, Handelsman DJ, Walters KA. Neuroendocrine androgen action is a key extraovarian mediator in the development of polycystic ovary syndrome. Proc Natl Acad Sci U S A. 2017;114:E3334–43.

21. Kawwass JF, Sanders KM, Loucks TL, Rohan LC, Berga SL. Increased cerebrospinal fluid levels of GABA, testosterone and estradiol in women with polycystic ovary syndrome. Hum Reprod. 2017;32:1450–6.

22. Pinola P, Morin-Papunen LC, Bloigu A, Puukka K, Ruokonen A, Järvelin MR, Franks S, Tapanainen JS, Lashen H. Anti-Müllerian hormone: correlation with testosterone and oligo- or amenorrhoea in female adolescence in a population-based cohort study. Hum Reprod. 2014;29:2317–25.

23. Cimino I, Casoni F, Liu X, Messina A, Parkash J, Jamin SP, Catteau-Jonard S, Collier F, Baroncini M, Dewailly D, Pigny P, Prescott M, Campbell R, Herbison AE, Prevot V, Giacobini P. Novel role for anti-Müllerian hormone in the regulation of GnRH neuron excitability and hormone secretion. Nat Commun. 2016;7:10055. https://doi.org/10.1038/ncomms10055.

24. Elting MW, Korsen TJ, Rekers-Mombarg LT, Schoemaker J. Women with polycystic ovary syndrome gain regular menstrual cycles when ageing. Hum Reprod. 2000;15:24–8.

25. Nikolaou D, Gilling-Smith C. Early ovarian ageing: are women with polycystic ovaries protected? Hum Reprod. 2004;19:2175–9.

26. Forslund M, Landin-Wilhelmsen K, Schmidt J, Brännström M, Trimpou P, Dahlgren E. Higher menopausal age but no differences in parity in women with polycystic ovary syndrome compared with controls. Acta Obstet Gynecol Scand. 2019;98:320–6.

27. Minooee S, Ramezani Tehrani F, Rahmati M, Mansournia MA, Azizi F. Prediction of age at menopause in women with polycystic ovary syndrome. Climacteric. 2018;21:29–34.

28. Hudecova M, Holte J, Olovsson M, Sundström PI. Long-term follow-up of patients with polycystic ovary syndrome: reproductive outcome and ovarian reserve. Hum Reprod. 2009;24:1176–83.

29. Mellembakken JR, Berga SL, Kilen M, Tanbo TG, Abyholm T, Fedorcsák P. Sustained fertility from 22 to 41 years of age in women with polycystic ovarian syndrome. Hum Reprod. 2011;26:2499–504.

30. Morford JJ, Wu S, Mauvais-Jarvis F. The impact of androgen actions in neurons on metabolic health and disease. Mol cell Endocrinol. 2018;465:92–102.

31. Navarro G, Allard C, Morford JJ, Xu W, Liu S, Molinas AJ, Butcher SM, Fine NH, Blandino-Rosano M, Sure VN, Yu S, Zhang R, Münzberg H, Jacobson DA, Katakam PV, Hodson DJ, Bernal-Mizrachi E, Zsombok A, Mauvais-Jarvis F. (2018). Androgen excess in pancreatic β cells and neurons predisposes female mice to type 2 diabetes. JCI Insight 3(12). Pii: 98607. https://doi.org/10.1172/jci.insight.98607.
32. Cahill L. His brain, her brain. Sci Am. 2005;292:40–7.
33. Goldstein JM, Seidman LJ, Horton NJ, Makris N, Kennedy DN, Caviness VS Jr, Faraone SV, Tsuang MT. Normal sexual dimorphism of the adult human brain assessed by in vivo magnetic resonance imaging. Cereb Cortex. 2001;11:490–7.
34. Cahill L, Uncapher M, Kilpatrick L, Alkire MT, Turner J. Sex-related hemispheric lateralization of amygdala function in emotionally influenced memory: an FMRI investigation. Learn Mem. 2004;11:261–6.
35. McCarthy MM, Arnold AP. Reframing sexual differentiation of the brain. Nat Neurosci. 2011;14:677–83.
36. Agrawal R, Sharma S, Bekir J, Conway G, Bailey J, Balen AH, Prelevic G. Prevalence of polycystic ovaries and polycystic ovary syndrome in lesbian women compared with heterosexual women. Fertil Steril. 2004;82:1352–7.
37. Bosinski HA, Peter M, Bonatz G, Arndt R, Heidenreich M, Sippell WG, Wille R. A higher rate of hyperandrogenic disorders in female-to-male transsexuals. Psychoneuroendocrinology. 1997;22:361–80.
38. Meyer-Bahlburg HF, Dolezal C, Baker SW, New MI. Sexual orientation in women with classical or non-classical congenital adrenal hyperplasia as a function of degree of prenatal androgen excess. Arch Sex Behav. 2008;37:85–99.
39. Pasterski V, Zucker KJ, Hindmarsh PC, Hughes IA, Acerini C, Spencer D, Neufeld S, Hines M. Increased cross-gender identification independent of gender role behavior in girls with congenital adrenal hyperplasia: results from a standardized assessment of 4- to 11-year-old children. Arch Sex Behav. 2015;44:1363–75.
40. Lentini E, Kasahara M, Arver S, Savic I. Sex differences in the human brain and the impact of sex chromosomes and sex hormones. Cereb Cortex. 2013;23:2322–36.
41. Savic I. Asymmetry of cerebral gray and white matter and structural volumes in relation to sex hormones and chromosomes. Front Neurosci. 2014;8:329. https://doi.org/10.3389/fnins.2014.00329. eCollection 2014
42. Savic I, Berglund H, Gulyas B, Roland P. Smelling of odorous sex hormone-like compounds causes sex-differentiated hypothalamic activations in humans. Neuron. 2001;31:661–8.
43. Berglund H, Lindström P, Savic I. Brain response to putative pheromones in lesbian women. Proc Natl Acad Sci U S A. 2006;103:8269–74.
44. Savic I, Berglund H, Lindström P. Brain response to putative pheromones in homosexual men. Proc Natl Acad Sci U S A. 2005;102:7356–61.
45. Savic I, Lindström P. PET and MRI show differences in cerebral asymmetry and functional connectivity between homo- and heterosexual subjects. Proc Natl Acad Sci U S A. 2008;105:9403–8.
46. Rees DA, Udiawar M, Berlot R, Jones DK, O'Sullivan MJ. White matter microstructure and cognitive function in young women with polycystic ovary syndrome. J Clin Endocrinol Metab. 2016;101:314–23.
47. Marsh CA, Berent-Spillson A, Love T, Persad CC, Pop-Busui R, Zubieta JK, Smith YR. Functional neuroimaging of emotional processing in women with polycystic ovary syndrome: a case-control pilot study. Fertil Steril. 2013;100:200–7.
48. Kawwass JF, Loucks T, Berga SL. An algorithm for treatment of infertile women with polycystic ovary syndrome. Middle East Fertil Soc J. 2010;15:231–9.

Adolescence: A High-Risk Period for PCOS Development?

2

Charles Sultan, Laura Gaspari, Samir Hamamah, and Françoise Paris

Polycystic ovary syndrome (PCOS) has long been considered "a riddle wrapped in a mystery inside an enigma" [1], and the relationships among genetic, endocrine, metabolic, environmental, and lifestyle factors in its development are indeed quite complex. Moreover, the underlying causes [2], diagnostic criteria, and recommendations for managing adolescent PCOS [3] remain controversial. The diagnostic features in adult women, such as hyperandrogenemia, obesity, and menstrual disorders, may be part of the normal pubertal process [4]. We thus propose the following three criteria (Fig. 2.1) to make a definitive diagnosis [5].

The prevalence of PCOS has been estimated to range between 0.6 and 12%. In a group of post-menarcheal obese adolescents, Ybarra et al. identified 18.4% cases [6]. Christiansen, in a cross-sectional study including a high number of adolescents between 15 and 19 years, reported a PCOS diagnosis in 3.8%, 10.2%, and 23.10% of the overweight, moderately obese, and extremely obese adolescents, respectively [7].

C. Sultan (✉)
CHU Montpellier, Univ Montpellier, Unité d'Endocrinologie-Gynécologie Pédiatrique, Service de Pédiatrie, Montpellier, France

L. Gaspari · F. Paris
CHU Montpellier, Univ Montpellier, Unité d'Endocrinologie-Gynécologie Pédiatrique, Service de Pédiatrie, Montpellier, France

CHU Montpellier, Univ Montpellier, Centre de Référence Maladies Rares du Développement Génital, Constitutif Sud, Hôpital Lapeyronie, Montpellier, France

Univ Montpellier, INSERM 1203, Développement Embryonnaire Fertilité Environnement, Montpellier, France

S. Hamamah
Univ Montpellier, INSERM 1203, Développement Embryonnaire Fertilité Environnement, Montpellier, France

CHU Montpellier, Univ Montpellier, Département de Biologie de la Reproduction, Biologie de la Reproduction/DPI et CECOS, Montpellier, France

© International Society of Gynecological Endocrinology 2021
A. R. Genazzani et al. (eds.), *Impact of Polycystic Ovary, Metabolic Syndrome and Obesity on Women Health*, ISGE Series,
https://doi.org/10.1007/978-3-030-63650-0_2

1. **Hirsutism (progressive)**

2. **Irregular menses / oligomenorrhea (2 years after menarche)**

3. **Testosterone concentration > 45-55 mg/dl (follicular phase)**

----

4. **PCO morphology (US)**
   - **Enlarged ovaries (> 10mL)**
     - **+/- increased stroma**
     - **+ multiple small peripheral cysts**

----

* **optional :**
  - **- abdominal obesity**
  - **- insulin-resistance**
  - **- AMH concentration > 6.26 ng/mL**
  - **- risk factors (genetics, SGA, early puberty, EDCs, ...)**

Fig. 2.1 Criteria for the diagnosis of PCOS in adolescence

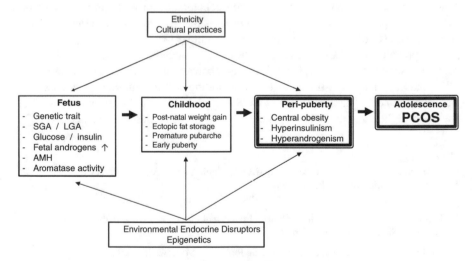

Fig. 2.2 Natural history of adolescent PCOS according to Louwers et al. [57]

Adolescent PCOS may have its origins in fetal life [8] (intrauterine growth retardation, hyperandrogenism) or before puberty (through premature pubarche, obesity, early puberty). In the last few years, evidence has clearly emerged showing that peri-puberty is a high-risk period for PCOS development (Fig. 2.2), through obesity, insulin resistance, metabolic syndrome, and hyperandrogenism (HA). In addition, androgens stimulate appetite, food craving, and recurrent binge eating (Fig. 2.3).

BRAIN	ABDOMINAL ADIPOSE	LIVER	PANCREAS
- GnRH / LH ↑	TISSUE	- Insulin sensitivity ↓	- Oxidative stress ↑
- Leptin sensitivity ↓	- Visceral fat ↑	- Inflammation ↑	
- Appetite ↑	- Adipocyte size ↑		
	- Adipokin release ↓		
	- Lipolysis ↓		

Fig. 2.3 Consequences of HA in women according to Rodriguez et al. [58]

PCOS is an obesity-related condition, with weight gain and obesity in adolescence contributing to its development [9]. In addition, the link between early adiposity rebound in childhood and obesity in adolescence has been established [10, 11].

Moreover, it is well known that the risk of developing a binge eating disorder increases around pubertal onset and continue to rise through adolescence, leading to overweight and obesity.

2.1 The Role of Peri-Pubertal Obesity

According to the ACOG, the prevalence of adolescent overweight and obesity is about 30% and 20%, respectively. The rising prevalence over the last few decades underscores the importance of recognizing its implication at different levels. Adolescent obesity merits special attention as its ramifications persist into adulthood by modulating endocrine, metabolic, and reproductive performances [12].

As obesity during pubertal development is a risk factor for endocrine and metabolic diseases, it has become critical to understand how this occurs [13]. Obesity is, for example, known to modulate pubertal development, as both cross-sectional and longitudinal studies have shown it is associated with earlier puberty [14].

How obesity impacts the relationship between sex steroids and glucose metabolism in early puberty is a matter of active research [13].

Besides, it is well known that girls show a "physiological" decrease in insulin sensitivity during puberty that begins in Tanner stage 2, reaches a nadir in mid to late puberty, and returns to pre-pubertal levels after puberty is completed. This "physiological" insulin resistance is thought to play a role in hyperinsulinemia. The association between childhood obesity and both insulin resistance and hyperinsulinemia has been well documented, especially in Tanner 1–3 girls. The concomitant elevation of insulin and testosterone suggests an interrelationship between these two hormones [15].

It was recently hypothesized that PCOS might be induced by eating disorders occurring at the onset of puberty and associated with stress, mood problems, and low self-esteem [16]. In addition, excessive nutrient intake and the subsequent peri-pubertal obesity can lead to abnormal endocrine and neuroendocrine activity during puberty, which may predispose to PCOS. High dietary intake of energy, proteins, and polyunsaturated fatty acids are risk factors for overweight and obesity and may exacerbate the hyperandrogenism (HA) occurring in most adolescents.

Even if obesity is evident in pubertal PCOS and increases with age, we still do not know if adolescents with PCOS have a predisposition to gain weight or whether PCOS and obesity are causally related [17].

A key question at this point is the following: Which factors mediate the effects of obesity on the development of PCOS?

In addition to genetic factors, insulin resistance and hyperinsulinemia are involved in androgen [18] biosynthesis by the ovary (in conjunction with LH), the development of metabolic syndrome, and the release of adipokines: adiponectin is lower in PCOS, contributing to insulin resistance [19]. Vistatin is increased and reinforces insulin resistance and metabolic dysfunction.

There is evidence that hyperinsulinemia can induce HA either by directly stimulating ovarian/adrenal production or by indirectly enhancing LH secretion, intensifying LH action on the ovary, or increasing bioavailability of testosterone through the reduction of liver SHBG production [20]. Insulin resistance is commonly associated with a higher prevalence of a chronic low-grade inflammatory state and hypoadiponectinemia, both of which negatively affect ovarian function. Lewi et al. reported profound metabolic derangements detected early in the course of PCOS, including a 50% reduction in peripheral tissue insulin sensitivity, hepatic insulin resistance, and compensatory HA in premenarcheal girls with PCOS [21].

Although the ovary is the major contributor to the hyperandrogenic state, increased circulating levels of DHEAS, an adrenal androgen, is present in 15–45% of PCOS girls. The cause of this increase may be adrenal hyperresponsiveness to ACTH, increased ACTH drive to androgens, or hyperinsulinemia, which is known to stimulate adrenal production of DHEAS.

In addition, it is generally accepted that obesity is a risk factor for the development of PCOS during the adolescence in girls who are genetically predisposed [22].

The amount of abdominal fat is recognized as a major contributor to the significant variation in the severity of PCOS phenotypes, with increased abdominal adiposity exacerbating the endocrine, metabolic, and psychological features of PCOS [23].

Abdominal obesity worsens HA, menstrual disorders, insulin-resistance, dyslipidemia, and metabolic syndrome. Notably, a large proportion of adolescents with PCOS are centrally obese [24].

In these adolescents, insulin resistance and its compensatory hyperinsulinism [25] are intrinsic factors that play a key role in producing hyperandrogenia in PCOS:

– Insulin excess can trigger insulin receptors in the pituitary gland to increase LH release and promote androgen secretion by both the ovary and adrenal gland.
– Increased insulin can inhibit the synthesis of hepatic SHBG and increase the level of free T.
– Enhanced activity of the IGF1 receptor in the ovary promotes androgen production by the thecal cells.

Insulin resistance/dyslipidemia, due to high level of free fatty acid and the inhibition of lipolysis, is the most common metabolic disorder [26].

Metabolic syndrome usually encompasses central obesity, insulin resistance, high fasting glucose, high fasting triglycerides, and low HDL cholesterol [27]. According to the Clinical Practice Guidelines from the American Academy of Pediatrics [28], metabolic syndrome is present when an adolescent meets three or more of the following criteria:

- Waist circumference in at least the 90th percentile for age.
- Systolic or diastolic blood pressure in at least the 90th percentile for age and height.
- HDL-C ≤ 40 mg/dl.
- Fasting triglycerides >110 mg/dl.
- Glucose sensitivity is usually increased on the OGTT, which is performed by measuring glucose before the administration of 75 g of oral dextrose and 30–60–90-120-180 minutes after.
  - Homeostatic model for insulin resistance (HOMA-IR).
  - Tissue sensitivity to insulin (HOMA-S).
  - β-cell function.

which are calculated using an online program [29].

2.2   Hyperandrogenism

Androgen excess is the cardinal feature of PCOS.

HA causes a series of endocrine changes, including insulin resistance, hyperinsulinemia, metabolic syndrome, dyslipidemia, and increased LH secretion.

The free androgen index (FAI) is approximately three times higher in pubertal girls with obesity compared with normal-weigh pubertal girls, reflecting early evidence of obesity-associated HA in early pubertal development.

Previous reports have actually documented an association between obesity and HA in pre- and early pubertal girls (Tanner B1-B3). McCartney et al. first emphasized that obesity was associated with HA in 66–94% of obese girls [30]. Knudsen et al. reported that morning LH and fasting insulin were significant predictors of free T in obese peri-pubertal girls, suggesting that abnormal LH secretion and hyperinsulinemia can promote HA in peri-pubertal girls with obesity [31].

Abdominal obesity has been positively correlated with androgen levels, suggesting that obesity plays an important role in PCOS. Androgens have actually been shown to induce abdominal adipocyte accumulation and may cause abdominal tissue dysfunction, including lipid accumulation, oxidative stress, and inflammation [32]. HA is also associated with the development of white adipose tissue dysfunction, which includes increased visceral adiposity and visceral and subcutaneous adipocyte hypertrophy.

What do we know about the genetic background of HA and PCOS? Approximately 40% of sisters of affected girls have elevated total and bioavailable T level, suggesting a genetic susceptibility to this phenomenon [33].

Pre-menarcheal first-degree relatives have HA, further pointing to a genetic susceptibility to PCOS, which has been confirmed by the evidence of elevated T levels, early metabolic syndrome, and β-cell dysfunction in daughters of women affected with PCOS [34]. Polymorphisms and splice variants in genes such as follistatin, fibrillin-3, CYP11A, insulin receptor, 17βHSDB6, androgen receptor, and 5αreductase have been linked to PCOS [35].

It is likely that gene variations resulting in HA during a key developmental window program the phenotypic feature of PCOS.

Recent studies in young female macaques have suggested that DNA methylation and RNA levels of the genes associated with pathways involved in inflammation, metabolic syndrome, and adipogenesis were involved in the regulation of the white adipose tissue (WAT) transcriptional profile [36]. This contributes to body fat distribution and the modulation of the pathophysiological response to obesity. In addition, these studies reported the synergistic effects of HA and the obesogenic Western-style diet on this process.

Lastly, animal studies currently reinforce the hypothesis that androgen excess plays a key role in the origin of PCOS.

In female monkeys, DHT exposure induces PCOS reproductive traits of cycle irregularity, ovulation dysfunction, and reduced follicular maturations. Simultaneously, a PCOS metabolic characteristic of increased adiposity, adipocyte hypertrophy, and hepatic steatosis was observed.

2.3   GnRH Dysregulation

PCOS is associated with a neuroendocrine abnormality characterized by increased GnRH and LH secretions. It has been reported that HA enhances the GnRH pulse frequency and the subsequently elevated LH secretion. Insulin may increase the frequency and amplitude of GnRH and LH pulse secretion. Insulin has also been reported to stimulate GnRH-mediated LH release from the pituitary.

A reduced dopaminergic tone along with low plasma norepinephrine and serum serotonin has been associated in PCOS women [37]. In a rat model of PCOS, Chaudhari et al. recently demonstrated that GnRH inhibitor neurotransmitter, serotonin, dopamine, GABA, and acetylcholine were reduced, whereas glutamate, an active stimulator of GnRH activity, was increased (Fig. 2.4) [38]. The kisspeptin/GPR54 system is also involved in this stimulation [39]. The dysregulated neurotransmission profile could explain the frequency of low self-esteem anxiety, depression, and mood disorders associated with PCOS adolescents. This neurotransmission dysregulation may be a key feature in PCOS development [40].

2.4   Brain Disorders

PCOS is associated with by psychological distress and episodes of overeating and/or dieting during puberty and adolescence, when body dissatisfaction and emotional problems are present [16].

Fig. 2.4 Hypothalamic-pituitary-ovarian axis in adolescent PCOS girls

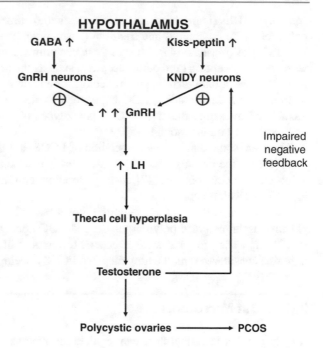

It is well known that eating disorders disturb endocrine pathways: bulimia can increase insulin level as well as stress. Binge-foods are usually high in fat or sugar and increase the insulin level. Binge-eating and stress induce hypercortisolism. Obesity is also associated with leptin resistance, leading to leptin overproduction. Ghrelin increases food intake and adiposity.

Even if PCOS is associated with psychological issues usually observed in obese girls, some investigators consider that pre-existent mental health problems may contribute to weight gain and the development of PCOS at the vulnerable age of puberty [41]. Screening for anxiety and repression is thus required, and the assessment of eating disorders should be considered in the peri-pubertal period of high-risk adolescents.

Moreover, activation of the hypothalamic-pituitary-ovarian axis during puberty can be epigenetically altered by psychological stressors, which are common during adolescence, and can thus lead to the development of PCOS [40].

Recent studies have revealed that the pathophysiology of PCOS also involves the gut-brain axis (GBA), which plays a critical role in the regulation of appetite, food intake, glucose metabolism, energy maintenance, and body weight.

Gastrointestinal hormones, including ghrelin, glucagon-like peptide, and cholecystokinin, are actually involved in insulin resistance and inflammation disorders.

2.5   Endocrine-Disrupting Chemicals

Within the past few decades, more than 1000 of the 100,000 environmental chemicals in the world have been documented as endocrine-disrupting chemicals (EDCs) [42]. These include diethylstilbestrol (DES), dioxin (herbicide), PCBs (electrical coolant), PBDEs (flame retardants), DTT (pesticide), atrazine (herbicide), alkylphenols (detergents), parabens and triclosan (cosmetics), phthalates (plastics, cosmetics), and BPA (plastics) [43]. Most of them can mimic estrogen action and interfere with nuclear receptors (and other receptors, such as the aryl-hydrocarbon receptor: AhR), transcriptional factors, growth factors, or enzymatic activity (aromatase).

In several animal studies, EDC exposure was shown to induce endocrine and metabolic expressions that fit the PCOS phenotype [44], including ovarian polycystic morphology on ultrasound [45].

There are some data on the association of PCOS and EDCs in women [46, 47]. According to the investigators, EDCs can modify neuroendocrine modulation [46], adipose tissue development [47], insulin secretion, and metabolic disorders, favoring PCOS development [48].

Very recently, Luo et al. reported novel associations between the UDP-glucuronosyltransferase polymorphisms and EDC concentrations in patients with PCOS, supporting the relevance of genetic differences in EDC metabolism, which might be considered a modulating factor of PCOS development [49].

2.6   Gut Microbiota

It is known that intestinal flora can regulate the synthesis and secretion of insulin, and a variety of endocrine and metabolic diseases are affected by the dynamics and structure of the gut microbiota. Tremelen et al. suggested that the high-sugar, high-fat, and low-fiber diet usually observed in adolescent girls may cause an imbalance in the intestinal flora, which then increases the permeability of the liposaccharides known to activate the immunological system, causing inflammation [50]. Recently, a potential two-way interaction between androgens and the intestinal flora was proposed [51, 52].

We should also consider the role of gut microbiota in addition to the epigenetic regulation of neurotransmitters. Recent studies have shown that dysbiosis of the gut microbiota may be associated with the PCOS phenotype [53]. Some groups have proposed that it may be a potential player in the development of PCOS (Fig. 2.5).

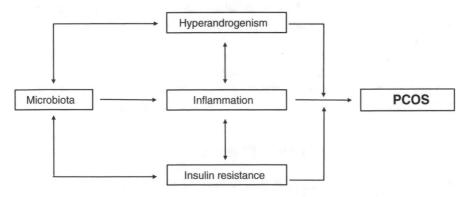

Fig. 2.5 The microbiota as a key factor in the development of PCOS

2.7 AMH

AMH is a new factor involved in the development of PCOS in obese girls. AMH is known to be secreted by the granulosa cells of the ovarian follicles.

Since polycystic ovaries have a larger number of follicles, they produce more AMH. High AMH concentration is considered a marker of adolescent PCOS, but it also contributes to the pathophysiology of PCOS [54]. Recent studies have suggested that AMH may play a role in the development of PCOS by increasing GnRH-dependent LH secretion and inhibiting aromatase activity within the ovary [22].

Previous studies found increased AMH levels in PCOS girls during early puberty, suggesting that an alteration in ovarian follicular genesis may begin early in development [55].

An AMH value of 6.26 ng/mL seems to be an optimal cut-off value in obese girls for predicting PCOS [56].

2.8 Conclusions

Several studies have outlined the multifactorial origin of PCOS, which includes genetic factors, obesity, neuroendocrine dysregulation and HA, metabolic dysfunctions, immune disorders, lifestyle, and psychological disorders. Insulin resistance is one of the main pathological changes (Fig. 2.6).

Although PCOS can manifest at any age in reproductive life, it often develops during adolescence, coincident with pubertal activation of the hypothalamic-pituitary-ovarian axis, eating disorders, and obesity. Identifying peri-pubertal girls at risk of PCOS may prevent that adulthood PCOS. One of the main future

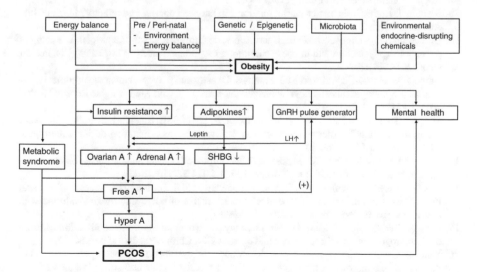

Fig. 2.6 Endocrine and metabolic disorders associated with peri-pubertal abdominal obesity

challenges will be to identify the environmental triggers of PCOS development during adolescence and manage them accordingly.

References

1. Padmanabhan V. Polycystic ovary syndrome--"a riddle wrapped in a mystery inside an enigma". J Clin Endocrinol Metab. 2009;94(6):1883–5.
2. Vassalou H, Sotiraki M, Michala L. PCOS diagnosis in adolescents: the timeline of a controversy in a systematic review. J Pediatr Endocrinol Metab. 2019;32(6):549–59.
3. Pena AS, Witchel SF, Hoeger KM, Oberfield SE, Vogiatzi MG, Misso M, et al. Adolescent polycystic ovary syndrome according to the international evidence-based guideline. BMC Med. 2020;18(1):72.
4. Dabadghao P. Polycystic ovary syndrome in adolescents. Best Pract Res Clin Endocrinol Metab. 2019;33(3):101272.
5. Sultan C, Paris F. Clinical expression of polycystic ovary syndrome in adolescent girls. Fertil Steril. 2006;86 Suppl 1:S6.
6. Ybarra M, Franco RR, Cominato L, Sampaio RB. Sucena da Rocha SM, Damiani D. polycystic ovary syndrome among obese adolescents. Gynecol Endocrinol. 2018;34(1):45–8.
7. Christensen SB, Black MH, Smith N, Martinez MM, Jacobsen SJ, Porter AH, et al. Prevalence of polycystic ovary syndrome in adolescents. Fertil Steril. 2013;100(2):470–7.
8. Rosenfield RL. Clinical review: identifying children at risk for polycystic ovary syndrome. J Clin Endocrinol Metab. 2007;92(3):787–96.
9. Yildiz BO. Polycystic ovary syndrome: is obesity a symptom? Womens Health (Lond). 2013;9(6):505–7.
10. Kang MJ. The adiposity rebound in the 21st century children: meaning for what? Korean J Pediatr. 2018;61(12):375–80.
11. Rolland-Cachera MF, Deheeger M, Bellisle F, Sempe M, Guilloud-Bataille M, Patois E. Adiposity rebound in children: a simple indicator for predicting obesity. Am J Clin Nutr. 1984;39(1):129–35.
12. Raperport C, Homburg R. The source of polycystic ovarian syndrome. Clin Med Insights Reprod Health. 2019;13:1179558119871467.
13. Reinehr T, Roth CL. Is there a causal relationship between obesity and puberty? Lancet Child Adolesc Health. 2019;3(1):44–54.
14. De Leonibus C, Marcovecchio ML, Chiavaroli V, de Giorgis T, Chiarelli F, Mohn A. Timing of puberty and physical growth in obese children: a longitudinal study in boys and girls. Pediatr Obes. 2014;9(4):292–9.
15. Barber TM, Hanson P, Weickert MO, Franks S. Obesity and polycystic ovary syndrome: implications for pathogenesis and novel management strategies. Clin Med Insights Reprod Health. 2019;13:1179558119874042.
16. Steegers-Theunissen RPM, Wiegel RE, Jansen PW, Laven JSE, Sinclair KD. Polycystic ovary syndrome: a brain disorder characterized by eating problems originating during puberty and adolescence. Int J Mol Sci. 2020;21(21).
17. Anderson AD, Solorzano CM, McCartney CR. Childhood obesity and its impact on the development of adolescent PCOS. Semin Reprod Med. 2014;32(3):202–13.
18. de Medeiros SF, Yamamoto MMW. Souto de Medeiros MA, Barbosa BB, Soares JM, Baracat EC. Changes in clinical and biochemical characteristics of polycystic ovary syndrome with advancing age. Endocr Connect. 2020;9(2):74–89.
19. Zeng X, Xie YJ, Liu YT, Long SL, Mo ZC. Polycystic ovarian syndrome: correlation between hyperandrogenism, insulin resistance and obesity. Clin Chim Acta. 2020;502:214–21.
20. Sanchez-Garrido MA, Tena-Sempere M. Metabolic dysfunction in polycystic ovary syndrome: pathogenic role of androgen excess and potential therapeutic strategies. Mol Metab. 2020;35:100937.

21. Lewy VD, Danadian K, Witchel SF, Arslanian S. Early metabolic abnormalities in adolescent girls with polycystic ovarian syndrome. J Pediatr. 2001;138(1):38–44.
22. Torchen LC, Legro RS, Dunaif A. Distinctive reproductive phenotypes in Peripubertal girls at risk for polycystic ovary syndrome. J Clin Endocrinol Metab. 2019;104(8):3355–61.
23. Carmina E, Bucchieri S, Esposito A, Del Puente A, Mansueto P, Orio F, et al. Abdominal fat quantity and distribution in women with polycystic ovary syndrome and extent of its relation to insulin resistance. J Clin Endocrinol Metab. 2007;92(7):2500–5.
24. McCartney CR, Prendergast KA, Chhabra S, Eagleson CA, Yoo R, Chang RJ, et al. The association of obesity and hyperandrogenemia during the pubertal transition in girls: obesity as a potential factor in the genesis of postpubertal hyperandrogenism. J Clin Endocrinol Metab. 2006;91(5):1714–22.
25. Friesen M, Cowan CA. Adipocyte metabolism and insulin signaling perturbations: insights from genetics. Trends Endocrinol Metab. 2019;30(6):396–406.
26. Li L, Feng Q, Ye M, He Y, Yao A, Shi K. Metabolic effect of obesity on polycystic ovary syndrome in adolescents: a meta-analysis. J Obstet Gynaecol. 2017;37(8):1036–47.
27. Jeanes YM, Reeves S. Metabolic consequences of obesity and insulin resistance in polycystic ovary syndrome: diagnostic and methodological challenges. Nutr Res Rev. 2017;30(1):97–105.
28. DeBoer MD. Assessing and managing the metabolic syndrome in children and adolescents. Nutrients. 2019;11(8).
29. Lim SS, Kakoly NS, Tan JWJ, Fitzgerald G, Bahri Khomami M, Joham AE, et al. Metabolic syndrome in polycystic ovary syndrome: a systematic review, meta-analysis and meta-regression. Obes Rev. 2019;20(2):339–52.
30. McCartney CR, Blank SK, Prendergast KA, Chhabra S, Eagleson CA, Helm KD, et al. Obesity and sex steroid changes across puberty: evidence for marked hyperandrogenemia in pre- and early pubertal obese girls. J Clin Endocrinol Metab. 2007;92(2):430–6.
31. Knudsen KL, Blank SK, Burt Solorzano C, Patrie JT, Chang RJ, Caprio S, et al. Hyperandrogenemia in obese peripubertal girls: correlates and potential etiological determinants. Obesity (Silver Spring). 2010;18(11):2118–24.
32. Lim SS, Norman RJ, Davies MJ, Moran LJ. The effect of obesity on polycystic ovary syndrome: a systematic review and meta-analysis. Obes Rev. 2013;14(2):95–109.
33. Legro RS, Bentley-Lewis R, Driscoll D, Wang SC, Dunaif A. Insulin resistance in the sisters of women with polycystic ovary syndrome: association with hyperandrogenemia rather than menstrual irregularity. J Clin Endocrinol Metab. 2002;87(5):2128–33.
34. Kahsar-Miller MD, Nixon C, Boots LR, Go RC, Azziz R. Prevalence of polycystic ovary syndrome (PCOS) in first-degree relatives of patients with PCOS. Fertil Steril. 2001;75(1):53–8.
35. Yalamanchi SK, Sam S, Cardenas MO, Holaday LW, Urbanek M, Dunaif A. Association of fibrillin-3 and transcription factor-7-like 2 gene variants with metabolic phenotypes in PCOS. Obesity (Silver Spring). 2012;20(6):1273–8.
36. Carbone L, Davis BA, Fei SS, White A, Nevonen KA, Takahashi D, et al. Synergistic effects of Hyperandrogenemia and obesogenic Western-style diet on transcription and DNA methylation in visceral adipose tissue of nonhuman primates. Sci Rep. 2019;9(1):19232.
37. Chaudhari N, Dawalbhakta M, Nampoothiri L. GnRH dysregulation in polycystic ovarian syndrome (PCOS) is a manifestation of an altered neurotransmitter profile. Reprod Biol Endocrinol. 2018;16(1):37.
38. Kawwass JF, Sanders KM, Loucks TL, Rohan LC, Berga SL. Increased cerebrospinal fluid levels of GABA, testosterone and estradiol in women with polycystic ovary syndrome. Hum Reprod. 2017;32(7):1450–6.
39. Tang R, Ding X, Zhu J. Kisspeptin and polycystic ovary syndrome. Front Endocrinol (Lausanne). 2019;10:298.
40. Coutinho EA, Kauffman AS. The role of the brain in the pathogenesis and physiology of polycystic ovary syndrome (PCOS). Med Sci (Basel). 2019;7(8).
41. Cooney LG, Lee I, Sammel MD, Dokras A. High prevalence of moderate and severe depressive and anxiety symptoms in polycystic ovary syndrome: a systematic review and meta-analysis. Hum Reprod. 2017;32(5):1075–91.

42. Kahn LG, Philippat C, Nakayama SF, Slama R, Trasande L. Endocrine-disrupting chemicals: implications for human health. Lancet Diabetes Endocrinol. 2020;8(8):703–18.
43. Schug TT, Johnson AF, Birnbaum LS, Colborn T, Guillette LJ Jr, Crews DP, et al. Minireview: endocrine disruptors: past lessons and future directions. Mol Endocrinol. 2016;30(8):833–47.
44. Mathew H, Mahalingaiah S. Do prenatal exposures pose a real threat to ovarian function? Bisphenol a as a case study. Reproduction. 2019;157(4):R143–R57.
45. Rutkowska AZ, Diamanti-Kandarakis E. Polycystic ovary syndrome and environmental toxins. Fertil Steril. 2016;106(4):948–58.
46. Akin L, Kendirci M, Narin F, Kurtoglu S, Hatipoglu N, Elmali F. Endocrine disruptors and polycystic ovary syndrome: phthalates. J Clin Res Pediatr Endocrinol. 2020;12(4):393–400.
47. Akgul S, Sur U, Duzceker Y, Balci A, Kizilkan MP, Kanbur N, et al. Bisphenol a and phthalate levels in adolescents with polycystic ovary syndrome. Gynecol Endocrinol. 2019;35(12):1084–7.
48. Barrett ES, Sobolewski M. Polycystic ovary syndrome: do endocrine-disrupting chemicals play a role? Semin Reprod Med. 2014;32(3):166–76.
49. Luo Y, Nie Y, Tang L, Xu CC, Xu L. The correlation between UDP-glucuronosyltransferase polymorphisms and environmental endocrine disruptors levels in polycystic ovary syndrome patients. Medicine (Baltimore). 2020;99(11):e19444.
50. Jobira B, Frank DN, Pyle L, Silveira LJ, Kelsey MM, Garcia-Reyes Y, et al. Obese adolescents with PCOS have altered biodiversity and relative abundance in gastrointestinal microbiota. J Clin Endocrinol Metab. 2020;105(6).
51. Tremellen K, Pearce K. Dysbiosis of Gut Microbiota (DOGMA)--a novel theory for the development of Polycystic Ovarian Syndrome. Medical Hypotheses. 2012;79(1):104–12.
52. Yurtdas G, Akdevelioglu Y. A new approach to polycystic ovary syndrome: the gut microbiota. J Am Coll Nutr. 2020;39(4):371–82.
53. He FF, Li YM. Role of gut microbiota in the development of insulin resistance and the mechanism underlying polycystic ovary syndrome: a review. J Ovarian Res. 2020;13(1):73.
54. Efthymiadou A, Bogiatzidou M, Kritikou D, Chrysis D. Anti-Mullerian hormone in girls with premature Adrenarche: the impact of polycystic ovary syndrome history in their mothers. J Pediatr. 2019;205:190–4.
55. Reinehr T, Kulle A, Rothermel J, Knop C, Lass N, Bosse C, et al. Weight loss in obese girls with polycystic ovarian syndrome is associated with a decrease in anti-Muellerian hormone concentrations. Clin Endocrinol. 2017;87(2):185–93.
56. Kim JY, Tfayli H, Michaliszyn SF, Lee S, Nasr A, Arslanian S. Anti-Mullerian hormone in obese adolescent girls with polycystic ovary syndrome. J Adolesc Health. 2017;60(3):333–9.
57. Louwers YV, Laven JSE. Characteristics of polycystic ovary syndrome throughout life. Ther Adv Reprod Health. 2020;14:2633494120911038.
58. Rodriguez Paris V, Bertoldo MJ. The Mechanism of androgen actions in PCOS etiology. Med Sci (Basel). 2019;7(9).

Toward Adolescent Prevention of Adult Anovulation in Polycystic Ovary Syndrome

3

Francis de Zegher and Lourdes Ibáñez

3.1 Definition, Origins, and Diagnosis of Adolescent PCOS

Recent changes in the paradigm of adolescent polycystic ovary syndrome (PCOS) are summarized in Table 3.1 [1].

Adolescent PCOS is defined by the co-presence of irregular menses (as proxy for oligo-anovulation) and androgen excess (clinical + biochemical evidence) at least 2 years after menarche, and by the exclusion of disorders such as an androgen-secreting tumor; ovarian morphology is not a criterion [2].

Worldwide, PCOS is the most prevalent endocrinopathy of adolescent girls (≈10%), and its prevalence is rising since, in essence, adolescent PCOS is the outcome of a mismatch between a relatively energy-sparing (epi)genetic background and a relatively energy-rich environment [3]. In any variant of such a mismatch, there is a chronic need to store more fat than is safely feasible in subcutaneous adipose tissue, and the lipid excess ends up being stored in ectopic depots, notably in liver and viscera (= hepato-visceral fat excess, or central obesity). Adolescent PCOS is typically driven by an ensemble including central obesity, insulin resistance, LH hypersecretion, and low concentrations of circulating high-molecular-weight (HMW) adiponectin, which is a key adipokine with insulin-sensitizing properties [2–4].

F. de Zegher
Department of Development & Regeneration, University of Leuven, Leuven, Belgium

L. Ibáñez (✉)
Centro de Investigación Biomédica en Red de Diabetes y Enfermedades Metabólicas Asociadas (CIBERDEM), ISCIII, Madrid, Spain

Endocrinology Department, Research Institute Sant Joan de Déu, University of Barcelona, Barcelona, Spain
e-mail: libanez@hsjdbcn.es

© International Society of Gynecological Endocrinology 2021
A. R. Genazzani et al. (eds.), *Impact of Polycystic Ovary, Metabolic Syndrome and Obesity on Women Health*, ISGE Series,
https://doi.org/10.1007/978-3-030-63650-0_3

Table 3.1 Adolescent PCOS: a changing paradigm

	Past	Present
The essence of PCOS	Highly heritable disorder of the hypothalamic-pituitary-ovarian axis	Mismatch disorder in obesogenic world: Absolute or relative excess of subc fat leads to ectopic adiposity and insulin resistance, on a background of genetic susceptibility (involving >19 genes)
Sequence	PCOS → fat excess	Fat excess → PCOS
Forerunners	Early androgen excess?	Upward mismatch between BW Z-score and subsequent BMI Z-score → early adrenarche/pubarche, → early puberty/menarche
Clinical presentation	Hirsutism, severe acne/seborrhea, irregular menses	
Diagnostic criteria • Androgen excess • Oligo-amenorrhea • Polycystic ovaries (US)	Presence of any 2 of the 3 criteria	Presence of the 2 upper criteria

Subc subcutaneous, *BMI* body mass index, *BW* birth weight, *US* ultrasound
Adapted from [1]

Adolescent PCOS is commonly heralded by an upward Z-score change from weight-at-birth to body mass index (BMI)-in-childhood; weight-at-birth tends to be below average in non-obese PCOS, but not in obese PCOS girls [5]. The magnitude of this Z-score increment is partly driven by genetic variants that control appetite and/or BMI [6]. A higher Z-score increment associates with more insulin resistance and with more central adiposity in childhood [7], and also with a faster maturation toward pubarche and menarche [8, 9].

Oligo-anovulation may result from an adaptive neuroendocrine response to a deficit of central fat (as in athletic amenorrhea) [10], or to an excess of central fat (as in obese PCOS and non-obese PCOS) [11, 12], and there is genetic variation in the hypothalamo-pituitary responsiveness to central adiposity. Girls genetically attuned to the harshest environments are nowadays the most vulnerable to develop PCOS under circumstances of physical inactivity and/or nutritional abundance [13, 14].

3.2 Treatment of Adolescent PCOS: Lifestyle, Estro-Progestagen, SPIOMET

There is still no EMA/FDA-approved treatment for adolescent PCOS. Given the crucial role of central fat excess, the prime aim should be a preferential loss of central fat. Such a loss can revert the entire PCOS phenotype, and it can be achieved with sustained lifestyle measures that involve multiple factors including diet, exercise, sleep, and biorhythm, all within an environment that may remain stubbornly obesogenic [15].

Failure to sustain these lifestyle measures is frequent, and the standard approach is then to add an oral estro-progestagen contraceptive [2, 16]. This adjunct silences the gonadotropic axis, reduces the androgen excess [in part via a pharmacological increment of circulating sex-hormone-binding globulin (SHBG)], and leads to regular and anovulatory pseudo-menses [2, 16], but it does not solve the core (or central-fat) problem, and thus channels the adolescent girl toward a post-treatment rebound of androgen excess and oligo-anovulation, in other words, toward adult PCOS [12].

Alternative adjuncts could aim at enhancing the effects of lifestyle measures, by switching fat from ectopic to eutopic depots, and/or by stimulating brown adipose tissue (BAT) activity, thereby increasing energy expenditure. A first example of such an alternative adjunct could be SPIOMET, which is a fixed low-dose combination of three old and safe generics that act through different pathways: spironolactone (only 50 mg/day), pioglitazone (only 7.5 mg/day), and metformin (only 850 mg/day).

Spironolactone has been used for >50 years as a mixed anti-androgen and anti-mineralocorticoid, and has recently been identified as a potent activator of BAT [17, 18], and thus as a potential driver of energy expenditure. There are no major safety concerns when spironolactone is dosed at only 50 mg/d ($\leq$1 mg/kg/day) in adolescent girls with PCOS [19].

Pioglitazone has been used for >20 years as an anti-diabetes medication, in four- to six-fold higher doses than in SPIOMET. The observation that low-dose pioglitazone (7.5 mg/day) raises the concentrations of circulating HMW adiponectin [20] suggests that such a low dose acts as an inhibitor of cyclin-dependent kinase 5 (CDK5)-mediated phosphorylation of peroxisome proliferator-activated receptor (PPAR)-Y rather than as an activator of PPAR-Y [21], also in the hypothalamus [22]. The uncertainty around a potential risk for bladder cancer in older male patients with diabetes and with long-term, high-dose pioglitazone treatment has recently been cleared: there is no evidence for this risk, which is now considered to have been "a red herring" [23].

Metformin has been known for >20 years to have normalizing effects on the endocrine-metabolic state [24] and on the ovulation rate [25] of adolescent girls with PCOS. Metformin monotherapy failed to reach the market for adolescent PCOS because it proved to be too cheap to be commercially viable [26]. The pharmacokinetics of metformin in girls compare to those in women [27]. Metformin is well tolerated by adolescent girls with PCOS [24, 25], and also by younger girls at high risk of developing PCOS [28].

SPIOMET components have partially overlapping benefits that are essentially present with low doses, and have different side effects that are essentially absent with low doses. Hence, the SPIOMET concept is to aim for the presence of cumulative effectiveness, and for the absence of safety concerns.

3.3   SPIOMET Experience in Adolescent Girls: Limited but Promising

So far, the effects of SPIOMET have only been investigated in two randomized controlled pilot studies (ISRCTN29234515 and ISRCTN11062950) that were based in Barcelona between 2012 and 2019 and were performed in non-obese girls with PCOS and with no need for contraception (total N = 62; mean age 16 year and BMI 24 Kg/m^2; treatment for 1 year; ovulation assessment during the post-treatment year). In these two studies, the effects of SPIOMET were compared to those of an oral contraceptive (OC; ethinylestradiol-levonorgestrel).

Proof-of-concept by ISRCTN29234515 has been reported in 2017 [12] and has recently been confirmed by ISRCTN11062950 [29]. Indeed, pooled results from both studies disclosed that SPIOMET has more normalizing effects than OC, notably on insulin sensitivity, visceral fat, and liver fat (Fig. 3.1); there were a mean threefold (and even a median fivefold) more ovulations post-SPIOMET than post-OC (Fig. 3.2); normovulation was only observed post-SPIOMET; anovulation was >ten-fold more frequent post-OC [29].

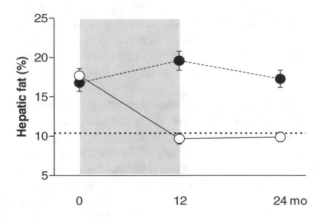

Fig. 3.1 Hepatic fat content (by magnetic resonance imaging) in non-obese adolescent girls with PCOS who were randomized to receive either an oral contraceptive (OC; N = 31; dark circles) for 12 months or a low-dose combination of spironolactone-pioglitazone-metformin (SPIOMET; N = 31; white circles) for 12 months; subsequently, both subgroups were untreated for 12 months. Body weight did not change in either subgroup. The dotted line indicates the average level in healthy control girls of similar age. Results are expressed as mean ± SEM. P < 0.0001 for on-treatment change between subgroups. Modified from Reference 29

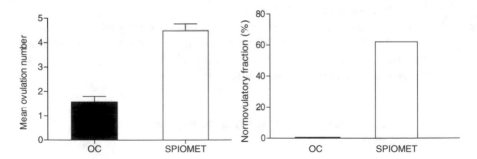

Fig. 3.2 Post-treatment ovulation results in adolescent girls with polycystic ovary syndrome who were randomized to receive an oral contraceptive (OC) or low-dose spironolactone + pioglitazone + metformin (SPIOMET) for 12 months and were subsequently followed for 12 months without treatment. Ovulations were assessed twice over 12 weeks, for a total of 24 weeks, between the study timepoints of 15–18 months (= post-treatment months 3–6) and 21–24 months (= post-treatment months 9–12). Both the ovulation number and the normovulatory fraction (%) were significantly higher ($p < 0.0001$) in girls receiving SPIOMET

3.4   Perspective

Adolescence may provide an early opportunity to normalize the PCOS phenotype, and to prevent subsequent oligo-anovulation, and its consequences and comorbidities (Fig. 3.3).

SPIOMET's efficacy and safety remain to be corroborated by a randomized, double-blind, multicenter study wherein the effects of SPIOMET (in a single tablet) are tested versus placebo, versus pioglitazone, and versus pioglitazone-plus-spironolactone, all on a background of standardized lifestyle measures, in larger study populations that are more diverse in genetic background and that span broader ranges of age and BMI.

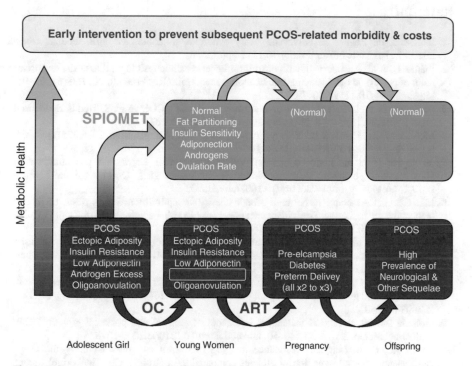

Fig. 3.3 Summary of how early SPIOMET treatment may prevent or reduce subsequent PCOS-related morbidity and costs. Adolescent girls with PCOS are rather unhealthy (= on the low/red side along the metabolic-health spectrum), and lifestyle measures are recommended for most of these girls, particularly when obese. Pharmacological treatment with an oral contraceptive (OC) reduces the androgen excess but fails to improve other markers of metabolic health. Post-OC oligo-anovulation may require the use of assisted reproductive technology (ART) in order to achieve a pregnancy. In turn, ART-induced pregnancies in women with PCOS are accompanied by a doubling-to-tripling of major complications, and followed by a higher prevalence of sequelae in the offspring. In contrast, pharmacological intervention with SPIOMET in adolescent girls with PCOS improves their metabolic health and leads to the virtual disappearance of the entire PCOS phenotype. The anticipation that there will be fewer complications in spontaneous post-SPIOMET pregnancies than in post-OC/ART pregnancies remains to be corroborated in future studies

The primary endpoint of clinical relevance could be ovulation rate, but this is cumbersome to assess in adolescent girls [12]. Circulating microRNA-451a, either alone [30], or together with fasting insulinemia [29], are simple candidate proxies to gauge the normalization of the underpinning PCOS condition. Indeed, circulating microRNA-451a was recently identified as a biomarker that associates closely to androgen excess, insulin resistance, hepato-visceral adiposity, and ovulation rate in adolescent girls with PCOS [30].

Acknowledgments The authors declare no conflict of interest.

This study was supported by the Ministerio de Ciencia, Innovación y Universidades, Instituto de Salud Carlos III, and the Fondo Europeo de Desarrollo Regional (FEDER) (PI15/01078).

References

1. Ibáñez L, de Zegher F. Polycystic ovary syndrome in adolescent girls. Pediatr Obes. 2020;15(2):e12586. https://doi.org/10.1111/ijpo.12586.
2. Ibáñez L, et al. An international consortium update: pathophysiology, diagnosis, and treatment of polycystic ovarian syndrome in adolescence. Horm Res Paediatr. 2017;88(6):371–95. https://doi.org/10.1159/000479371.
3. de Zegher F, et al. Central obesity, faster maturation, and 'PCOS' in girls. Trends Endocrinol Metab. 2018;29(12):815–8. https://doi.org/10.1016/j.tem.2018.09.005.
4. McCartney CR, Marshall JC. Polycystic ovary syndrome. N Engl J Med. 2016;375(1):54–64. https://doi.org/10.1056/NEJMcp1514916.
5. de Zegher F, et al. Reduced prenatal weight gain and/or augmented postnatal weight gain precedes polycystic ovary syndrome in adolescent girls. Obesity (Silver Spring). 2017;25(9):1486–9. https://doi.org/10.1002/oby.21935.
6. Elks CE, et al. Associations between genetic obesity susceptibility and early postnatal fat and lean mass: an individual participant meta-analysis. JAMA Pediatr. 2014;168(12):1122–30. https://doi.org/10.1001/jamapediatrics.2014.1619.
7. de Zegher F, et al. Towards a simple marker of hepato-visceral adiposity and insulin resistance: the Z-score change from weight-at-birth to BMI-in-childhood. Pediatr Obes. 2019;14(10):e12533. https://doi.org/10.1111/ijpo.12533.
8. Ong KK, et al. Opposing influences of prenatal and postnatal weight gain on adrenarche in normal boys and girls. J Clin Endocrinol Metab. 2004;89(6):2647–51. https://doi.org/10.1210/jc.2003-031848.
9. Sloboda DM, et al. Age at menarche: influences of prenatal and postnatal growth. J Clin Endocrinol Metab. 2007;92(1):46–50. https://doi.org/10.1210/jc.2006-1378.
10. Frisch RE, et al. Magnetic resonance imaging of overall and regional body fat, estrogen metabolism, and ovulation of athletes compared to controls. J Clin Endocrinol Metab. 1993;77(2):471–7. https://doi.org/10.1210/jcem.77.2.8345054.
11. Kuchenbecker WK, et al. In women with polycystic ovary syndrome and obesity, loss of intraabdominal fat is associated with resumption of ovulation. Hum Reprod. 2011;26(9):2505–12. https://doi.org/10.1093/humrep/der229.
12. Ibáñez L, et al. Normalizing ovulation rate by preferential reduction of hepato-visceral fat in adolescent girls with polycystic ovary syndrome. J Adolesc Health. 2017;61(4):446–53. https://doi.org/10.1016/j.jadohealth.2017.04.010.
13. Boyle JA, et al. Prevalence of polycystic ovary syndrome in a sample of indigenous women in Darwin. Aust Med J Aust. 2012;196:62–6. https://doi.org/10.5694/mja11.10553.
14. Wijeyaratne CN, et al. Phenotype and metabolic profile of south Asian women with polycystic ovary syndrome (PCOS): results of a large database from a specialist endocrine clinic. Hum Reprod. 2011;26(1):202–13. https://doi.org/10.1093/humrep/deq310.

15. Lass N, et al. Effect of lifestyle intervention on features of polycystic ovarian syndrome, metabolic syndrome, and intima-media thickness in obese adolescent girls. J Clin Endocrinol Metab. 2011;96(11):3533–40. https://doi.org/10.1210/jc.2011-1609.
16. Teede HJ, et al. Recommendations from the international evidence-based guideline for the assessment and management of polycystic ovary syndrome [published correction appears in hum Reprod. 2019;34(2):388]. Hum Reprod 2018;33(9):1602–1618. https://doi.org/10.1093/humrep/dey256.
17. Thuzar M, et al. Mineralocorticoid antagonism enhances brown adipose tissue function in humans: a randomized placebo-controlled cross-over study. Diabetes Obes Metab. 2019;21(3):509–16. https://doi.org/10.1111/dom.13539.
18. García-Beltran C, et al. (2019) Reduced circulating levels of chemokine CXCL14 in adolescent girls with polycystic ovary syndrome: normalization after insulin sensitization. BMJ Open Diab Res & Care. 2020; 8(1):e001035. https://doi.org/10.1136/bmjdrc-2019-001035.
19. Armstrong PW. Aldosterone antagonists--last man standing? N Engl J Med. 2011;364(1):79–80. https://doi.org/10.1056/NEJMe1012547.
20. Ibáñez L, et al. Pioglitazone (7.5 mg/day) added to flutamide-metformin in women with androgen excess: additional increments of visfatin and high molecular weight adiponectin. Clin Endocrinol. 2008;68(2):317–20. https://doi.org/10.1111/j.1365-2265.2007.03137.x.
21. Choi JH, et al. Anti-diabetic drugs inhibit obesity-linked phosphorylation of PPARgamma by Cdk5. Nature. 2010;466(7305):451–6. https://doi.org/10.1038/nature09291.
22. Ryan KK, et al. A role for central nervous system PPAR-γ in the regulation of energy balance. Nat Med. 2011;17(5):623–6. https://doi.org/10.1038/nm.2349.
23. Ryder REJ, DeFronzo RA. Pioglitazone: inexpensive; very effective at reducing HbA1c; no evidence of bladder cancer risk; plenty of evidence of cardiovascular benefit. Diabet Med. 2019;36(9):1185–6. https://doi.org/10.1111/dme.14053.
24. Ibáñez L, et al. Sensitization to insulin in adolescent girls to normalize hirsutism, hyperandrogenism, oligomenorrhea, dyslipidemia, and hyperinsulinism after precocious pubarche. J Clin Endocrinol Metab. 2000;85(10):3526–30. https://doi.org/10.1210/jcem.85.10.6908.
25. Ibáñez L, et al. Sensitization to insulin induces ovulation in nonobese adolescents with anovulatory hyperandrogenism. J Clin Endocrinol Metab. 2001;86(8):3595–8. https://doi.org/10.1210/jcem.86.8.7756.
26. https://cordis.europa.eu/project/rcn/110171/reporting/en.
27. Sánchez-Infantes D, et al. Pharmacokinetics of metformin in girls aged 9 years. Clin Pharmacokinet. 2011;50(11):735–8. https://doi.org/10.2165/11593970-000000000-00000.
28. Ibáñez L, et al. Early metformin therapy (age 8-12 years) in girls with precocious pubarche to reduce hirsutism, androgen excess, and oligomenorrhea in adolescence. J Clin Endocrinol Metab. 2011;96(8):E1262–7. https://doi.org/10.1210/jc.2011-0555.
29. Ibáñez L, et al. Toward a treatment normalizing ovulation rate in adolescent girls with polycystic ovary syndrome. J Endocr Soc. 2020 Mar 14;4(5):bvaa032. https://doi.org/10.1210/jendso/bvaa032.
30. Díaz M, et al. Low circulating levels of miR-451a in girls with polycystic ovary syndrome: different effects of randomized treatments. J Clin Endocrinol Metab. 2020; 105(3):dgz204. http://doi.org/10.1210/clinem/dgz204.

Environmental Factors Responsible for Obesity and Insulin Resistance in Polycystic Ovary Syndrome

4

Andrzej Milewicz, Alina Urbanovych, and Anna Brona

Polycystic ovary syndrome (PCOS) is an important public health concern with reproductive, metabolic, and psychological features. PCOS is one of the most common endocrine disorders in reproductive-aged women affecting 8–13% of them [1]. Except meeting the diagnostic criteria, women with PCOS present with metabolic disturbances including insulin resistance (IR), metabolic syndrome, prediabetes, type 2 diabetes (DM2), and cardiovascular risk factors [1]. The prevalence of insulin resistance ranges from 50 to 70% [2].

Obesity is associated with deterioration of reproductive and metabolic status in women with PCOS. Hence, it is necessary to address any factor that increase the risk of obesity in PCOS. Among environmental factors endocrine-disrupting chemicals (EDCs), advanced glycated end products (AGEs), and vitamin D are proposed to have an impact on obesity and insulin resistance in polycystic ovary syndrome.

Exposure to environmental toxins, EDCs and AGEs, may lead to endocrine, metabolic, and reproductive disruption resulting in development of different PCOS phenotypes and adverse health effects. Metabolic disorders include increase in insulin resistance, oxidative stress, and inflammation that result in increased adipogenesis and finally leads to obesity [3]. Vitamin D deficiency has been postulated to play a role in the pathogenesis of insulin resistance and to be related to metabolic risk factors in PCOS [4, 5].

A. Milewicz (✉) · A. Brona
Department of Endocrinology, Diabetes and Isotope Therapy, Wroclaw Medical University, Wrocław, Poland
e-mail: andrzej.milewicz@umed.wroc.pl

A. Urbanovych
Department of Endocrinology, Lviv National Medical University, Lviv, Ukraine

© International Society of Gynecological Endocrinology 2021
A. R. Genazzani et al. (eds.), *Impact of Polycystic Ovary, Metabolic Syndrome and Obesity on Women Health*, ISGE Series,
https://doi.org/10.1007/978-3-030-63650-0_4

4.1   Endocrine-Disrupting Chemicals

A 2000 report documented 2300 pesticide exposures in American schools from 1993 to 1996.

In 2004, levels of polybrominated diphenyl ethers (PBDEs) were about 40 higher in North American women than in Swedish women, based on samples of breast milk. A 2001 study showed that 96% of the pregnant women surveyed tested positive for bisphenol A (BPA).

As of October 2013, there are nearly 1000 endocrine-disrupting chemicals on The Endocrine Disruption Exchange's (TEDX) list. A 2008 study showed that 19 out of 20 children tested had PBDE levels an average of 3.2 times higher than their mothers [6].

Most of the 2000 chemicals that come on the market each year don't go through even simple tests to determine toxicity [6].

An endocrine-disrupting chemical (EDC) is an exogenous chemical, or mixture of chemicals, than can interfere with any aspect of hormone action. It is suggested that EDCs influence hormone action in different ways. EDCs or their metabolites can influence hormone metabolism in tissues-specific manner, and may directly interfere with hormone action only in those tissues where they are generated. EDCs or their metabolites may also interact with hormone receptors in a tissue-specific manner and exert direct agonist or antagonist effects, either because some tissues exhibit greater receptor density or because different receptor isoforms are expressed in different tissues [7].

4.1.1   Bisphenol A

One of EDCs, bisphenol A is considered to interfere with the endocrine system and play a role in the development of insulin resistance and obesity with major contributors being modern human diet and genomic composition.

Bisphenol A (BPA) is one of the most common plasticizers; it was first synthesized in 1891 and was discovered to be estrogenic in 1936. The xenoestrogen PBA is especially prevalent as a component used in rigid plastic products such as compact discs, dental materials, cosmetics, food and beverage containers, food and formula can linings, and glossy paper receipts. The BPA from food containers can leach into foods when they are heated or scratched and then be ingested [8]. More BPA is produced annually that any other chemicals (EDCs) with 15 billion pounds produced in 2013.

In the human urine, BPA was detected in 52 up to 100% of participants [9]. These findings indicate broad human exposure to BPA. The Environmental Protection Agency (EPA) in the USA has established the tolerable daily intake (TDI) for BPA at 50 mg per kg (body weight) per day in 1988 [10]. In January 2015, European Food Safety Authority has reduced TDI for BPA from 50 to 4 mg per kg (body weight) per day [10].

BPA exert diabetogenic and obesogenic effects. BPA contributes to insulin action in several mechanisms. It has an impact on insulin synthesis and release by b-pancreatic cells, and insulin signaling within liver, muscle, adipose tissues [11].

BPA has been shown to act through variety of receptors, such as the estrogen receptors alpha and beta, ERa and ERb, membrane receptor G-protein-coupled receptor 30 (GPR30), and the estrogen-related receptor gamma ERRγ [12].

It was reported that BPA between 1 and 10 nmol/l concentrations interferes with adipocyte metabolism by increasing oxidative stress and contributing to inflammation due to inhibition of adiponectin release and stimulation of interleukin 6 and tumor necrosis factor release [13]. Additionally, Wells et al. suggested a relation between BPA exposure and central obesity. They observed higher BPA concentrations in individuals with higher waist-to-hip ratio [14].

BPA acts as a xenoestrogen, thus binding to estrogen receptors. However, the interaction of BPA with ER receptors is relatively weak, ranging 2–3 orders of magnitude lower compared to estrogens [10].

It has been well described that all three estrogen receptors (ERa, ERb, and the G protein coupled ER (GPER)) are present on rodent and human b cells [10]. It has been reported that BPA mimics the action of estradiol and exerts effects on energy balance and glucose homoeostasis [15]. In vitro, BPA increased the frequency of glucose-induced ionized calcium oscillations in pancreatic beta cells and enhanced insulin secretion. In vivo, male mice taking daily doses of BPA presented higher insulin concentration in pancreatic beta cells and enhanced insulin secretion in comparison with control mice [15]. These changes result in hyperinsulinemia.

It is also known that BPA binds estrogen receptors in both adipocytes and pancreatic beta cells, and BPA-exposed cells develop lipid accumulation [15].

BPA acts in human tissues through ER receptors alpha, beta, and gamma resulting in gene expression. Additionally, BPA binds to membrane receptors resulting in non-genomic effects. Gene transcription depends on ER confirmation induced by BPA. Conformation alterations are responsible for recruitment of transcriptional co-regulators [10].

Other than the proposed ER-activation mechanism that involves binding to nuclear receptors, it has been suggested that BPA may exert its effects through rapid non-genomic pathways [10]. Binding to membrane ER receptor promotes rapid influx of calcium ion [10]. BPA causes membrane depolarization followed by alteration of conformation of voltage-dependent calcium channels. These changes do not require high BPA concentration; they occur at picomolar and at nanomolar concentrations [10].

In the animal study of Jayashree et al. [16], it has been demonstrated that after BPA administration glucose oxidation and glycogen content in the liver were decreased [11]. Another factor promoting hepatic insulin resistance – decreased Akt phosphorylation – was also reported. Additionally, decreased phosphorylation of Akt and GSK3b in skeletal muscle was found. It may explain how BPA contributes to insulin resistance in the muscle. Menale et al. [17] showed that BPA decrease the expression of PCSK1 gene in human pancreatic cell line [11]. PCSK1 contributes to insulin synthesis. The BPA action on adipose tissue was also investigated [11]. BPA administration caused increase in circulating inflammatory factors and local inflammation in the white adipose tissue. In addition higher plasma leptin levels were detected.

Decreased glucose utilization and phosphorylation of insulin receptor contributes to impaired insulin action in 3T3-L1 cells [11]. It has been demonstrated that BPA induced adipogenesis in 3T3-L1 preadipocytes [8]. Its actions comprise enhanced mRNA expression and increased enzymatic activity of 11β-hydroxysteroid dehydrogenase type 1 (11-βHSD type 1). 11-βHSD type 1 induces adipogenesis in human adipose tissue [8]. It suggests that BPA contributes to obesity susceptibility [8].

Also from an epidemiologic point of view, there are several studies to investigate positive correlation between exposure to PBA and obesity. In 3390 Chinese adults aged 40 year or older BPA were was positively associated with generalized obesity, abdominal obesity, and insulin resistance [18]. Another study provided evidence for a positive association between urinary BPA concentrations and waist circumference in the group of 1030 Korean adults [19]. In the National Health and Nutritional Examination Survey (NHANES) 2003–2008, the association between urinary BPA levels and obesity in the US population was reported [20]. Moreover, Hong et al. found that higher urinary BPA levels are associated with obesity and insulin resistance in Korean reproductive-aged women [15].

It is known that BPA promotes hyperandrogenism state, impairs oocyte development and folliculogenesis, and has a negative impact on metabolic parameters such as insulin resistance, obesity, oxidative stress, and inflammation [4]. Additionally, another studies have been conducted to investigate relationship between metabolic disturbances in PCOS and BPA. That is, a case control study of 71 women with PCOS and 100 women without PCOS showed positive association between BPA and insulin resistance. Moreover, higher serum BPA concentration was found in PCOS women [21].

Authors of meta-analysis have also demonstrated that BPA levels in PCOS women were significantly higher than controls. They found that high BPA levels were significantly associated with high BMI and high HOMA-IR [22]. Several mechanisms have been proposed to explain BPA action on insulin resistance. Findings from different studies pointed to changes of the structures and metabolism of pancreas leading to impaired insulin secretion. They also showed changes of insulin signaling in liver and muscles [22]. Studies in women with PCOS did not reveal the exact mechanisms for impact of BPA on insulin resistance [22], but there are numerous studies conducted in animals or cell culture elucidating these mechanisms (as described before).

4.2 Advanced Glycation End Products

Advanced glycation end products (AGEs) are derivatives of nonenzymatic glucose–protein, glucose–lipids, and glucose–nucleic acids reactions [23]. They are the end products of a chemical procedure called Maillard reaction [23]. These processes are irreversible. Aging, hyperglycemia, obesity, oxidative stress, and hypoxia accelerate the generation of their precursors [24]. AGEs are formed exogenously from thermally processed foods that are rich in proteins and reducing sugars. It is known that 10% of ingested AGEs are absorbed [25]. It has been reported that AGEs play a role in the pathogenesis of different diseases by causing oxidative stress, altering enzymatic activities, affecting cytotoxic pathways, or damaging nucleic acids.

It has been shown that serum AGEs are elevated in women with PCOS [26]. In another study increased serum levels of AGEs and upregulation in advanced glycation end products receptor (RAGE) expression in circulating monocytes in women with PCOS with insulin resistance without hyperglycemia had been found [26]. AGEs have also been reported to correlate with insulin, HOMA, and waist-to-hip ratio in these women [27]. Elevated serum AGEs levels were also found in lean women with PCOS without insulin resistance [27].

AGEs group includes over 20 heterogeneous compounds [11]. They bind to receptor or form crosslinks with extracellular matrix [24]. The AGE receptor (RAGE) binds also other molecules/ligands (i.e., amyloid b peptide) [24]. When ligands bind to RAGE, they activate signaling pathways (the PI3K/AKT pathways or the mitogen-activated protein kinase (MAPK) signaling pathways), and finally, genes associated with inflammation and apoptosis are transcribed [24]. The AGE–RAGE binding activates also JAK-2/STAT-1, another signaling pathway that contributes to inflammation and cytokine production. This signaling pathway is associated with the composition and activity of proteasomal subunits [24].

Physiological role of RAGE is yet not well understood, but it displays a role in immune or inflammatory response. Cytokines (IL-1, IL-6, IL-8) and chemokines are formed after AGE binding to RAGE which leads to the activation of inflammatory processes. Then through NADPH oxidase, as well as activation of the transcription factor NF-kB, excess oxidative stress is generated [24]. The excessive reactive oxygen species (ROS) production leads to upregulation in RAGE expression [24].

Insulin resistance and hyperinsulinemia are found in approximately 50 up to 70% of women with PCOS. Oxidative stress and inflammation contribute to hyperinsulinemia and insulin resistance [24]. It is suggested that excessive oxidative stress is one of the features of PCOS and it cannot be compensated by the antioxidant mechanisms [24].

Increased AGEs level is associated with inflammatory markers such as high-sensitivity C-reactive protein (CRP), fibrinogen, 8-isoprostanes (a marker of lipid peroxidation), TNF-a, and vascular adhesion molecule-1 (VAM-1) [28].

There is a system of glyoxalases that protects cells from damage caused by cytotoxic metabolites such as AGEs [24]. This is the glyoxalase detoxification system. It comprises two glyoxalases GLO-I and GLO-II [24]. Significant reduction of ovarian GLO activity has been reported in PCOS animal study. Animals fed a high-AGE diet had lower ovarian GLO activity than animals fed a low-AGE diet [24].

AGEs change insulin cell signaling and modify glucose transporters and glucose metabolism in insulin-sensitive cells, also in ovarian cells. That is, RAGE overexpression led to a decrease in GLUT-4 gene expression and attenuation of insulin signaling in adipocytes and caused morphological changes of adipocytes [24]. Women with PCOS presented impaired action of GLUT-4 [24]. Insulin resistance (IR) in PCOS has complex molecular pathophysiology. It includes different mechanisms: a post-binding receptor defect, low levels of IRS-1 expression, impaired IRS-1 phosphorylation, reduced activity of the serine/threonine kinase AKT2, and altered glucose transporter GLUT-4 translocation to the plasma membrane [24]. Hence, it is suggested that AGEs impair insulin signaling and glucose metabolism through several mechanisms.

Thera are different studies presenting the effect of AGEs on glucose metabolism. In one study the effect of human glycated albumin (HGA) on glucose transport in the human granulosa KGN cell in the presence of insulin was investigated [24]. Inhibition of insulin-mediated AKT phosphorylation was found in these cells. HGA also inhibited insulin-induced GLUT-4 translocation from the cytoplasm to the membrane compartments of KGN cells [24]. In skeletal muscle cells the phosphatidylinositol 3-kinase (PI3K)/protein kinase B (PKB) pathway (part of insulin signaling cascade) was suppressed by HGA [24]. HGA activated PKCa that caused an increase in serine/threonine phosphorylation of IRS and ultimately altered insulin metabolic signals [24]. In addition, it has been reported that AGEs cause b cell malfunction in animals [24].

Obesity is also commonly observed in women with PCOS, in 30–75% of cases [23]. Recent studies have shown how AGEs contribute to the development of obesity [27]. For example, in animal studies, weight gain in mice fed with high-AGE diet and low-AGE diet was compared. Animals on H-AGE diet had a significant weight gain in comparison to control group [27].

The effect of high-AGE diet on hormonal and metabolic parameters in human was also investigated. Low-AGE diet in comparison with high-AGE diet resulted in lower testosterone levels, HOMA-IR, and improved oxidative stress status in women with PCOS [25]. Results suggest a novel treatment strategy for ovarian dysfunction by decreasing AGEs in diet to attenuate AGEs effects.

In another study association between AGEs/soluble receptor of advanced glycation end products (AGEs/sRAGE) and anthropometric parameters in reproductive-aged PCOS patients was investigated. Positive correlation between serum levels of AGEs and BMI was found. On the contrary serum levels of sRAGE were decreased along with increased BMI [23].

There is evidence that AGEs induced the production of inflammatory mediators in adipocytes and macrophages via RAGE activation [29]. It has been found that MG stimulated adipogenesis by the upregulation of Akt signaling (increased the phosphorylation of Akt1) [30]. MG treatment increased also the phosphorylation of p21 and p27. P21 and p27 are the major regulators of the cell cycle. The increased phosphorylation of p21 and p27 activates their degradation and leads to the entry of cells to S phase that enhance cell proliferation [30].

Studies have also shown that women with PCOS have increased serum CML (carboxymethyl-lysine, one of the AGEs) in comparison to the control group, independently of obesity and insulin resistance [25].

4.2.1 Vitamin D

Vitamin D receptors are expressed in 2776 genomic positions and modulate the expression of 229 genes in more than 30 different tissues, such as skeleton, brain, breast, pancreas, parathyroid glands, immune cells, cardiomyocytes, and ovaries [2].

Women with PCOS are likely to have an increased risk of vitamin D deficiency (VDD). The prevalence of vitamin D deficiency among the general adult population is estimated about 20–48% [2], while among women with PCOS approximately 67–85% [31].

Vitamin D affects glucose metabolism. It contributes to increased insulin secretion, increased insulin sensitivity, increased glucose uptake, and expression of insulin receptor [32]. Multiple cellular and molecular mechanisms have been proposed to explain this. 1,25-dihydroxyvitamin D enhance insulin release from β-cells, transcriptional activation of the human insulin receptor gene, and suppression of the release of proinflammatory cytokines that are involved in insulin resistance [33]. Vitamin D may also exert effect on insulin action due to the regulation of extracellular calcium concentration and normal calcium influx across cell membranes [34].

Vitamin D deficiency was observed in obese individuals. In a large study comprising 42,024 persons, 10% increase of BMI was associated with 4% decrease of serum vitamin D [35]. The National Health and Nutrition Examination Survey (2001–2004) showed that abdominal obesity was associated with vitamin D deficiency [36]. Drincic et al. recommend 2–3 times higher daily dose of vitamin D supplementation in obese persons in comparison to normal (2.5 IU/kg) [37].

In Tsakova et al.'s study, higher prevalence of vitamin D deficiency in obese women with PCOS than in lean women with PCOS (70% vs. 60%) was found [38].

In obese individuals, a higher proportion of vitamin D, which is fat soluble, is sequestered in adipose tissues; and hence, bioavailability of the vitamin is lowered [5].

There is an evidence that vitamin D level plays an important role in insulin sensitivity and glucose metabolism.

Negative correlation between serum vitamin D levels and waist circumference, triglycerides, fasting glucose, and HOMA-IR were found [39]. It has been reported that PCOS patients with vitamin D deficiency were more likely to have increased levels of fasting glucose and HOMA-IR compared to those without vitamin D deficiency [2].

Inverse association between vitamin D concentration and HOMA-IR, glucose, CRP, and triglycerides have been found in many studies [2]. These studies have also shown positive correlation between vitamin D concentration and HDL-C or QUICKI.

It has been demonstrated that both intrinsic and extrinsic factors contribute to insulin resistance in PCOS women [40]. Impaired serine phosphorylation of the insulin receptor-1 is the intrinsic factor [40]. Ngo et al. investigated the potential role of vitamin D and NO responsiveness (defined as platelet response to NO donor) as extrinsic factors [40]. They found on multivariate analysis that NO responsiveness and 25(OH)D3 levels were significantly associated with QUICKI. Low vitamin D levels and low platelet response to NO donor correlated with low QUICKI in the whole study group.

Another prospective study investigated effects of calcium and vitamin supplementation on serum insulin level, HOMA-IR, and QUICKI [41]. The 8 weeks supplementation in PCOS women with vitamin D deficiency led to a significant reduction in serum insulin levels, HOMA-IR score, and a significant elevation in QUICKI index.

Li et al. reported that severe vitamin D deficiency correlated with insulin resistance and was independent of BMI and waist-to-hip ratio in women with PCOS. They also showed higher insulin levels in women without PCOS but with severe vitamin D deficiency [5].

It was proposed by Irani et al. that vitamin D attenuates the effects of the AGE–RAGE system in vitamin D-deficient women with PCOS due to increase of serum sRAGE levels. sRAGE acts as an anti-inflammatory factor. It binds circulating AGEs and blocks the intracellular events following the AGE–RAGE binding [42]. It has been demonstrated that vitamin D3 supplementation significantly increased serum sRAGE levels [42]. It was also observed that serum sRAGE was inversely correlated with BMI.

It has been shown that environmental factors play a role in the development of obesity and insulin resistance in PCOS women. There is a bulk of evidence that endocrine-disrupting chemicals, advanced glycated end products, and vitamin D deficiency contribute to these disorders. The results of in vitro and in vivo studies have demonstrated different mechanisms involved in the development of these conditions. They suggest new ways of treatment. In addition, they point to the importance of avoidance of exposure to deleterious environmental factors.

References

1. International evidence based guideline for the assessment and management of polycystic ovary syndrome. Copyright Monash University, Melbourne Australia; 2018.
2. He C, Lin Z, Robb SW, Ezeamama AE. Serum vitamin D levels and polycystic ovary syndrome: a systematic review and meta-analysis. Nutrients. 2015;7(6):4555–77. https://doi.org/10.3390/nu7064555.
3. Rutkowska AZ, Diamanti-Kandarakis E. Polycystic ovary syndrome and environmental toxins. Fertil Steril. 2016;106(4):948–58. https://doi.org/10.1016/j.fertnstert.2016.08.031.
4. Patra SK, Nasrat H, Goswami B, Jain A. Vitamin D as a predictor of insulin resistance in polycystic ovarian syndrome. Diabetes Metab Syndr. 2012;6(3):146–9. https://doi.org/10.1016/j.dsx.2012.09.006.
5. Li HW, Brereton RE, Anderson RA, Wallace AM, Ho CK. Vitamin D deficiency is common and associated with metabolic risk factors in patients with polycystic ovary syndrome. Metabolism. 2011;60(10):1475–81. https://doi.org/10.1016/j.metabol.2011.03.002.
6. Endo News April 2015.
7. Gore AC. Endocrine-disrupting chemicals. JAMA Intern Med. 2016;176(11):1705–6. https://doi.org/10.1001/jamainternmed.2016.5766.
8. Gore AC, Chappell VA, Fenton SE, et al. EDC-2: the Endocrine Society's second scientific statement on endocrine-disrupting chemicals. Endocr Rev. 2015;36(6):E1–E150. https://doi.org/10.1210/er.2015-1010.

9. Vandenberg LN, Hauser R, Marcus M, Olea N, Welshons WV. Human exposure to bisphenol a (BPA). Reprod Toxicol. 2007;24(2):139–77. https://doi.org/10.1016/j.reprotox.2007.07.010.
10. Pjanic M. The role of polycarbonate monomer bisphenol-a in insulin resistance. PeerJ. 2017;5:e3809. https://doi.org/10.7717/peerj.3809.
11. Le Magueresse-Battistoni B, Multigner L, Beausoleil C, Rousselle C. Effects of bisphenol a on metabolism and evidences of a mode of action mediated through endocrine disruption. Mol Cell Endocrinol. 2018;475:74–91. https://doi.org/10.1016/j.mce.2018.02.009.
12. Le Magueresse-Battistoni B, Labaronne E, Vidal H, Naville D. Endocrine disrupting chemicals in mixture and obesity, diabetes and related metabolic disorders. World J Biol Chem. 2017;8(2):108–19. https://doi.org/10.4331/wjbc.v8.i2.108.
13. Ben-Jonathan N, Hugo ER, Brandebourg TD. Effects of bisphenol a on adipokine release from human adipose tissue: implications for the metabolic syndrome. Mol Cell Endocrinol. 2009;304(1–2):49–54. https://doi.org/10.1016/j.mce.2009.02.022.
14. Wells EM, Jackson LW, Koontz MB. Association between bisphenol a and waist-to-height ratio among children: National Health and nutrition examination survey, 2003-2010. Ann Epidemiol. 2014;24(2):165–7. https://doi.org/10.1016/j.annepidem.2013.06.002.
15. Hong SH, Sung YA, Hong YS, et al. Urinary bisphenol a is associated with insulin resistance and obesity in reproductive-aged women. Clin Endocrinol. 2017;86(4):506–12. https://doi.org/10.1111/cen.13270.
16. Jayashree S, Indumathi D, Akilavalli N, Sathish S, Selvaraj J, Balasubramanian K. Effect of Bisphenol-A on insulin signal transduction and glucose oxidation in liver of adult male albino rat. Environ Toxicol Pharmacol. 2013;35(2):300–10. https://doi.org/10.1016/j.etap.2012.12.016.
17. Menale C, Piccolo MT, Cirillo G, Calogero RA, Papparella A, Mita L, Del Giudice EM, Diano N, Crispi S, Mita DG. Bisphenol A effects on gene expression in adipocytes from children: association with metabolic disorders. J Mol Endocrinol. 2015;54(3):289–303. https://doi.org/10.1530/JME-14-0282.
18. Wang T, Li M, Chen B, et al. Urinary bisphenol a (BPA) concentration associates with obesity and insulin resistance. J Clin Endocrinol Metab. 2012;97(2):E223–7. https://doi.org/10.1210/jc.2011-1989.
19. Ko A, Hwang MS, Park JH, Kang HS, Lee HS, Hong JH. Association between urinary bisphenol a and waist circumference in Korean adults. Toxicol Res. 2014;30(1):39–44. https://doi.org/10.5487/TR.2014.30.1.039.
20. Teppala S, Madhavan S, Shankar A. Bisphenol a and metabolic syndrome: results from NHANES. Int J Endocrinol. 2012;2012:598180. https://doi.org/10.1155/2012/598180.
21. Kandaraki E, Chatzigeorgiou A, Livadas S, et al. Endocrine disruptors and polycystic ovary syndrome (PCOS): elevated serum levels of bisphenol a in women with PCOS. J Clin Endocrinol Metab. 2011;96(3):E480–4. https://doi.org/10.1210/jc.2010-1658.
22. Hu Y, Wen S, Yuan D, et al. The association between the environmental endocrine disruptor bisphenol a and polycystic ovary syndrome: a systematic review and meta-analysis. Gynecol Endocrinol. 2018;34(5):370–7. https://doi.org/10.1080/09513590.2017.1405931.
23. Liao Y, Huang R, Sun Y, et al. An inverse association between serum soluble receptor of advanced glycation end products and hyperandrogenism and potential implication in polycystic ovary syndrome patients. Reprod Biol Endocrinol. 2017;15(1):9. https://doi.org/10.1186/s12958-017-0227-8.
24. Merhi Z, Kandaraki EA, Diamanti-Kandarakis E. Implications and future perspectives of AGEs in PCOS pathophysiology. Trends Endocrinol Metab. 2019;30(3):150–62. https://doi.org/10.1016/j.tem.2019.01.005.
25. Tantalaki E, Piperi C, Livadas S, et al. Impact of dietary modification of advanced glycation end products (AGEs) on the hormonal and metabolic profile of women with polycystic ovary syndrome (PCOS). Hormones (Athens). 2014;13(1):65–73. https://doi.org/10.1007/BF03401321.

26. Diamanti-Kandarakis E, Piperi C, Kalofoutis A, Creatsas G. Increased levels of serum advanced glycation end-products in women with polycystic ovary syndrome. Clin Endocrinol. 2005;62(1):37–43. https://doi.org/10.1111/j.1365-2265.2004.02170.x.
27. Garg D, Merhi Z. Relationship between advanced glycation end products and steroidogenesis in PCOS. Reprod Biol Endocrinol. 2016;14(1):71. https://doi.org/10.1186/s12958-016-0205-6.
28. Uribarri J, Cai W, Peppa M, et al. Circulating glycotoxins and dietary advanced glycation end-products: two links to inflammatory response, oxidative stress, and aging. J Gerontol A Biol Sci Med Sci. 2007;62(4):427–33. https://doi.org/10.1093/gerona/62.4.427.
29. Gaens KH, Stehouwer CD, Schalkwijk CG. Advanced glycation endproducts and its receptor for advanced glycation endproducts in obesity. Curr Opin Lipidol. 2013;24(1):4–11. https://doi.org/10.1097/MOL.0b013e32835aea13.
30. Jia X, Chang T, Wilson TW, Wu L. Methylglyoxal mediates adipocyte proliferation by increasing phosphorylation of Akt1. PLoS One. 2012;7(5):e36610. https://doi.org/10.1371/journal.pone.0036610.
31. Thomson RL, Spedding S, Buckley JD. Vitamin D in the aetiology and management of polycystic ovary syndrome. Clin Endocrinol. 2012;77(3):343–50. https://doi.org/10.1111/j.1365-2265.2012.04434.x.
32. Rojas-Rivera J, De La Piedra C, Ramos A, Ortiz A, Egido J. The expanding spectrum of biological actions of vitamin D. Nephrol Dial Transplant. 2010;25(9):2850–65. https://doi.org/10.1093/ndt/gfq313.
33. Teegarden D, Donkin SS. Vitamin D: emerging new roles in insulin sensitivity. Nutr Res Rev. 2009;22(1):82–92. https://doi.org/10.1017/S0954422409389301.
34. Pittas AG, Lau J, Hu FB, Dawson-Hughes B. The role of vitamin D and calcium in type 2 diabetes. A systematic review and meta-analysis. J Clin Endocrinol Metab. 2007;92(6):2017–29. https://doi.org/10.1210/jc.2007-0298.
35. Vimaleswaran KS, Berry DJ, Lu C, et al. Causal relationship between obesity and vitamin D status: bi-directional Mendelian randomization analysis of multiple cohorts. PLoS Med. 2013;10(2):e1001383. https://doi.org/10.1371/journal.pmed.1001383.
36. Scragg R, Sowers M. Bell C; third National Health and nutrition examination survey. Serum 25-hydroxyvitamin D, diabetes, and ethnicity in the third National Health and nutrition examination survey. Diabetes Care. 2004;27(12):2813–8. https://doi.org/10.2337/diacare.27.12.2813.
37. Drincic A, Fuller E, Heaney RP, Armas LA. 25-Hydroxyvitamin D response to graded vitamin D_3 supplementation among obese adults. J Clin Endocrinol Metab. 2013;98(12):4845–51. https://doi.org/10.1210/jc.2012-4103.
38. Tsakova AD, Gateva AT, Kamenov ZA. 25(OH) vitamin D levels in premenopausal women with polycystic ovary syndrome and/or obesity. Int J Vitam Nutr Res. 2012;82(6):399–404. https://doi.org/10.1024/0300-9831/a000137.
39. Forouhi NG, Luan J, Cooper A, Boucher BJ, Wareham NJ. Baseline serum 25-hydroxy vitamin d is predictive of future glycemic status and insulin resistance: the Medical Research Council Ely prospective study 1990-2000. Diabetes. 2008;57(10):2619–25. https://doi.org/10.2337/db08-0593.
40. Ngo DT, Chan WP, Rajendran S, et al. Determinants of insulin responsiveness in young women: impact of polycystic ovarian syndrome, nitric oxide, and vitamin D. Nitric Oxide. 2011;25(3):326–30. https://doi.org/10.1016/j.niox.2011.06.005.
41. Asemi Z, Foroozanfard F, Hashemi T, Bahmani F, Jamilian M, Esmaillzadeh A. Calcium plus vitamin D supplementation affects glucose metabolism and lipid concentrations in overweight and obese vitamin D deficient women with polycystic ovary syndrome. Clin Nutr. 2015;34(4):586–92. https://doi.org/10.1016/j.clnu.2014.09.015.
42. Irani M, Minkoff H, Seifer DB, Merhi Z. Vitamin D increases serum levels of the soluble receptor for advanced glycation end products in women with PCOS. J Clin Endocrinol Metab. 2014;99(5):E886–90. https://doi.org/10.1210/jc.2013-4374.

Pathogenesis of PCOS: From Metabolic and Neuroendocrine Implications to the Choice of the Therapeutic Strategy

5

Alessia Prati, Andrea R. Genazzani, and Alessandro D. Genazzani

5.1 Introduction

Polycystic ovary syndrome (PCOS) is a heterogeneous condition affecting between 5 and 20% of fertile women [1]. It is the most common cause of anovulation and therefore of infertility, characterized by hyperandrogenism with the arrest of follicular development, esthetic problems (acne, hirsutism, alopecia), and frequently associated with metabolic alterations such as insulin resistance or overweight/obesity.

Although several diagnostic criteria have been proposed (Rotterdam, Androgen Excess and PCOS Society, National Institutes of Health), the diagnosis of PCOS is still based on the Rotterdam criteria (2003) [2], which require the presence of two out of three main features of the syndrome: chronic anovulation that means oligo–/amenorrhea, hyperandrogenism (clinical and/or bio-humoral), and polycystic ovaries at ultrasound [3].

Over the years a very variable spectrum of clinical manifestations has been highlighted, variously combined in different patterns, so that four different possible phenotypes can be identified (Table 5.1).

The common features of these patients are the well-known presence of an inappropriate gonadotropin secretion, often characterized by elevated LH levels compared to FSH levels, this last reduced up to lower than 30%, and an increased LH/FSH ratio (>2.5), due to the increased amplitude of LH pulses, this being the cause

A. Prati · A. D. Genazzani
Center of Endocrinological Gynecology, Obstetric and Gynecological Clinic, University of Modena and Reggio Emilia, Modena, Italy

A. R. Genazzani (✉)
Center of Endocrinological Gynecology, Obstetric and Gynecological Clinic, University of Modena and Reggio Emilia, Modena, Italy

Department of Obstetrics and Gynecology, University of Pisa, Pisa, Italy

© International Society of Gynecological Endocrinology 2021
A. R. Genazzani et al. (eds.), *Impact of Polycystic Ovary, Metabolic Syndrome and Obesity on Women Health*, ISGE Series,
https://doi.org/10.1007/978-3-030-63650-0_5

43

Table 5.1 Adult Diagnostic Criteria (Rotterdam)

1. Phenotype 1 (classic PCOS)
(a) Clinical and/or biochemical evidence of hyperandrogenism
(b) Evidence of oligo-anovulation
(c) Ultrasonographic evidence of a polycystic ovary
2. Phenotype 2 (Essential NIH Criteria)
(a) Clinical and/or biochemical evidence of hyperandrogenism
(b) Evidence of oligo-anovulation
3. Phenotype 3 (ovulatory PCOS)
(a) Clinical and/or biochemical evidence of hyperandrogenism
(b) Ultrasonographic evidence of a polycystic ovary
4. Phenotype 4 (nonhyperandrogenic PCOS)
(a) Evidence of oligo-anovulation
(b) Ultrasonographic evidence of a polycystic ovary

of ovarian hyperandrogenism. In addition to the well-known clinical symptoms, PCOS is also characterized by a series of metabolic problems such as obesity, present in 25–50% of the patients, and hyperinsulinemia that occurs in up to 50% of subjects. Indeed, extensive literature has shown that insulin resistance is very common in PCOS, independently from BMI.

Insulin resistance is a biological compensatory event that induces the elevation of insulin concentrations (hyperinsulinemia) in order to keep the glycemic values within the normal range. It is present in 50–80% of women with PCOS and obesity and in 15–30% of PCOS with normal weight [4, 5, 6]. During pregnancy, women with PCOS have a greater risk of incurring complications such as gestational diabetes, hypertensive disorders, preeclampsia, HELLP syndrome, and preterm birth, especially if they have a compensatory hyperinsulinism [7].

5.2 Physiopathology of the PCOS Patients

5.2.1 Weight and Metabolism

It is well-known how reproductive axis and body weight are tightly linked. Depending on the bodily disposition of the fat, obesity is classified into gynoid obesity, in which the fat is distributed in the lower part of the body, i.e., buttocks and thighs, and android obesity, in which the fat is located centrally at abdominal, mesenteric, and visceral level [8]. The substantial difference of this different conformation relies in the fact that the adipose tissue accumulated at the abdominal level is metabolically more active, more sensitive to catecholamines and less to insulin, and releases higher amount of triglycerides, and this is considered a direct index of cardiovascular risk. In fact, the Waist Hip Ratio determination (WHR) is an excellent index to assess the degree of obesity, quantifying the amount of intra-abdominal fat. In a subject with BMI > 25 kg/m^2, a ratio greater than 0.80 is a clear sign of android obesity, while a ratio lower than 0.75 is an index of gynoid obesity. The waist circumference, more than BMI, is directly correlated with the risk of developing Metabolic Syndrome (MS); in fact it is included among the diagnostic criteria for MS drawn up by the Adult Treatment Panel III (ATIII), which considers as a risk factor a waist circumference equal or greater than 102 cm in males and 88 cm in women [8].

As a result of this excess of weight, in particular in women, an alteration of reproductive capacity is frequently observed. The adipose tissue is not inert, but it is a real endocrine organ, with effects at both peripheral and central level, which unlike the other endocrine systems is poorly controlled and modulated in its action by the hypothalamic area or by other endocrine systems: in fact, fat cells are able not only to aromatize androgens into estrogens but also to release hormonal signals (adiponectin, leptin), acting directly on the CNS and regulating food intake, energy expenditure, and reproductive function. An excessive intake of food influences the balance of our metabolic and endocrine systems up to modulating the hypothalamus, which is the control unit that regulates and coordinates the whole metabolic-hormonal system, with consequent abnormal release of hypothalamic tropins and irregular menstrual cycle, from oligomenorrhea and anovulation, up to amenorrhea. In the brain all the signals relating to the nutritional state, such as the excess as well as the weight defect, are recorded and processed as function of time and quite often are negatively recorded. The metabolic signals arriving at the hypothalamic level are transmitted by leptin and adiponectin (both hormones produced in adipocytes), Ghrelin, and many other neurotransmitters, modulating the release of hypothalamic GnRH. When the hypothalamic function is negatively affected, functional disorders result (i.e., PCOS, hypothalamic amenorrhea, etc.). In humans and nonhuman primates, the majority of hypothalamic GnRH neurons are located more dorsally in the medial basal hypothalamus, in the infundibulum, and in the periventricular region. They are surrounded by the centers that control the sleep-wake rhythm, thermoregulation, hunger/satiety, and glycemic control: modifications of the function of these centers, induced by peripheral signals, lead to an alteration in the production and pulsatile release of GnRH that affects the reproductive function, triggering oligomenorrhea, anovulation, and/or amenorrhea.

5.2.2 Hyperandrogenism

Although PCOS is a syndrome, we have always tried to understand where hyperandrogenism is triggered: abnormalities of the metabolic control (diabetes, thyroid diseases), malfunctioning at ovarian level (ovarian cysts, atresic follicles), or hyperandrogenism caused by endocrine diseases such as those of adrenal gland (exaggerated adrenarche, Cushing's syndrome, adrenal hyperplasia). However, only 3% of PCOS hyperandrogenism is due to an isolated adrenal disease [9] (Table 5.2).

Table 5.2 Differential diagnosis of hyperandrogenemia

A. Physiologic adolescent anovulation
B. Functional gonadal hyperandrogenism
1. PCOS: Primary FOH (Functional Ovarian Hyperandrogenism) (common form of PCOS)
2. Secondary FOH
a. Virilizing congenital adrenal hyperplasia
b. Adrenal rests of the ovary
c. Ovarian steroidogenic blocks
d. Insulin resistance syndromes
e. Acromegaly
f. Epilepsy (valproic acid therapy)
3. Disorders of sex development
4. Pregnancy-related hyperandrogenism
C. FAH (Functional Adrenal Hyperandrogenism)
1. PCOS: primary FAH (uncommon form of PCOS)
2. Virilizing congenital adrenal hyperplasia
3. Other glucocorticoid-suppressible FAH
a. Hyperprolactinemia
b. Cortisone RD deficiency (and apparent RD deficiency)
c. Apparent DHEA sulfotransferase deficiency
4. Glucocorticoid-nonsuppressible FAH
a. Cushing's syndrome
b. Glucocorticoid resistance
D. Peripheral androgen metabolic disorders
1. Obesity
2. Idiopathic hyperandrogenism
3. Portohepatic shunting
E. Virilizing tumors
F. Androgenic drugs

Androgens and its precursors are normally produced at ovarian and adrenal level in approximately equal amounts, respectively, under LH and ACTH control. Androgens, however, do not have a negative feedback or a neuroendocrine mechanism that directly regulates/controls their production. In fact, the androgenic production from the ovary has intra-ovarian mechanisms, in order to optimize the synthesis of androgens, estrogens, and folliculogenesis: androgens are obviously the substrate for the production of estrogens, but if they are present in exaggerated amount, they block ovulation. The ovarian androgenic hypersecretion, typical of PCOS patients, appears to be caused by a mechanism of desensitization of thecal cells to LH, which however limit excessive androgenic production; on the other hand, the amount of androgens produced is under paracrine control, which essentially acts on the activity of the cytochrome p450c17 that limits the formation of steroid hormones.

Whatever triggers PCOS, the aromatase activity at ovarian level is altered. It is well-known that in the ovaries the production of estradiol is linked to the correct aromatization of androgens in estrogens: whenever a metabolic factor, such as a compensatory hyperinsulinemia, induced by peripheral insulin resistance, alters this equilibrium, androgen production increases, and aromatase activity is abnormally reduced.

The failure of the conversion of androgens to estradiol and the resulting hyperandrogenism induce reduced hepatic SHBG synthesis, promoting the increase of plasmatic free androgens levels and a higher bioactive availability, thus promoting the onset of clinical signs such as hirsutism and acne [6]. Furthermore, the excess of androgens negatively modulates the function of insulin in the liver and at peripheral level: in fact it has been shown that testosterone negatively modulates the transmission of the intracellular insulin signal, reducing both the number and the efficiency of glucose transporters (GLUT-4), generating/improving insulin resistance mechanisms [10]. All such facts in women with PCOS promote also an excess of IGF-1 other than of insulin, with a further increase of androgens' levels, caused by the aromatase deficiency and by SHBG levels decrease, with the consequent increase of the amount of free androgens, which are biologically active and deeply affecting the reproductive axis. The importance of nutritional status for the proper functioning of the reproductive axis is thus further emphasized.

5.2.3   Insulin Resistance

Insulin, as already mentioned, plays a role on the synthesis of androgens modulating the cytochrome P450-17alpha, and its levels correlate with glycemia. When performing the oral glucose tolerance test (OGTT) in a patient with a suspect of insulin resistance, we must not focus on blood glucose levels only since the metabolic homeostasis reacts to control blood glucose levels inducing the release of insulin up to 10 times the amount of insulin normally necessary. Prevention is therefore the most powerful tool we have. Through a correct lifestyle and the use of insulin-sensitizers (like Metformin), we can be helpful in managing these conditions.

Insulin resistance and hyperinsulinemia are the elements that most frequently determine the clinical and biochemical difference between PCOS patient with overweight/obesity from those with normal weight. When obesity and insulin resistance occur together with an android-type distribution of adipose tissue, despite having absolute values of androgens only moderately increased, SHBG levels are reduced, and the clinical signs of hyperandrogenism become more evident. In PCOS without insulin resistance, the amount of free androgens is lower, and the clinical manifestations linked to hyperandrogenism are less marked.

In this context, the data obtained from the OGTT becomes essential. Similar to other endocrine diseases, such as in girls with hypo-GH, we find an insulin response to the glucose load similar to that observed in obese patients: in fact, the GH deficiency triggers a compensatory mechanism modifying both cortisol and insulin secretions, in order to compensate the lack of GH, thus inducing a compensatory hyperinsulinemia. The result of this is an insulin response to glucose load in normal-weight patients with GH deficiency paradoxically similar to that observed in obese or PCOS patients.

Another important aspect recently investigated is the involvement of liver in this endo-metabolic framework. The well-known NAFLD (Nonalcoholic Fatty Liver Disease) is the result of insulin resistance, which leads to an accumulation of fat in the liver; it has been recently shown that the liver produces two hormones, HGF (Hepatocyte Growth Factor) and betatrophin, both involved in a system that modulates the compensatory response of beta-pancreatic cells to insulin resistance. Betatrophin modulates in a direct way the proliferation of beta cells in case of insulin resistance in order to increase the amount of insulin and thus to obtain a better control of glycemia and glucose uptake from the plasmatic circulation [11]; HGF is a growth factor that plays a key role in the connection, via the opioidergic and neuroaminergic pathways, of the brain-liver-pancreas axis, modulating the adaptive response of the pancreas to insulin resistance [11].

Studies on animal models have hypothesized that insulin receptors are also present at central level, in particular localized on kisspeptin-secreting neurons that stimulate GnRH neurons. Under compensatory hyperinsulinemia, an excessive activity of kisspeptin-secreting neurons has been observed, thus inducing an increase of GnRH release. Neuroendocrinology of obese patients, therefore, described a direct link between CNS and metabolism, and in particular, there is a metabolic-induced modulation of several neuroendocrine activities [12].

It is well-known that insulin resistance is due to several conditions that can act already during the prenatal period, such as gestational diabetes and obesity during pregnancy, or that can act after birth as in case of children with IUGR (Intrauterine Growth Restriction), where hyperinsulinemia represents a compensatory defensive mechanism that allows the low-in-weight infants to store energy, survive, and thus reach quickly a more appropriate body weight. Insulin resistance may also be linked to receptor or signal transduction defects or to genetic factors such as familial diabetes, but when obesity occurs during adulthood the mechanism triggering the gain of weight is clear [11].

5.3   New Perspectives in the Pathogenesis of PCOS

A recent review collected the results from several studies on animal models and rationally hypothesized a primarily neuroendocrine origin of PCOS [13]: in particular, since hyperandrogenism is present in 60% of PCOS patients, the effects of high androgen levels have been assessed. In these animal models the exposure to high androgen levels during prenatal life or during the first months of life induces the onset of the typical features of PCOS: clinical manifestations of hyperandrogenism, hypersecretion of LH, ultrasonographic evidence of polycystic ovaries, ovulatory dysfunction, increased amount of fat mass, hypertrophy of fat cells, and also insulin resistance. Probably the androgen receptor (AR) plays an essential role in the pathogenesis of PCOS: AR is expressed in the structures of the hypothalamic-pituitary-ovarian axis, as well as in adipocytes and in hepatocytes. However, the role played

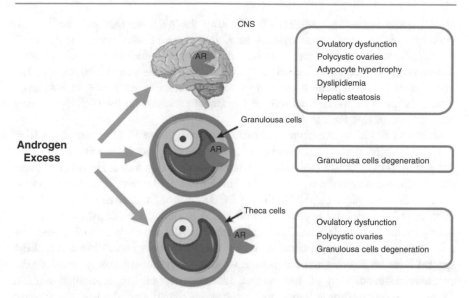

Fig. 5.1 Different sites of AR action in generating the characteristic features of PCOS. In particular, silencing AR at the level of the CNS and generating states of hyperandrogenism in the rats did not induce the reproductive and metabolic traits of PCOS; therefore the loss of central AR function protects from the onset of PCOS more than the loss of function of AR in the ovaries (modified from [13])

by androgens in central nervous system (CNS) is probably predominant, since in knock-out animal model for AR in the brain and undergoing to states of hyperandrogenism a much more marked reduction in the typical manifestations of PCOS has been observed compared to the knock-out model for AR only at ovarian level [13] (Fig. 5.1).

A frequent characteristic of the PCOS patient is the increased frequency and amplitude of LH pulse. This reflects the increased stimulation of GnRH neurons: on animal models it has been observed that these neurons do not express receptors for androgens, progesterone, and alpha-estrogens. Interestingly the negative and positive feedback at central level is not played on GnRH neurons, and these mechanisms are indirect. In fact, recently two neuronal groups have been identified: kisspeptin/neurokinin B/dynorphin neurons (KNDy), which act with a mechanism depending on the levels of circulating estrogens, and the GABAergic neurons of the arcuate nucleus, which guarantee a stimulatory effect on the GnRH-secreting neurons [14]. The kisspeptin-secreting neurons have two locations: one group is in anteroventral periventricular nucleus (AVPV) and is sensitive to low levels of circulating estrogens, generating a positive feedback on GnRH-secreting neurons; the other is in the arcuate nucleus and is activated by high levels of estrogen, thus playing the negative feedback on the GnRH pulse generator.

On such basis, androgen receptors have been proposed as potential modulator of the KNDy system [15]: in fact, it has been observed that prenatal exposure to hyperandrogenic states leads to a drop of innervation by the KNDy system on

GnRH-secreting neurons, negatively affecting the negative feedback action. On such basis, it has been postulated that the KNDy system could become a "putative" therapeutic target to modulate the activity of the pulse generator GnRH/LH, in order to reduce the frequency of LH pulse, the circulating levels of LH, and testosterone [15]. In contrast, hyperandrogenism in the prenatal life generates an increased innervation of GABAergic neurons of the arcuate nucleus on the GnRH-secreting neurons, increasing their activity.

A model linked to adipocyte dysfunction as a trigger of PCOS pathophysiology has also been proposed, and a role of androgen receptors at the ovarian level in the development of the PCOS reproductive tracts cannot be excluded. However, the role that androgens play at the central level is emblematic in the development and pathogenesis of the typical characteristics of PCOS, although it obviously remains to determine how prenatal exposure to androgens in humans modifies the pathways acting on the hypothalamus. This experimental model lets us postulate a potential role of those molecules blocking androgen receptors, thus generating again at the central level an equilibrium among the various neurotransmitters/systems for the reactivation/resumption of the correct functionality of the reproductive axis. Certainly, the exposure to hyperandrogenic states during prenatal life is a relevant epigenetic cofactor for the triggering and development of PCOS.

5.4   Genetics, Metabolism, and PCOS

Data regarding genetic mutations directly linked to the onset of PCOS are particularly scarce. A 2017 study conducted on animal models with a selective mutation of the PTEN gene (*phosphatase and TENsin homolog*) in ovarian theca cells showed the occurrence of numerous reproductive characteristics typical of PCOS, including alteration of menstrual cyclicity, anovulation, high levels of circulating androgens, and characteristic PCO-like ovarian aspect. We recall that in the absence of the PTEN protein, which takes part to the cascade of insulin signaling, the correct mechanism of glucose transporters is altered [16]. Considering the frequency of insulin resistance in PCOS, attention was given to carbohydrate metabolism and, in particular, to the epimerase, responsible for the transformation of myo-inositol (MYO) into D-chiro-inositol (DCI), which has been reported to reduce functionality or expression in patients with hyperinsulinemia and PCOS, especially in those who have familial diabetes [17]. There are two main isoforms of inositols working in the transmission of the metabolic signal of numerous peptide hormones. Other than insulin, also TSH and FSH have inositols as element of the post-receptor signaling. Whereas inositol participates and promotes glucose transport into the cells, glucose oxidative use, and glycogen storage, it is well worth considering the possibility of inositols' integrative use in PCOS as well as in diabetes. The amount of MYO present inside the cells is in balance with all other inositol isoforms and when required is transformed into DCI by the epimerase which is expressed in a tissue-specific way and guarantees the conversion in the various districts [18]. In diabetic patients or in case of insulin resistance, a lower amount of DCI was found in urine reflecting a lower insulin-sensitivity than in the general population, supporting the hypothesis that there may be an anomalous function/expression of the epimerase which should guarantee the synthesis of DCI, inducing the worsening of insulin resistance and a compensatory hyperinsulinemia [19].

It has been proposed that the *primum movens* of PCOS was a dysfunctional ovarian hyperandrogenism, caused by a lack of regulation in androgen secretion. Recently it has been shown that this characteristic occurs in two thirds of PCOS patients, who show an excessive production of 17OH-P in response to gonadotropin stimulation [20]. The third remaining is a population of atypical and heterogeneous PCOS, in which hyperandrogenism has an adrenal origin, associated or not with obesity [20]. Approximately half of the women with PCOM (polycystic ovarian morphology) have a dysfunctional ovarian hyperandrogenism related to a defect of steroidogenesis [20]: in fact in vitro theca cells of women with PCOS show an intrinsic dysregulation of steroidogenesis, compatible with what observed in vivo, with a high expression of steroidogenetic enzymes and in particular of the cytochrome p450c17, an enzyme responsible for androgens production in case of excessive synthesis, present at gonadal and adrenal levels. Recently DENND1A.V2, a protein promoting steroidogenesis, has been identified in androgen-producing cells, differentially expressed in neoplastic and normal cells, which in normal theca cells reproduced the PCOS phenotype observed in vitro [20].

The etiology of dysfunctional ovarian hyperandrogenism certainly remains multifactorial: as already mentioned, it seems to be triggered by a complex interaction between predisposing congenital factors and promoting environmental factors such as insulin resistance and obesity, both characterized by an inheritance component. In fact, obesity is associated with the increased ovarian androgenic production, primarily due to systemic conditions of hyperinsulinemia, but also to an increased production of inflammatory cytokines. Metabolic syndrome related to obesity and insulin resistance occurs in about half of women with PCOS and compensatory hyperinsulinemia that is classically observed with tissue-specific effects, creating the worsening of hyperandrogenism.

In fact, PCOS evolves from the interaction between various genetic and environmental factors: among hereditary factors, we include PCOM, hyperandrogenism, insulin resistance, and defects in insulin secretion; the environmental factors include prenatal exposure to a hyperandrogenic environment, reduced fetal growth (IUGR), small for gestational age (SGA) newborn, and acquired obesity. The great variety of biological processes involved in glucose metabolism and steroidogenesis, associated to many possible environmental conditions, makes the pathogenesis multifactorial and the syndrome particularly heterogeneous. Therefore, other studies are needed to understand the exact triggers of the pathophysiology of PCOS in order to act on hyperandrogenism, anovulation, and hyperinsulinemia [20, 21].

Since 1968, studies have suggested an important role of genetics in the etiology of PCOS [22]: in fact first-degree relatives of patients with PCOS have an increased risk of being themselves affected compared to the general population [23], and it has been observed a greater correspondence of pathology between monozygotic twins compared to heterozygotes [24], concluding that the genetic component contributes more than 70% to the pathogenesis. However, studies based on the genes candidate for the pathogenesis of PCOS did not lead to concrete results. To date, numerous new loci and genes have been identified as candidates for the pathogenesis of PCOS through the Genome-Wide Association Studies (GWAS), which is a new approach to the study of the genome to understand the genetic basis of many complex diseases, using a survey of the variations of genes observed in patients affected by the same disease. Unfortunately these loci identified by the GWAS explained less than 10% of the genetic component of PCOS, because this method allows studying only the most common variants, while the less frequent and rarer variants, which however could have a big impact in generating the syndrome and the various possible phenotypes, are not yet detectable [25].

Certainly this disease cannot be explained by a limited number of variants [26]: in this context, a process of massive sequencing of the genome has begun, probably leading to its complete analysis, looking for rare genetic variants that contribute to the pathogenesis of PCOS and mapping the genetic variants that generate the different phenotypes of the syndrome [26]. More genetic knowledge, in association with epigenetic studies on PCOS, could help us to understand more clearly the pathogenesis of this syndrome, creating practical implications as a simpler and earlier diagnosis of the patient's specific phenotype, which would allow treating and preventing the possible associated pathologies in an extremely personalized way.

5.5   The Management of Infertility in PCOS Patients

Since up to now the etiology of PCOS has not been completely defined, the therapeutic options are not specifically organized, and many treatments remain today off-label. Up to now, several approaches and attempts have been tested to induce ovulation in PCOS patient: we will discuss the main and most commonly used methods.

5.5.1   Lifestyle Modification

Obesity obviously has a negative impact on the fertility of women with PCOS: it decreases the chances of conception because of the reduced number of spontaneous ovulatory cycles and the high percentage of spontaneous abortions, as well as the risk of complications during pregnancy and adverse perinatal outcomes. Lifestyle modification therefore is the first and most basic therapeutic approach, which includes the combination of a hypocaloric diet, constant physical activity to improve metabolic and anthropometric features (body weight, WHR, and fat mass/lean mass ratio), and a psychological support if it is necessary [27]. Furthermore, the reduction of both insulin and androgens plasma levels favors the restoration of menstrual and ovulatory cycles, improving reproductive outcomes in PCOS women.

Diet and regular exercise should therefore be always recommended as the first line of treatment for patients with PCOS with BMI > 25 kg/m^2, in particular in case of obesity [28], but these issues seem to be effective even in normal-weight PCOS patients, independently from the body weight and even if there is no concrete weight loss, since it simply improves the metabolic risk factors associated with PCOS [29].

The lifestyle modification therefore starts from a hypocaloric diet (500–1000 fewer calories per day) in association with physical exercise (20–60 min of physical activity a day, from 3 to 5 times a week) for 6 months. Any doctor who takes care of this patient has to lead to a change of the lifestyle with an adequate counseling, making the patient understand that the ultimate purpose is the good health as well as the restoration of the reproductive function. If the patient's compliance is poor, it has to be considered the opportunity to have a psychological support.Despite the appropriate lifestyle changes, in case of strong hyperinsulinemia or extreme difficulty in weight loss, it is possible to introduce Metformin for 6 months or more, which has been shown to favor the decline in BMI, with an important reduction of subcutaneous fat and the recovery of menstrual cyclicity, better than a correct lifestyle associated with placebo [30].

It is essential to investigate the insulin response to the oral glucose tolerance test (OGTT), at least at times 0 and 90′, to understand the relationship between blood glucose and insulin response and to evaluate how they change after meals. Weight loss is the driving force, even if modest, but sufficient to reduce the metabolic risk. In women with PCOS, lifestyle changes improve body composition and reduce hyperandrogenism and insulin resistance [28].

To underline the importance of lifestyle change regardless of any therapy, a well-established study has evaluated the effect of treatment with Metformin (850 mg/day) or only of lifestyle change (weight loss of 7% and physical activity for 150 min per week) in a group of subjects with impaired glucose tolerance [29]: for each subject the presence of metabolic syndrome was evaluated before and after the observational period. The results of this study show that the lifestyle change allows more positive effects on reduction of glucose plasma levels and of the risk of metabolic syndrome, both in terms of prevention of the development of the disease and improvement of basic metabolic conditions. Treatment with Metformin has been shown to be effective in preventing or delaying the onset of diabetes, but with less efficacy than having a different lifestyle.

Therefore, any pharmacological treatment that aims to improve the metabolic setting must be associated to an intervention of lifestyle correction. Women with overweight and PCOS show, other than a greater incidence of menstrual cycle alterations (oligo–/amenorrhea, anovulation, polymenorrhea), various metabolic alterations (hyperinsulinemia, diabetes, abdominal obesity), and they are also more exposed to the risk of developing cardiovascular diseases in young age, or in any case within 50 years: in fact insulin resistance and hyperinsulinemia have a negative impact at vascular level where they interact with the vasoactive factors, such as endothelin and nitric oxide, generating processes of alteration of vasodilation, predisposing to hypertension. In practice, nutrition and metabolic features are closely linked with the neuroendocrine world, compromising the reproductive function of any young woman with PCOS predisposing to pathologies that occur during adult or pre-menopausal period such as diabetes and cardiovascular diseases up to estrogen-dependent cancers.

5.5.2 Bariatric Surgery

Current guidelines suggest that bariatric surgery should be considered only in cases of grade III obesity, i.e., with BMI ≥ 40 kg/m^2, or ≥ 35 kg/m^2 in association with comorbidity who have failed to lose weight after 6 months of correct diet and regular physical activity [31]. This type of surgery is effective for weight loss, improves fertility outcomes in obese patients with PCOS, restores menstrual cycle and ovulation, and reduces hyperandrogenism and insulin resistance [31]. Obviously patients must be informed that there are risks related to this type of surgery, both linked to the surgery itself and to the onset of numerous possible complications during a pregnancy that arose after such surgery, which should be considered at high risk for preterm delivery, small-for-gestational age infants, stillbirth, or neonatal death, while the risk of gestational diabetes and of large-for-gestational age infants is reduced [32]. Therefore, bariatric surgery has to be considered as the last possible therapeutic option, exposing the body to a sudden weight loss associated with the onset of possible intestinal malabsorption. It is evident that bariatric surgery is only an "extrema ratio" for the management of PCOS patients, and the omen is that it will never become necessary.

5.5.3 Metformin

Metformin, a synthetic biguanide, is an oral hypoglycemic agent, considered the first-line treatment in type 2 diabetes mellitus. It works by reducing hepatic glucose production and intestinal glucose uptake, while increasing glucose uptake at peripheral level by skeletal muscle and liver. Being therefore an insulin-sensitizing agent, it is used in PCOS to reduce serum insulin concentrations and thus improve the metabolic setting in these patients, favoring the recovery of ovulatory cycles. In our clinical practice the starting dose is 250 mg twice a day 15 min before lunch and dinner, which can be increased up to 500–1000 mg after 15 days, with a gradual increase in dosage to avoid common gastrointestinal side effects. Although lifestyle modification is by far the first line of treatment in obese patients with PCOS and infertility, Metformin can be a valuable support in achieving weight loss. A recent meta-analysis [30] including 12 studies for a total of 608 patients has shown that the combination of Metformin and lifestyle modification in PCOS patients is more effective in weight loss than diet and physical activity alone [30]. A recent Cochrane review [33] that included 42 trials evaluating the beneficial effects of Metformin in women with PCOS has shown an increase in ovulatory cycles and pregnancy rates in the Metformin arm compared to placebo.

Although in this type of patients Metformin induces a higher rate of ovulatory cycles than placebo [34], it should not be considered the first-line treatment of chronic anovulation, since there are specific ovulation inducers, such as Clomiphene Citrate (CC) and Letrozole that both induce better results in terms of ovulation rate, number of pregnancies, and live births [35].However, the association between Metformin and CC, which should be considered for those patients not responding to treatment with CC alone, reported by a Cochrane review [33], provides only limited evidences on the efficacy of the association of these two products. To confirm this data, two meta-analyses [36, 37] have also been done on PCOS patients undergoing ART, and the administration of Metformin has been reported not to increase the pregnancy rate but to reduce the risk of the ovarian hyperstimulation syndrome (OHSS).

In conclusion, Metformin represents an important tool in the management of obese PCOS patients, being an insulin-sensitizing agent that acts by improving the metabolic profile and favoring weight loss; however, there are only relative effects on the increase in the pregnancy rate and live births. However, it remains a low-cost therapy, with good tolerability, though some gastrointestinal side effects that are dose-dependent and a good safety profile. It does not require a constant monitoring and does not induce multiple pregnancies. We might consider its prescription in association with supplements therapy, such as inositols and alpha-lipoic acid, which can further improve its effectiveness.

5.5.4 Clomiphene Citrate

Clomiphene citrate is a "selective estrogen receptor modulator" (SERM) that competes with endogenous estrogens on their receptor-binding sites. It is characterized by an anti-estrogenic effect that modifies the cervical mucus composition and endometrial receptivity, events that could favor implantation or conception after correctly inducing ovulation. It is anyway considered the treatment of choice in anovulatory PCOS patients. The starting dose is 50 mg a day for 5 days (from the third–fourth to the seventh–eighth day of the menstrual cycle depending on the protocols) and can be increased up to a maximum of 150 mg a day. However, resistance to Clomiphene is a very frequent event, which occurs in 15–40% of women with PCOS [38]. The percentage of ovulation in women with PCOS after CC administration is approximately 75–80%, while pregnancy is observed in 22% of cases [39]. This discrepancy of about 40% between the percentage of ovulation and pregnancy is probably due to the hypoestrogenic effect of CC on the endometrium and cervical changes of mucus.

Treatment with CC is generally suggested for a period not exceeding 6 months. Observations referred to a cumulative rate of success for the whole treatment cycle up to 65% [39].

In a large meta-analysis [40], including 57 trials and 8082 women, the most common ovulation induction protocols have been compared: all pharmacological treatments such as CC, Metformin, CC in association with Metformin, Letrozole, Tamoxifen, ovarian drilling, and follicle stimulating hormone (FSH) have been shown to be more effective than placebo in terms of ovulation or pregnancy rates. Compared to Letrozole, Clomiphene alone has shown lower rates of ovulation, pregnancy, and live births, probably due to its endometrial anti-proliferative effect.

A recent systematic review [41], focused on the effects of CC and other ovulation-inducing agents in women with anovulatory cycles, confirmed these results. Obviously,

CC has shown lower efficacy in terms of reproductive outcomes compared to exogenous gonadotropins [42], considered a second-line intervention in anovulatory PCOS women if the starting treatments were ineffective, since their use is expensive, requires constant monitoring, and may be associated with side effects such as multiple pregnancies and/or ovarian hyperstimulation syndrome (OHSS).To date, CC remains the most widely used treatment worldwide for ovulation induction in PCOS patients [39, 43]: it is taken orally, and it is cheap, effective, and safe, substantially free of side effects, even if literature reports same cases of multiple pregnancies.

5.5.5   Letrozole

Letrozole is an aromatase inhibitor and is commonly used to induce ovulation, generally as an alternative treatment to Clomiphene, especially in CC-resistant women. Its use as ovulation inducer is off-label or even prohibited in some countries of the world: in some studies, it has been associated with teratogenic effects on the fetus [44] and is burdened by important side effects linked to hypoestrogenism, typical of premenopausal symptoms. The mechanism of action consists in the inhibition of the aromatase enzyme, which converts androgens into estrogens at the ovarian level, peripheral tissues, and brain levels. As there is no estrogen receptor antagonism, it acts through a negative feedback mechanism at the central level, which generally determines the growth of a single dominant follicle. The starting dose is 2.5 mg a day for 5 days, from the third to the seventh day of the menstrual cycle. The dose can be increased up to a maximum of 7.5 mg for 5 days.

Despite the important side effects of Letrozole, numerous clinical trials have demonstrated the higher efficacy compared to Clomiphene, in terms of ovulation, pregnancy rate, and live birth rates [45]. In a large multicenter study of 750 women with PCOS and infertility [46], who received Letrozole or CC, the greater efficacy of Letrozole in terms of ovulation rate (61.7 vs 48.35%; $p < 0.001$) and higher cumulative live birth rate (27.5 vs 19.1%; $p = 0.007$) has been demonstrated compared to women treated with CC, except for a subgroup of women with BMI <30 kg/m^2, in which both treatments showed the same efficacy in terms of live birth rate. The greater efficacy of Letrozole could be probably explained since it has no direct antiestrogen effects on cervical mucus and on the endometrium and by its short half-life [46].

In conclusion, Letrozole can be considered as a potential therapeutic option for ovulation induction, even more effective than Clomiphene especially in obese PCOS patients, but certainly characterized by greater side effects.

5.5.6   Ovarian Drilling

Laparoscopic ovarian drilling can be considered a second-line treatment for PCOS patients with CC-resistant infertility [39]. Usually it is suggested to make 3 to 8 small perforations on the surface of each ovary with a depth and a diameter of about

1–2 mm using either heat (monopolar or bipolar electrocautery) or laser with comparable outcomes [47]. With this procedure, there is a partial destruction of the ovarian cortex and a sharp drop in the levels of androgens produced by this area, with a fall in LH and an increase in FSH plasma levels, thus inducing a correct follicular recruitment up to ovulation [48].

In a recent meta-analysis conducted on 484 participants, comparing the effects of unilateral vs bilateral ovarian drilling, there were no differences between the two techniques in terms of ovulation, pregnancy rate, number of live births, or abortion rate, with no differences in serum AMH concentrations after 6 months of surgical treatment, which therefore support the fact of not to have a negative impact on the ovarian reserve.

In the last Cochrane review [49], there were no differences in terms of live birth rate comparing the surgical technique, the use of exogenous gonadotropins, or aromatase inhibitors. This surgical technique is therefore indicated in patients resistant to CC or Letrozole and especially if a diagnostic laparoscopy is needed for other indications, such as the evaluation of tubal patency. However, similar to any surgical procedure, it can be associated with numerous post-operative complications, including the formation of intra-abdominal adhesions and the reduction of the ovarian reserve if the procedure is not performed correctly.

5.5.7 Gonadotropins and IVF

Gonadotropins (Follicle Stimulating Hormone (FSH) or Human Menopausal Gonadotropin (HMG)) represent a good putative treatment for patients with PCOS and anovulation, in which Clomiphene or Letrozole has not been effective. Such treatments are classically performed in ART (Assisted Reproductive Techniques).

Exogenous gonadotropins work by increasing circulating FSH levels and stimulating directly follicular growth. The recommended starting dose in PCOS patients to avoid hyperstimulation is 37.5–75 IU/day [39]; in particular the identification of the optimal dose is generally obtained after a few stimulation cycles following several attempts. Subsequently, when the follicles reach an average diameter of 18 mm, a single dose of hCG-r 250 μg or hCG-u 5000 IU is used to trigger ovulation. If the recruited follicles are too numerous (3 or more follicles greater than 14 mm in diameter), the hCG is not administered to avoid the risk of ovarian hyperstimulation or multiple pregnancies. The treatment should be repeated up to a maximum of 6 cycles. Using low-dose step-up protocols, the ovulation of a single follicle rate is nearly 70%, while pregnancy rate is 20% per cycle [39].

A recent Cochrane review [50] compared the effectiveness of various gonadotropin preparations in women with PCOS resistant to Clomiphene and showed no differences in terms of live birth rates or incidence of OHSS (urinary FSH, recombinant FSH, or HMG), demonstrating that outcomes are linked more on the administered dose of gonadotropins than on the preparation used. Combination therapy with Metformin has been shown to be effective in improving the effects of gonadotropins, increasing the live birth rates compared to administration of gonadotropins alone (OR 2.46, 95% CI 1.36 to 4.46) [51].

Exogenous gonadotropins are clearly more effective in promoting pregnancy than Clomiphene; however they are particularly expensive drugs with possible side effects (OHSS, multiple pregnancies); therefore they should be administered under strict ultrasound monitoring.Ovarian stimulation associated with IVF techniques is considered the third-line treatment in PCOS patients with chronic anovulation, especially recommended if other infertility factors are associated such as tubal pathologies, male subfertility, advanced woman age, and severe endometriosis [39].Single embryo-transfer procedure is essential to reduce the risk of multiple pregnancies, which is one of the most frequent complications when using gonadotropins.

Despite the high number of cycles suspended in PCOS patients, pregnancy and live births rate is comparable to those of non-PCOS women [52]. The use of GnRH antagonists also reduces the risk of ovarian hyperstimulation syndrome (OHSS), whose incidence is significantly higher in PCOS patients (15% vs 3%) [53].

5.5.8 Inositols

Recently the approach to PCOS has considered the possibility to treat the insulin resistance with specific integrative compounds that can counteract the metabolic impairment(s) that trigger anovulation and/or menstrual irregularities. In this perspective, inositols, in particular myo-inositol (MI) and D-chiro-inositol (DCI), the two most important isoforms, have become widely used in these last years.

Inositol is a molecule structurally similar to glucose. It is involved in numerous biological processes including transmission of insulin post-receptor signaling as well as in other protein hormones such as TSH and FSH [17]. It can be either taken with diet or synthesized by the human body. Both myo-inositol and D-chiro-inositol have the same chemical structure and differ only in the position of the hydroxyl group: in vivo, DCI is synthesized starting from MI by an epimerase, whose functionality or expression is probably reduced in hyperinsulinemic PCOS patients especially in case of familial diabetes [17]. In fact supplementation with MI or DCI or a combination of these products significantly improves the metabolic profile in PCOS patients, but in presence of diabetic relatives DCI seems to be more effective [17, 54].

Myo-inositol can be synthesized starting from glucose-6-phosphate, which is isomerized and then dephosphorylated [55], but the greater portion comes from the diet. At the intracellular level myo-inositol is transformed into phosphatidyl-myo-inositol, a precursor of inositol 3-phosphate, which acts as a intracellular second messenger in the cascade triggered by various peptide hormones [56, 57, 58]: in fact, the inositols are second messengers not only of the intracellular insulin signaling pathway, to reduce plasma levels via a greater cellular glucose uptake especially in the liver and skeletal muscles, but also of other protein hormones such as TSH and FSH [17, 59]. This aspect is relevant, since inositol administration can also improve the hormonal profile in terms of reproductive capacity, thanks to a better transduction of the FSH signal at the ovarian level.

Inositols take part in different ways in the post-receptor insulin-induced signal. There are two main routes in transmission of the metabolic signal of insulin: one is phosphatidyl-inositol 3-phosphate pathway, which through various steps activates a protein kinase PKB/Akt, allowing the translocation of GLUT-4 vesicles to the plasma membrane, to increase glucose transport into the cells through a facilitated diffusion mechanism, essentially in skeletal and cardiac muscle and in adipose tissue [60]; the other pathway is mediated by the G protein, which triggers a series of steps that lead to the release of a DCI molecule, which favors the glycogen storage in the cytosol and glucose oxidative use in the mitochondria. Therefore, the action of the two main inositol isoforms is very relevant in the control of numerous peptide hormone signals, as well as a diet that guarantees an adequate intake and a good MYO-to-DCI conversion mechanism through the epimerase activity [60]. Considering that inositol promotes mechanisms of glucose transport into the cells, glucose oxidative use, and glycogen storage, it is necessary to consider the possibility of its integrative use in diabetes and in PCOS (Fig. 5.2).

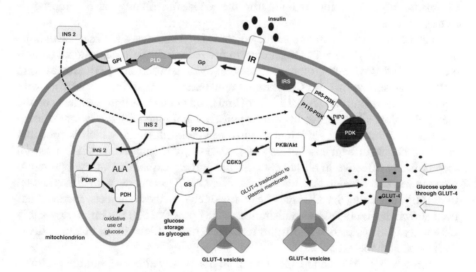

Fig. 5.2 Schematic representation of insulin signaling proposed by Larner et al. (modified from [17]). The insulin binding to its receptor (IR) activates a signal via two different and parallel pathways. In the first pathway, the substrates of the insulin receptor (IRS) activate various proteins (PI3K, PDK, PKB/Akt) in order to activate PKB/Akt and induce glucose transporter 4 (GLUT-4) translocation to the plasma membrane to upload glucose. The second pathway IR via G protein (Gp) causes the hydrolysis of glycosylphosphatidylinositol (GPI), which releases an inositol phosphoglycan containing D-chiro-inositol, which acts as second messenger of insulin (INS-2). INS-2 enhance glucose storage (GS) as glycogen in the cytosol and also glucose oxidative use in the mitochondria. Relevant the fact that mitochondria synthetize alpha lipoic acid (ALA) that activates PKB/Akt independently from insulin signal. (modified from [17]). *GSK3* Glycogen synthase kinase 3, *PDH* pyruvate dehydrogenase, *PDHP* pyruvate dehydrogenase phosphatase, *PDK* phosphoinositide-dependent kinase, *PI3K* phosphoinositide 3 kinase, *PKB/Akt* protein kinase B/Akt, *PP2Ca* phosphoprotein phosphatase 2C alpha

The amount of MYO present inside the cells is in balance with the other isoforms and when required is transformed as previously described into DCI by an epimerase which acts in a tissue-specific manner and therefore guarantees the useful conversion in the various districts [18]. In diabetes or insulin resistance, a lower amount of DCI was found in urine and in insulin-sensitive tissues than in the general population, thus demonstrating that an abnormal epimerase function/expression may exist, contributing to the worsening of insulin resistance and compensatory hyperinsulinemia [19]. In 1999 Nestler administered 1200 mg/day of DCI to obese PCOS patients for 8 weeks and demonstrated an improvement of insulin sensitivity and reduced circulating levels of androgens; subsequently it was shown that DCI increased the occurrence of ovulatory cycles and was also effective in normal-weight PCOS [61]. Other authors have subsequently shown a predominant role of MYO at ovarian level, positively correlating with oocyte quality and estradiol concentration in the follicular fluid [62]; in fact, in PMA cycles MYO improves oocytes and embryos qualities [63], so certainly the ovarian metabolic and endocrine pattern does not require high concentrations of DCI [64]. However, most of the organs like liver, skeletal muscle, and kidneys need DCI, since it plays a role for the correction of insulin resistance, fundamental for the good functioning of the reproductive system.

In 2012 Unfer [63] summarized the outcomes of 21 studies and observed that the administration of MYO in PCOS patients improved metabolic and hormonal parameters, reduced BMI, and promoted menstrual cycle and fertility [63]. However, in 2012 it was shown that MYO, when administered to obese PCOS patients with regular fasting insulin values (<12 microU/ml), did not induce improvements on the metabolic profile in terms of insulin response to oral glucose load, demonstrating that obesity alone is not sufficient to justify hyperinsulinemia, which is probably due to a deficit of synthesis/release of DCI-IPG [65], suggesting MYO was not metabolically effective in all patients. So the activity/expression of the epimerase enzyme was suspected to be altered in diabetic or PCOS patients with diabetic relatives [66], suggesting that DCI may be more effective in these subjects. Indeed it has been shown that daily DCI administration at the dosage of 500 mg improves insulin sensitivity in all patients with insulin resistance more efficiently in PCOS patients with familial diabetes [67, 68].

Therefore both MYO and DCI seem to be potentially effective, but the presence of diabetic relatives must be discriminant in the choice of their use, as in these subjects the conversion of MYO to DCI may not be optimal [67, 68]. Since DCI has strong metabolic effects, while MYO perform an important action in ovary, in some cases it could be useful to supplement a combination of both. A recent Consensus Conference proposed the use of a combination of them, close to their physiological plasma concentrations, guaranteeing systemic and ovarian benefits [69] and the prevention of the metabolic syndrome as well the risk of gestational diabetes.A recent meta-analysis, including 10 RCTs and 601 women [70], showed that supplementation with inositol improves the ovulatory rate and frequency of menstrual cycle compared to placebo. However, a recent review denies these data in terms of reproductive outcomes [71]: inositol, administered to PCOS patients undergoing ICSI cycles, does not improve oocyte quality and pregnancy rates, while DCI seems to have controversial role.

In conclusion, there are numerous evidences that demonstrate the efficacy of these integrative products and that both are able to modulate the reproductive and metabolic function in PCOS patients: according to a recent review [17] anamnestic data might be relevant to the choice of inositol integration, so we have to investigate diabetes predisposition and/or familial diabetes. It is advisable to evaluate this therapeutic option especially considering that it has no side effects and can be associated with lifestyle modification, and in combination with Metformin or ovulation induction treatments.

5.5.9   Alpha-Lipoic Acid

Recently another product was reported to be of great interest in the management of insulin resistance in PCOS patients, that is, alpha-lipoic acid (ALA). In animal models ALA modulates and increases the use of glucose via the activation of AMPK (adenosine monophosphate-activated protein kinase) in skeletal muscle and favoring the activation of GLUT-4 [72, 73]. Recently it has also been proposed as an adjuvant therapy in several endocrinopaties including diabetes [74, 75].

We recently reported that the administration of 400 mg of ALA per day was able to improve insulin sensitivity in obese PCOS patients, regardless of the presence of diabetic relatives [76]. In fact ALA induced a significant reduction in insulin levels after oral glucose load both in patients with or without diabetic relatives. Recent studies have shown that the lipoic acid synthase (LASY), responsible for the lipoic acid synthesis at the mitochondrial level in mammals as well as in humans, is poorly expressed in case of type I and II diabetes [77, 78]. The endogenous ALA modulates the use of glucose, activating the enzyme AMPK in skeletal muscle [17], which in turn activates GLUT-4, the main glucose transporter into the cells [73], reducing the amount of insulin necessary to maintain correct blood glucose levels (Fig. 5.2). Indeed we have shown that the exogenous administration of ALA, probably through the above described mechanism, corrects insulin resistance in PCOS patients. Our data showed that insulin sensitivity improves after treatment with ALA in all PCOS patients, especially in patients with diabetic relatives, probably because in these patients there is a defect of endogenous synthesis of ALA due to the defect of the enzyme responsible for its production, as previously discussed [77, 78].

Interestingly only in patients with diabetic relatives, a significant reduction of plasma triglyceride and transaminase levels was observed. These last are generally at the higher limits of normality, thus supporting the hypothesis that ALA has its own specific efficacy in the liver, in particular reducing the risk of steatosis classically described as NAFLD (nonalcoholic fatty liver disease). It should be observed that under treatment with ALA no changes in hormonal parameters were observed, that is, no change in terms of gonadotropin or androgen plasma levels, consequently no improvement in hormonal and reproductive profiles.

However, it remains a product of great importance for the correction of metabolic impairments of PCOS patients, improving insulin sensitivity and protecting liver function, thus preventing the onset of NAFLD and diabetes. It is therefore a useful strategy to combine ALA with MYO or DCI, as recently reported in our recent studies, which demonstrated the high metabolic and endocrine/reproductive efficiency of both the associations [79, 80]. Indeed, considering that innumerable studies have nowadays demonstrated inositol efficacy in the correction of metabolic status, hormonal values, and therefore fertility, it is advisable to evaluate the integrative option of the association with alpha-lipoic acid, evaluating anamnestic history, in particular the presence of diabetic relatives.

5.6   Conclusions

The available options to induce ovulation in PCOS patients are a lot and various: side effects, costs, and compliance of the patients need to be attentively evaluated, to have a personalized tailored choice, considering the clinical history and previous attempts, but also carefully evaluating the clinical and familial story, BMI, and PCOS phenotype. Considering the specific physiopathological characteristics of PCOS, it is essential that physicians take them in great consideration to make the best choice of treatment for the PCOS patient.

References

1. Norman RJ, Dewailly D, Legro RS. Polycystic ovary syndrome. Lancet. 2007; 370(9588):685–97.
2. Teede HJ. Recommendations from the international evi-dence-based guideline for the assessment and management of polycystic ovary syndrome. Hum. Reprod. Published online July 19, 2018. 2018; https://doi.org/10.1093/humrep/dey256.
3. Rotterdam ESHRE/ASRM-Sponsored PCOS Consensus WorkshopGroup. Revised 2003 consensus on diagnostic criteria and long-term health risks related to polycystic ovary syndrome. Fertil. Steril. 2004; 81(1): p. 19–25.
4. Ciampelli M, Fulghesu AM, Cucinelli F, Pavone V, Ronsisvalle E, Guido M, Caruso A, Lanzone A. Impact of insulin and body mass index on metabolic and endocrine variables in polycystic ovary syndrome. Metabolism. 1999;48:167–72.
5. Fauser BC, Tarlatzis BC, Rebar RW, Legro RS, Balen AH, Lobo R, Carmina E, Chang J, Yildiz BO, Laven JS, Boivin J, Petraglia F, Wijeyeratne CN, Norman RJ, Dunaif A, Franks S, Wild RA, Dumesic D, Barnhart K. Consensus on women's health aspects of polycystic ovary syndrome (PCOS): the Amsterdam ESHRE/ASRM-sponsored 3rd PCOS consensus workshop group. Fertil Steril. 2012;97:28–38.
6. Genazzani AD, Ricchieri F, Lanzoni C. Use of metformin in the treatment of polycystic ovary syndrome. Womens Health (Lond). 2010;6:577–93.
7. Joham AE, et al. Polycystic ovary syndrome, obesity, and pregnancy. Semin Reprod Med. 2016;34:93–101.
8. Genazzani AD, Vito G, Lanzoni C, Strucchi C, Mehmeti H, Ricchieri F, Mbusnum MN. La Sindrome metabolica Menopausale. Giorn. It. Ost. Gin. 2005;11/12:487–93.
9. The Pathogenesis of Polycystic Ovary Syndrome (PCOS): The Hypothesis of PCOS as Functional Ovarian Hyperandrogenism Revisited. Robert L. Rosenfield and David A. Ehrmann. Endocrine Reviews, October 2016, 37(5):467–520.

10. Ciaraldi TP, el Roeiy A, Madar Z, Reichart D, Olefsky JM, Yen SS. Cellular mechanisms of insulin resistance in polycystic ovarian syndrome. J Clin Endocrinol Metab. 2002; 75:577–83.
11. Araùjo TG, Oliveira AG, Saad MJ. Insulin-resistance-associated compensatory mechanisms of pancreatic Beta cells: a current opinion. Front Endocrinol (Lausanne). 2013;4:146.
12. Sliwowska JH, Fergani C, Gawałek M, Skowronska B, Fichna P, Lehman MN. Insulin: its role in the central control of reproduction. Physiol Behav. 2014;133:197–206. Epub 2014 May 27
13. Walters KA, Gilchrist RB, Ledger WL, Teede HJ, Handelsman DJ, Campbell RE. New perspectives on the pathogenesis of PCOS: neuroendocrine origins. Trend in Endocrinology and metabolism. in press
14. Navarro VM. New insights into the control of pulsatile GnRH release: the role of Kiss1/neurokinin B neurons. Front Endocrinol (Lausanne). 2012;3:48.
15. Walters KA, et al. The role of central androgen receptor actions in regulating the hypothalamic–pituitary–ovarian axis. Neuroendocrinology. 2018;106:389–400.
16. Lan ZJ, Krause MS, Redding SD, Li X, Wu GZ, Zhou HX, Bohler HC, Ko C, Cooney AJ, Zhou J, Lei ZM. Selective deletion of Pten in theca-interstitial cells leads to androgen excess and ovarian dysfunction in mice. Mol Cell Endocrinol. 2017;444:26–37. Epub 2017 Jan 28
17. Genazzani AD. Inositol as putative integrative treatment for PCOS. Reprod Biomed Online. 2016;33:770–80.
18. Larner J. D-chiro-inositol: its functional role in insulin action and its deficit in insulin resistance. Int J Exp Diabetes Res. 2002;3:47–60.
19. Baillargeon JP, Nestler JE. Commentary: polycystic ovary syndrome: a syndrome of ovarian hypersensitivity to insulin? J Clin Endocrinol Metab. 2006;91:22–4.
20. Rosenfield RL, Ehrmann DA. The pathogenesis of polycystic ovary syndrome (PCOS): the hypothesis of PCOS as functional ovarian Hyperandrogenism revisited. Endocr Rev. 2016;37(5):467–520.
21. Raiane P. Crespo, Tania A. S. S. Bachega, Berenice B. Mendonça, Larissa G. Gomesl. An update of genetic basis of PCOS pathogenesis. Arch Endocrinol Metab. 2018;62/3.
22. Cooper HE, Spellacy WN, Prem KA, Cohen WD. Hereditary factors in the stein-Leventhal syndrome. Am J Obstet Gynecol. 1968;100(3):371–87.
23. Kahsar-Miller MD, Nixon C, Boots LR, Go RC, Azziz R. Prevalence of polycystic ovary syndrome (PCOS) in first-degree relatives of patients with PCOS. Fertil Steril. 2001; 75(1):53–8.
24. Vink JM, Sadrzadeh S, Lambalk CB, Boomsma DI. Heritability of polycystic ovary syndrome in a Dutch twin-family study. J Clin Endocrinol Metab. 2006;91(6):2100–4.
25. Manolio TA, Collins FS, Cox NJ, Goldstein DB, Hindorff LA, Hunter DJ, et al. Finding the missing heritability of complex diseases. Nature. 2009;461(7265):747–53.
26. de Bruin C, Dauber A. Insights from exome sequencing for endocrine disorders. Nat Rev Endocrinol. 2015;11(8):455–64.
27. Moran LJ, Hutchison SK, Norman RJ, Teede HJ. Lifestyle changes in women with polycystic ovary syndrome. Cochrane Database Syst Rev. 2011;7:CD007506.
28. Balen AH, Morley LC, Misso M, Franks S, Legro RS, Wijeyaratne CN, et al. The management of anovulatory infertility in women with polycystic ovary syndrome: an analysis of the evidence to support the development of global WHO guidance. Hum Repr Update. 2016;22:687–708.
29. Poehlman ET, Dvorak RV, DeNino WF, Brochu M, Ades PA. Effects of resistance training and endurance training on insulin sensitivity in nonobese, young women: a controlled randomized trial. The Journal of Clinical Endocrinol and Metab. 2000;85:2463–8.
30. Naderpoor N, Shorakae S, de Courten B, Misso ML, Moran LJ, Teede HJ. Metformin and lifestyle modification in polycystic ovary syndrome: systematic review and meta-analysis. Hum Reprod Update. 2015;21:560–74.
31. Malik SM, Traub ML. Defining the role of bariatric surgery in polycystic ovarian syndrome patients. World J Diabetes. 2012;3:71–9.
32. Johansson K, Cnattingius S, Näslund I, Roos N, Trolle-Lagerros Y, Granath F, et al. Outcomes of pregnancy after bariatric surgery. N Engl J Med. 2015;372:814–24.

33. Morley LC, Tang T, Yasmin E, Norman RJ, Balen AH. Insulin-sensitising drugs (metformin, rosiglitazone, pioglitazone, D-chiro-inositol) for women with polycystic ovary syndrome, oligo amenorrhoea and subfertility. Cochrane Database Syst Rev. 2017;11:CD003053.
34. Practice Committee of the American Society for Reproductive Medicine. Role of metformin for ovulation induction in infertile patients with polycystic ovary syndrome (PCOS): a guideline. Fertil Steril. 2017; 108(3).
35. Siebert TI, Viola MI, Steyn DW, Kruger TF. Is metformin indicated as primary ovulation induction agent in women with PCOS? A systematic review and metaanalysis. Gynecol Obstet Investig. 2012;73:304–13.
36. Palomba S, Falbo A, La Sala GB. Effects of metformin in women with polycystic ovary syndrome treated with gonadotrophins for in vitro fertilisation and intracytoplasmic sperm injection cycles: a systematic review and meta-analysis of randomised controlled trials. BJOG. 2013;120(3):267–76.
37. Huang X, Wang P, Tal R, Lv F, Li Y, Zhang X. A systematic review and metaanalysis of metformin among patients with polycystic ovary syndrome undergoing assisted reproductive technology procedures. Int J Gynaecol Obstet. 2015;131:111–6.
38. Abu Hashim H, Foda O, Ghayaty E. Combined metformin clomiphene in clomiphene-resistant polycystic ovary syndrome: a systematic review and metaanalysis of randomized controlled trials. Acta Obstet Gynecol Scand. 2015;94:921–30.
39. Thessaloniki ESHRE/ASRM-Sponsored PCOS Consensus Workshop Group. Consensus on infertility treatment related to polycystic ovary syndrome. Hum. Reprod. 2008; 23: p. 462–77.
40. Wang R, Kim BV, van Wely M, Johnson NP, Costello MF, Zhang H, et al. Treatment strategies for women with WHO group II anovulation: systematic review and network meta-analysis. BMJ. 2017;356:j138.
41. Gadalla MA, Huang S, Wang R, Norman RJ, Abdullah SA, El Saman AM, et al. Effect of clomiphene citrate on endometrial thickness, ovulation, pregnancy and live birth in anovulatory women: systematic review and meta-analysis. Ultrasound Obstet Gynecol. 2018;51(1):64–76.
42. Brown J, Farquhar C. Clomiphene and other antioestrogens for ovulation induction in polycystic ovarian syndrome. Cochrane Database Syst Rev. 2016;12:CD002249.
43. Fields E, Chard J, James D, Treasure T. Guideline Development Group. Fertility (update): summary of NICE guidance. BMJ. 2013; 346: p. 650.
44. Tulandi T, Martin J, Al-Fadhli R, Kabli N, Forman R, Hitkari J, Librach C, Greenblatt E, Casper RF. Congenital malformations among 911 newborns conceived after infertility treatment with letrozole or clomiphene citrate Fertil Steril. 2006;85(6):1761–5. Epub 2006 May 2.
45. Hu S, Yu Q, Wang Y, Wang M, Xia W, Zhu C. Letrozole versus clomiphene citrate in polycystic ovary syndrome: a meta-analysis of randomized controlled trials. Arch Gynecol Obstet. 2018;297(5):1081–8.
46. Legro RS, Brzyski RG, Diamond MP, Coutifaris C, Schlaff WD, Casson P, et al. NICHD reproductive medicine network. Letrozole versus clomiphene for infertility in the polycystic ovary syndrome. N. Engl. J. Med. 2014;371(2):119–29.
47. Hueb CK, Dias-Junior JA, Abrão MS, Filho EK. Drilling: medical indications and surgical technique. Rev Assoc Med Bras. 2015;61:530–5.
48. Seow KM, Juan CC, Hwang JL, Ho LT. Laparoscopic surgery in polycystic ovary syndrome: reproductive and metabolic effects. Semin Reprod Med. 2008;26(1):101–10.
49. Farquhar C, Brown J, Marjoribanks J. Laparoscopic drilling by diathermy or laser for ovulation induction in anovulatory polycystic ovary syndrome. Cochrane Database Syst Rev. 2012;6:CD001122.
50. Weiss NS, Nahuis M, Bayram N, Mol BW, Van der Veen F, van Wely M. Gonadotropins for ovulation induction in women with polycystic ovarian syndrome. Cochrane Database Syst Rev. 2015;9:CD010290.
51. Bordewijk EM, Nahuis M, Costello MF, Van der Veen F, Tso LO, Mol BW, et al. Metformin during ovulation induction with gonadotrophins followed by timed intercourse or intrauterine insemination for subfertility associated with polycystic ovary syndrome. Cochrane Database Syst Rev. 2017;24(1):CD009090.

52. Li HW, Lee VC, Lau EY, Yeung WS, Ho PC, Ng EH. Cumulativen live-birth rate in women with polycystic ovary syndrome or isolated polycystic ovaries undergoing in-vitro fertilisation treatment. J Assist Reprod Genet. 2014;31:205–11.
53. Soave I, Marci R. Ovarian stimulation in patients in risk of OHSS. Minerva Ginecol. 2014;66(2):165–78.
54. Baillargeon JP, Diamanti-Kandarakis E, Ostlund RE Jr, Apridonidze T, Iuorno MJ, et al. Altered d-chiro-inositol urinary clearance in women with polycystic ovary syndrome. Diabetes Care. 2006;29:300–5.
55. Loewus MW, Wright RW Jr, Bondioli KR, Bedgar DL, Karl A. Activity of myo-inositol-1-phosphate synthase in the epididymal spermatozoa of rams. J Reprod Fertil. 1983;69:215–20.
56. Buttner J. Johann Joseph von Scherer (1814–69). The early history of clinical chemistry. J Clin Chem Clin Biochem. 1978;16:478–83.
57. Thomas RM, Nechamen CA, Mazurkiewicz JE, Ulloa-Aguirre A, Dias JA. The adapter protein APPL1 links FSH receptor to inositol 1,4,5-trisphosphate production and is implicated in intracellular Ca2_ mobilization. Endocrinology. 2011;152:1691–701.
58. Unfer V, Proietti S, Gullo G, Porcare G, Carlomagno G, Bizzarri M. Polycystic ovary syndrome: features, diagnostic criteria and treatments. Endocrinol Metab Synd. 2014;3:2. https://doi.org/10.4172/2161-1017.1000136.
59. Thomas RM, Nechamen CA, Mazurkiewicz JE, Ulloa-Aguirre A, Dias JA. The adapter protein APPL1 links FSH receptor to inositol 1,4,5-trisphosphate production and is implicated in intracellular ca(2+) mobilization. Endocrinology. 2011;152:1691–701.
60. Croze ML, Soulage CO. Potential role and therapeutic interests of myo-inositol in metabolic diseases. Biochimie. 2013;95:1811–27.
61. Iuorno MJ, Jakubowicz DJ, Baillargeon JP, Dillon P, Gunn RD, Allan G, Nestler JE. Effects of d-chiroinositol in lean women with the polycystic ovary syndrome. Endocr Pract. 2002;8:417–23.
62. Chiu TT, Rogers MS, Law EL, Briton-Jones CM, Cheung LP, Haines CJ. Follicular fluid and serum concentrations of myo-inositol in patients undergoing IVF: relationship with oocyte quality. Hum Reprod. 2002;17:1591–6.
63. Unfer V, Carlomagno G, Dante G, Facchinetti F. Effects of myo-inositol in women with PCOS: a systematic review iof randomized controlled trials. Gynecol Endocrinol. 2012;28:509–15.
64. Rosalbino I, Raffone E. Does ovary need D-chiroinositol? J Ovarian Res. 2012;5:14.
65. Cheang KI, Baillargeon JP, Essah PA, Ostlund RE Jr, Apridonize T, Islam L, Nestler JE. Insulin-stimulated release of D-chiro-inositol-containing inositolphosphoglycan mediator correlates with insulin sensitivity in women with polycystic ovary syndrome. Metab Clin Exp. 2008;57:1390–7.
66. Larner J, Brautigan DL, Thorner MO. D-chiro-inositol glycans in insulin signaling and insulin resistance. Mol Med. 2010;16:543–52.
67. Genazzani AD, Santagni S, Rattighieri E, Chierchia E, Despini G, Marini G, Prati A, Simoncini T. Modulatory role of D-chiro-inositol (DCI) on LH and insulin secretion in obese PCOS patients. Gynecol Endocrinol. 2014b;30:438–43.
68. La Marca A, Grisendi V, Dondi G, Sighinolfi G, Cianci A. The menstrual cycle regularization following D-chiro-inositol treatment in PCOS women: a retrospective study. Gynecol Endocrinol. 2015;31:52–6.
69. Facchinetti F, Bizzarri M, Benvenga S, D'Anna R, Lanzone A, Soulage C, et al. Results from the international consensus conference to on myo-inositol and dchiroinositol in obstetrics and gynecology: the link between metabolic syndrome and PCOS. European Journal of Obstet., Gynecol., Reprod. Biol. 2015; 195: p. 72e6.
70. Pundir J, Psaroudakis D, Savnur P, Bhide P, Sabatini L, Teede H, et al. Inositol treatment of anovulation in women with polycystic ovary syndrome: a meta-analysis of randomised trials. BJOG. 2018;125(3):299–308.
71. Mendoza N, Pérez L, Simoncini T, Genazzani A. Inositol supplementation in women with polycystic ovary syndrome undergoing intracytoplasmicsperm injection: a systematic review and meta-analysis of randomized controlled trials. Reprod Biomed Online. 2017;35(5):529–35.

72. Lee WJ, Song KH, Koh EH, Won JC, Kim HS, et al. Alphalipoic acid increases insulin sensitivity by activating AMPK in skeletal muscle. Biochem Biophys Res Commun. 2005;332:885–91.
73. Shen QW, Zhu MJ, Tong J, Ren J, Du M. Ca2+/calmodulindependent protein kinase kinase is involved in AMP-activated protein kinase activation by alpha-lipoic acid in C2C12 myotubes. Am J Physiol Cell Physiol. 2007;293:C1395–403.
74. Gomes MB, Negrato CA. Alpha-lipoic acid as a pleiotropic compound with potential therapeutic use in diabetes and other chronic diseases. Diabetol Metab Syndr. 2014;6(1):80. https://doi.org/10.1186/1758-5996-6-80.
75. Scaramuzza A, Giani E, Radaelli F, Ungheri S, Macedoni M, Giudici V, Bosetti A, Ferrari M, Zuccotti GV (2015) Alpha-lipoic acid and antioxidant diet help to improve endothelial dysfunction in adolescents with type 1 diabetes: a pilot study. J Diabetes Res. https://doi.org/10.1155/2015/474561.
76. Genazzani AD, Shefer K, Della Casa D, Prati A, Napolitano A, Manzo A, Despini G, Simoncini T. Modulatory effects of alpha-lipoic acid (ALA) administration on insulin sensitivity in obese PCOS patients. J Endocrinol Investig. https://doi.org/10.1007/s40618-017-0782-z.
77. Morikawa T, Yasuno R, Wada H. Do mammalian cells synthesize lipoic acid? Identification of a mouse cDNA encoding a lipoic acid synthase located in mitochondria. FEBS Lett. 2001;498:16–21.
78. Padmalayam I, Hasham S, Saxena U, Pillarisetti S. Lipoic acid synthase (LASY): a novel role in inflammation, mitochondrial function, and insulin resistance. Diabetes. 2009;58:600–8.
79. Genazzani AD, Prati A, Santagni S, Ricchieri F, Chierchia E, Rattighieri E, Campedelli A, Simonicini T, Artini PG. Differential insulin response to myo-inositol administration in obese polycystic ovary syndrome patients. Gynecol Endocrinol. 2012 Dec;28(12):969–73. https://doi.org/10.3109/09513590.2012.685205.
80. Genazzani AD, Prati A, Simoncini T, Napolitano A. Modulatory role of D-chiro-inositol and alpha lipoic acid combination on hormonal and metabolic parameters of overweight/obese PCOS patients. Eur Ginecol Obstet. in press

Polycystic Ovary Syndrome: Considerations About Therapeutic Strategies Choices from Fertile Life to Menopause

6

Alessandro D. Genazzani, Ambrosetti Fedora, Despini Giulia, Manzo Alba, Caroli Martina, Arnesano Melania, Petrillo Tabatha, Tomatis Veronica, and Andrea R. Genazzani

6.1 Introduction

Polycystic ovary syndrome (PCOS) is a very frequent endocrine disorder in women since it occurs in as many as 8–10% of women of reproductive age [1, 2]. Due to the multiple heterogeneity of the syndrome [3], there has been no agreement on the criteria on which to base the diagnosis of PCOS.

At the beginning, diagnostic criteria proposed by the NIH for PCOS were the presence of hyperandrogenism and chronic anovulation with clear exclusion of related ovulatory or other androgen excess disorders (i.e., hyperprolactinemia, thyroid diseases, androgen-secreting tumors, and adrenal dysfunction/hyperplasia) [4]. These criteria did not include the presence of polycystic ovaries at ultrasound examination because it was observed that polycystic ovaries could also be present in healthy eumenorrheic women [5]. A few years later the diagnostic criteria were expanded, and PCOS was considered as present when at least two of three features were diagnosed: oligo- or anovulation, clinical/biochemical hyperandrogenism, and polycystic ovaries as assessed by ultrasound examination [6]. This evolution was relevant because it permitted the inclusion of women with PCOS who were excluded by previous criteria: those with polycystic ovaries affected by hyperandrogenism and ovulatory cycles, or chronic anovulation and normal androgen levels. After

A. D. Genazzani · A. Fedora · D. Giulia · M. Alba · C. Martina · A. Melania · P. Tabatha
T. Veronica
Department of Obstetrics and Gynecology, Gynecological Endocrinology Center, University of Modena and Reggio Emilia, Modena, Italy
e-mail: algen@unimo.it; fedora.ambrosetti01@universitadipavia.it

A. R. Genazzani (✉)
Department of Obstetrics and Gynecology, University of Pisa, Pisa, Italy

© International Society of Gynecological Endocrinology 2021
A. R. Genazzani et al. (eds.), *Impact of Polycystic Ovary, Metabolic Syndrome and Obesity on Women Health*, ISGE Series,
https://doi.org/10.1007/978-3-030-63650-0_6

assessing this, we have then to clarify that PCOS is completely different from PCO. PCO means polycystic ovary and refers only to the morphological aspect of the ovary at ultrasound examination, that's it. Indeed, PCOS can be found in many other disendocrinopathies such as hyperprolactinemia, thyroid dysfunction, and stress-induced amenorrhea.

As a major feature, in this last decade, a new parameter has been introduced and taken into account to better approach not only the diagnosis but mainly the therapeutic choice, that is, insulin resistance (IR).

6.2   Endocrine Profile of PCOS

PCOS is characterized by higher plasma concentrations of ovarian and adrenal androgens, increased luteinizing hormone (LH) levels, high estrogen levels (especially estrone) due to extra-glandular conversion from androgens, lower levels of sex hormone-binding globulin (SHBG), and higher levels of prolactin and insulin, the latter often in presence of overweight or obesity.

Although the pathogenesis of PCOS is still controversial [7–9], PCOS typically shows elevated LH and normal or relatively low FSH secretion so that almost 50–60% of PCOS patients show a high LH/FSH ratio (>2.5) [7, 8], an exaggerated LH response to gonadotropin-releasing hormone (GnRH) stimulation test [7, 8], and a higher frequency of LH pulsatile release from pituitary [4, 7, 8, 10] that induces a higher stimulation on theca cells and an excess of androgen secretion as well as impaired follicular development [4].

Excess of androgens is classical of the syndrome, although it is not constant [7] and it is in great part of ovarian production with an adrenal contribution, since a certain percentage of PCOS patients might show a mild steroidogenetic defect in adrenal glands (such as for 21-hydroxylase) or just a higher adrenal hyper-activation due to stress [11]. Androstenedione and testosterone are the best markers of ovarian androgen secretion, while dehydroepiandrosterone sulfate (DHEAS) is the best marker of adrenal secretion. Most testosterone is derived from peripheral conversion of androstenedione and from direct ovarian production. In addition, adrenal glands contribute in part to testosterone although in hyperandrogenic PCOS the main source of androgens usually comes from the ovaries. Since cytochrome p450c17 is the androgen-forming enzyme in both the adrenal glands and the ovaries, whatever changes or increases its activity triggers the pathogenic mechanism underlying hyperandrogenism in PCOS [4]. In addition, in the presence of 5α-reductase, testosterone is converted within the cell to the more biologically potent androgen, namely, dihydrotestosterone. Excess or normal 5α-reductase activity in the skin determines the presence or absence of hirsutism [12]. Additionally, plasma levels of estrone, a weak estrogen with biological activity 100-times less than estradiol, are increased as a result of peripheral conversion of androstenedione by aromatase activity – more active in PCOS than in healthy controls – while estradiol levels are normal or low because of the frequent anovulatory cycles. All this results in a chronic hyperestrogenic state with the reversal of the estrone: estradiol ratio that might predispose to endometrial proliferation and to a possible increased risk for endometrial cancer [13, 14]. Another relevant aspect is the fact that normally less than 3% of testosterone circulates as unbound in the serum. In fact, most circulating androgens are bound to SHBG, thus being biologically inactive. Any condition that decreases the levels of SHBG (such as excess of circulating androgens) inducing a reduced hepatic synthesis induces a relative excess of free circulating androgens. In PCOS, hirsutism usually occurs with decreased SHBG levels and obesity [4].

6.3   Insulin Resistance (IR) and Compensatory Hyperinsulinism

The presence of increased insulin plasma level is a very frequent feature in PCOS patients, especially in those that show overweight or obesity. Indeed, overweight/obesity, depending on the geographical location, might be present in 50–70% of patients with PCOS. And this is not all. Another relevant feature is the presence of familial diabetes. It has been demonstrated that the presence of familial diabetes in first grade relatives (parents and/or grandparents) is a risk factor not only for the occurrence of IR but mainly for the high percentage of risk of occurrence of gestational diabetes and diabetes in late adulthood [15].

Such familial factors have always been evaluated through a quite detailed anamnestic investigation. In fact a risk factor of IR occurrence is not the presence of a familial diabetes only, but also the fact that the PCOS patients might be born as small for gestational age (SGA) and/or as after a IUGR (Intrauterine Growth Retardation) or may be born after a pregnancy during which a gestational diabetes occurred [16, 17].

Such kind of background(s) might predispose, at a higher grade, to the occurrence of insulin resistance due to specific genetic factors related to the familial predisposition to diabetes and also due to specific epigenetic factors that might be able to trigger the onset of a compensatory hyperinsulinemia [17].

It is clear that the presence of a familial diabetes predisposes to a less efficient post-receptor signalling driven by inositols not only for the insulin signal but also for FSH (on granulosa cells) and for TSH (on thyroid cells) [15, 18]. Also alpha-lipoic acid (ALA), a potent insulin sensitizer produced by mitochondrion, is impaired in case of diabetes or simply of predisposition to diabetes [19, 20].

In addition, androgen excess may both directly and indirectly induce alterations in glucose metabolism, ultimately being an additional cause of abnormal insulin sensitivity. Androgens may directly inhibit peripheral and hepatic insulin action. In fact, testosterone could induce insulin resistance in women with PCOS acting on the post-binding signal, in particular by reducing the number and efficiency of glucose transport proteins, such as the type 4 glucose transporter (GLUT-4), especially in muscle and fat tissues [21]. In addition, it has also been reported that women with central obesity, typical of obese PCOS, have higher free androgen levels and exhibit significantly higher levels of insulin insensitivity compared to weight-matched controls and show increased free fatty acids [4].

6.4   How to Manage and What to Do in PCOS?

The real target in PCOS patients is to teach them be aware of the great risk they have with such a disease. The real risk is not the anovulation or hyperandrogenism or hyperinsulinemia but the maintenance of such combination for a long time (quite often years!) so that that their biology is epigenetically induced to try to find "alternatives" to such a functional discomfort. The compensatory hyperinsulinemia is one of such biological solutions and is for sure a quite risky one since it is well known that it is a predisposition factor for metabolic syndrome in young as well as in adult or aged women.

The main solution is to take care of feeding, the choice of food, exercise, and, in case pregnancy is not an actual desire, a good choice of estro-progestin pill to overcome the hyperandrogenism that most of PCOS patients have. So, the putative question to a PCOS patient is: are you trying to be pregnant? If the answer is NO, all the solutions can be proposed, mainly a contraceptive pill; if the answer is YES, then contraception is absolutely skipped, and all integrative/anti-hyperinsulinemic treatment might be proposed together with a drastic lifestyle change especially overweight/obesity is present!

What is relevant to say is the fact that whatever is the biological situation that triggers PCOS and mainly the IR, the real risk is to maintain such abnormal condition up to the perimenopausal period when a lot of biological changes will occur, first of all a physiological increase of the insulin resistance. It is quite clear that a PCOS patient has to improve her metabolic health years before the occurrence of the perimenopausal transition. If not doing so, an increased risk of metabolic syndrome and of all cardiovascular risks up to death will take place.

6.5   Estrogen-Progestin Preparations and PCOS

Generally speaking, we can say that all combined estrogen-progestogen preparations are able to solve more or less the clinical complaints of any PCOS patient. This is due to the fact that such preparations block the ovary and suppress androgen production and improve SHBG synthesis thus reducing the circulating free androgens that are biologically effective on the target tissues such as skin, sebaceous glands, and hair follicles [22, 23].

Since it is well known that the estrogenic compound of the contraceptive pill (i.e., ethinyl estradiol) has only an ovario-static activity (no direct antiandrogenic effect), the antiandrogenic action has to be modulated by the progestogen compound. At present there are four progestogens with specific antiandrogenic activity: cyproterone acetate, dienogest, drospirenone, and chlormadinone acetate [22]. Cyproterone acetate is the progestogen with the highest antiandrogenic activity though being able to induce a relative higher rate of side effects such as cephalea, but all the others are able to induce similar positive effects [23]. The contraceptive pill administration is able not only to improve the clinical signs of the androgenization but also to normalize the ovarian size and morphology, typically impaired in

PCOS patients [24]. As additional effect, estrogen-progestogen preparations protect for both follicular and corpus luteum cysts occurrence [23].

The efficacy of contraceptive preparations on the signs of hyperandrogenism (i.e., acne, hirsutism, seborrhea, and alopecia) is determined as function of time since the biological evolution of the skin and of all its annexes is more or less 110–120 days. This means that the youngest cells of the epithelium of the skin become old and superficial in more or less 4 months. Whatever is the contraceptive pill administered, the minimum treatment interval has to be 4–5 months, eventually up to 12 months, at least. Better results are obtained when such pills are administered for longer interval and/or coupled with anti-androgen compounds such as flutamide [25] or finasteride.

Most of the clinicians agree on the fact that treatment of dysendocrinopathy of PCOS supports greatly the psycho-emotional recovery of almost all the PCOS patients. Moreover, the use of the contraceptive pill, also for a long time, protects the patient from being victim of the recrudescence of the hyperandrogenism and of its induced diseases, mainly chronic anovulation and infertility. In fact, the use of estrogen-progestogen preparation has been reported to improve the chance of conception [26], and there is no difference in this kind of beneficial protective effect on ovarian function between progestin-only pill and combined oral contraceptives. After 12 months of discontinuation of the treatment to conceive, the conception rate was 95–99% in those using the pill versus 70–81% conception rate for those patients using depot medroxyprogesterone acetate (DMPA) injections or Norplant (levonorgestrel implants) [26].

If the rationale is correct and all the data we have in regards PCOS are true [27], environmental and genetic factors are able to induce the starting of the PCOS disease and will mark as "affected" that patient up to the menopause. This means that predisposition to all the clinical problems will be quiescent up to the moment the patient undergoes a treatment and will appear aging (more or less evident) soon after the discontinuation.

6.6   No Contraception but Let's Overcome Dysmetabolism!

One of the main complaints of PCOS patients is the lack of ovulation and thus a consistent reduction of fertility. Obviously, the therapeutic use of the contraceptive pill is usually discarded but not so often. Indeed it might be proposed to use the pill for a certain amount of months during which correct lifestyle, i.e., diet and physical activity, is applied together with specific insulin sensitizers, such as metformin [2] and/or inositols and alpha-lipoic acid [19, 28–32]. The reduction of body weight is an essential feature for a good chance not only to recover a normal ovulatory function but also, if pregnancy starts, to have a controlled body mass that does not trigger a greater pregnant-induced insulin resistance that can trigger gestational diabetes.

Lots of studies have demonstrated that a correct lifestyle together with a correct treatment based on metformin and/or inositols and ALA greatly improves the chance of pregnancy, also while undergoing fertility programs [33, 34]. The clinical relevance of all these treatments is that they are all able to positively modulate the impaired and frequent compensatory hyperinsulinemia of PCOS patients, in particular in those that show a normal BMI [31], but the application of a correct lifestyle is the substrate for the best achievement of the desired result [35].

6.7   Long-Term Consideration for PCOS!

Since during the perimenopausal and postmenopausal transition there is a relevant modification of the endocrine profile in all women, those who have POCS during fertile life are more predisposed to have severe symptoms such as those related to behavior, mood, sleep, anxiety, as well as those related to metabolism, in particular insulin resistance and compensatory hyperinsulinemia. Menopausal transition induces, as a natural event, an insulin resistance that together with the hypoestrogenism and the lack of progesterone causes a greater tendency to gain body weight. There are convincing data that this metabolic link has to be considered as relevant when discussing about menopause with our ex-PCOS perimenopausal patients [36].

Substantially the menopausal transition might worsen a previously not perfect metabolic condition. Since both estrogens and progesterone are able to modulate the glucose metabolism, as soon as the perimenopausal modifications of the ovarian function take place and within few months/years menopause begins [37, 38], abnormalities of the metabolic pathways may be more relevant than expected if during fertile life abnormal metabolic function(s) were present, such as insulin resistance with overweight or obesity.

Though it cannot be generalized, the use of hormone replacement therapy is crucial and important for 1000 aims at the moment of the menopausal transition, being clear that the patient has no contraindications to it. It is relevant to maintain an adequate steroidal milieu so that biological pathways and in particular the metabolic ones are not crushed by the overlapping phenomena of menopause plus aging [39].

In conclusion lifestyle, good and healthy feeding, and the right amount of physical exercise are relevant in PCOS patients during fertile life, with or without the use of oral contraceptives, but when fertile life finishes and menopausal transition takes place all of the above need to be coupled with an adequate hormone replacement therapy to counteract the higher risk for PCOS-menopausal women to face higher rate diseases mainly cardiovascular diseases and dismetabolic/diabetes risks.

References

1. Carmina E, Lobo RA. Polycystic ovary syndrome: arguably the most common endocrinopathy is associated with significant morbidity in women. J Clin Endocrinol Metab. 1999;84(1897–1899):4.

2. Genazzani AD, Ricchieri F, Lanzoni C. Use of metformin in the treatment of polycystic ovary syndrome. Women's Health (Lond Engl). 2010;6:577–93.
3. Carmina E. Genetic and environmental aspects of polycystic ovary syndrome. J Endocrinol Investig. 2003;26:1151–9.
4. Zawadzki JK, Dunaif A: Diagnostic criteria for polycystic ovary syndrome: towards a rational approach. In: Polycystic Dunaif A, Givens JR, Haseltine FP, Merriam GR (Eds). Ovary Syndrome. Blackwell, MA, USA, 337–384 (1992).
5. Polson DW, Adams J, Wadsworth J, Franks S. Polycystic ovaries-a common finding in normal women. Lancet. 1988;1:870–2.
6. The Rotterdam ESHRE/ASRM-Sponsored PCOS Consensus Workshop Group. Revised 2003 consensus on diagnostic criteria and long-term health risks related to polycystic ovary syndrome (PCOS). Hum Reprod. 2004;19:41–7.
7. Hirschberg AL. Polycystic ovary syndrome, obesity and reproductive implications. Womens Health. 2009;5:529–40.
8. Doi SA. Neuroendocrine dysfunction in PCOS: a critique of recent reviews. Clin Med Res. 2008;6:47–53.
9. Vrbikova J, Hainer V. Obesity and polycystic ovary syndrome. Obes Facts. 2009;2:26–35.
10. Kalro BN, Loucks TL, Berga SL. Neuromodulation in polycystic ovary syndrome. Obstet Gynecol Clin N Am. 2001;28:35–62.
11. Genazzani AD, Petraglia F, Pianazzi F, Volpogni C, Genazzani AR. The concomitant release of androstenedione with cortisol and luteinizing hormone pulsatile releases distinguishes adrenal from ovarian hyperandrogenism. Gynecol Endocrinol. 1993;7:33–41.
12. Plouffe L Jr. Disorders of excessive hair growth in the adolescent. Obstet Gynecol Clin N Am. 2000;27:79–99.
13. Vrbikova J, Cibula D. Combined oral contraceptives in the treatment of polycycstic ovary syndrome. Hum Reprod Update. 2005;11:277–91.
14. Cibula D, Gompel A, Mueck AO, La Vecchia C, Hannaford PC, Skouby SO, Zikan M, Dusek L. Hormonal contraception and risk of cancer. Hum Reprod Update. 2010;16:631–50.
15. Genazzani AD. Inositol as putative integrative treatment for PCOS. Reprod Biomed Online. 2016;33:770–80. https://doi.org/10.1016/j.rbmo.2016.08.024.
16. de Melo AS, Dias SV, Cavalli Rde C, Cardoso VC, Bettiol H, Barbieri MA, Ferriani RA, Vieira CS. Pathogenesis of polycystic ovary syndrome: multifactorial assessment from the foetal stage to menopause. Reproduction. 2015 Jul;150(1):R11–24.
17. Ibáñez L, Potau N, Francois I, de Zegher F. Precocious pubarche, hyperinsulinism, and ovarian hyperandrogenism in girls: relation to reduced fetal growth. J Clin Endocrinol Metab. 1998;83:3558–62.
18. Berridge MJ, Irvine RF. Inositol trisphosphate, a novel second messenger in cellular signal transduction. Nature. 1984;312(5992):315–21.
19. Genazzani AD, Shefer K, Della Casa D, Prati A, Napolitano A, Manzo A, Despini G, Simoncini T. Modulatory effects of alpha-lipoic acid (ALA) administration on insulin sensitivity in obese PCOS patients. J Endocrinol Invest. 2018 May;41(5):583–90.
20. Padmalayam I, Hasham S, Saxena U, Pillarisetti S. Lipoic acid synthase (LASY): a novel role in inflammation, mitochondrial function, and insulin resistance. Diabetes. 2009;58:600–8.
21. Ciaraldi TP, El-Roeiy A, Madar Z, et al. Cellular mechanisms of insulin resistance in polycystic ovarian syndrome. J Clin Endocrinol Metab. 2002;75:577–83.
22. Schindler AE. Non-contraceptive use of hormonal contraceptives for women with various medical problems. J Pediat Obstet Gynecol. 2008;34:183–200.
23. Schindler AE. Non-contraceptive benefits of oral hormonal contraceptives. In J Endocrinol Metab. 2013;11:41–7.
24. Falsetti L, Gambera A, Tisi G. Efficacy of the combination ethinyl oestradiol and cyproterone acetate on endocrine, clinical and ultrasonographic profile in polycystic ovarian syndrome. Hum Reprod. 2001;16(1):36–42.
25. Paradisi R, Fabbri R, Battaglia C, Venturoli S. Ovulatory effects of flutamide in the polycystic ovary syndrome. Gynecol Endocrinol. 2013;29:391–5.

26. Barnhart KT, Schreiber CA. Return to fertility following discontinuation of oral contraceptives. Fertil Steril. 2009;91:659–63.
27. Franks S, Berga SL. Does PCOS have developmental origins? Fertil Steril. 2012;97:2–6.
28. Genazzani AD, Prati A, Simoncini T, Napolitano A. Modulatory role of D-chiro-inositol and alpha lipoic acid combination on hormonal and metabolic arameters of overweight/obese PCOS patients. European Gynecology and Obstetrics. 2019;1(1):29–33.
29. Genazzani AD, Despini G, Santagni S, Prati A, Rattighieri E, Chierchia E, Simoncini T. Effects of a combination of alpha lipoic acid and myo-inositol on insulin dynamics in overweight/obese patients with PCOS. Endocrinol Metab Synd. 2014;3:3. https://doi.org/10.4172/2161-1017.1000140.
30. Genazzani AD, Santagni S, Rattighieri E, Chierchia E, Despini G, Marini G, Prati A, Simoncini T. Modulatory role of D-chiro-inositol (DCI) on LH and insulin secretion in obese PCOS patients. Gynecol Endocrinol. 2014;30(6):438–43.
31. Genazzani AD, Santagni S, Ricchieri F, Campedelli A, Rattighieri E, Chierchia E, Marini G, Despini G, Prati A, Simoncini T. Myo-inositol modulates insulin and luteinizing hormone secretion in normal weight patients with polycystic ovary syndrome. J Obstet Gynaecol Res. 2014;40(5):1353–60.
32. Genazzani AD, Prati A, Santagni S, Ricchieri F, Chierchia E, Rattighieri E, Campedelli A, Simoncini T, Artini PG. Differential insulin response to myo-inositol administration in obese polycystic ovary syndrome patients. Gynecol Endocrinol. 2012;28:969–73.
33. Artini PG, Di Berardino OM, Papini F, et al. Endocrine and clinical effects of myo-inositol administration in polycystic ovary syndrome. A randomized study. Gynecol Endocrinol. 2013;29:375–9.
34. Zheng X, Lin D, Zhang Y, Lin Y, Song J, Li S, Sun Y. Inositol supplement improves clinical pregnancy rate in infertile women undergoing ovulation induction for ICSI or IVF-ET. Medicine 2017;96:49(e8842).
35. Tieu J, Shepherd E, Middleton P, Crowther CA. Dietary advice interventions in pregnancy for preventing gestational diabetes mellitus. Cochrane Database of Systematic Reviews 2017, Issue 1. Art. No.: CD006674.
36. Puurunen J, Piltonen T, Morin-Papunen L, Perheentupa A, Jarvela I, Ruokonen A, Tapanainen JS. Unfavorable hormonal, metabolic, and inflammatory alterations persist after menopause in women with PCOS. J Clin Endocrinol Metab. 2011;96:1827–34.
37. Dos Reis CM, de Melo NR, Meirelles ES, Vezozzo DP, Halpern A. Body composition, visceral fat distribution and fat oxidation in postmenopausal women using oral or transdermal oestrogen. Maturitas. 2003 Sep 25;46(1):59–68.
38. Davis SR, Castelo-Branco C, Chedraui P, Lumsden MA, Nappi RE, Shah D, Villaseca P; Writing Group of the International Menopause Society for World Menopause Day 2012. Understanding weight gain at menopause. Climacteric 2012;15(5):419–29.
39. Cagnacci A, Zanin R, Cannoletta M, Generali M, Caretto S, Volpe A. Menopause, estrogens, progestins, or their combination on body weight and anthropometric measures. Fertil Steril. 2007 Dec;88(6):1603–8.

Impact of Polycystic Ovary Syndrome, Metabolic Syndrome, Obesity, and Follicular Growth Arrest in Women Health

7

Claudio Villarroel, Soledad Henríquez, Paulina Kohen, and Luigi Devoto

7.1   Introduction

Polycystic ovary syndrome (PCOS) is the most common endocrine disorder in women in reproductive age. Depending on the diagnostic criteria used, the prevalence varies between 8% and 13% [1–4]. This syndrome was initially defined as a reproductive disease characterized by the presence of hyperandrogenism (HA), ovulatory dysfunction, and polycystic ovaries. However, growing data have shown the strong association with metabolic dysfunction. Although PCOS has been recognized clinically for more than 80 years, there has been an evolving set of diagnostic criteria and definition of PCOS phenotypes. In 1990, the National Institutes of Health (NIH) criteria defined PCOS diagnosis based on the presence of clinical or biochemical HA and chronic oligo-anovulation (OA) [1]. Subsequently, Rotterdam Consensus Criteria (2003) established a new diagnostic definition, including HA, OA, and polycystic ovarian morphology (PCOM) diagnosed by transvaginal ultrasound. This consensus introduced two new phenotypes: hyperandrogenic ovulatory (HA + PCOM) or non-hyperandrogenic anovulatory phenotypes (OA + PCOM), not previously considered [2]. The Androgens Excess and PCOS Society (2006) proposed an amendment to Rotterdam Consensus criteria: clinical or biochemical androgen excess was compulsory, including oligo-anovulation and polycystic ovarian morphology as secondary criteria [3]. Finally, new modifications were introduced by International PCOS Network (2018) about PCOM definition [4]. These different criteria have amplified the PCOS phenotype spectrum in a 30-year period of time.

C. Villarroel (✉) · S. Henríquez · P. Kohen · L. Devoto
Faculty of Medicine, Institute for Mother and Child Research (IDIMI), University of Chile, Santiago, Chile
e-mail: cvillarroel@uchile.cl

© International Society of Gynecological Endocrinology 2021
A. R. Genazzani et al. (eds.), *Impact of Polycystic Ovary, Metabolic Syndrome and Obesity on Women Health*, ISGE Series,
https://doi.org/10.1007/978-3-030-63650-0_7

Ovulatory dysfunction, defined by the presence of oligo-anovulation and PCOM, is observed in up to 75% of the PCOS women [5]. These features are the clinical expression of disrupted folliculogenesis, characterized by follicular arrest [6, 7], follicle stockpiling [8, 9], and alteration in the follicle dominance mechanism [10, 11], which occurs within the ovary environment.

Follicular growth arrest is one of the main features of folliculogenesis disruption. It leads to the classical PCOM characterized follicle stockpiling of less than 10 mm in diameter in the ovarian cortex. This phenomenon underlies an impaired selection of one dominant follicle, despite the presence of an excess number of selectable follicles [8, 10, 12]. The current understandings of the mechanisms underlying follicular growth arrest in PCOS are limited. Recent data suggest that defective follicle selection occurs due to extra-ovarian mechanisms such as FSH/LH pituitary secretion and defective action over theca and granulosa cells [13–15], and intraovarian mechanism such as increase androgen thecal cell secretion, and higher anti-müllerian hormone (AMH) expression by granulosa cells [11, 14, 16, 17], and defective angiogenesis which may impair follicular development [6, 18–20].

In the present chapter, we will review the possible extra-ovarian and intraovarian mechanisms involved in follicle growth arrest PCOS and its relation with metabolic syndrome.

7.2 PCOS and Metabolic Syndrome Linkage

Metabolic syndrome (MS) is present in 24–43% of women with PCOS [21]. Multiple studies show that women with classic PCOS phenotypes (HA + OA + PCOM or HA + OA) have higher insulin levels, insulin resistance, obesity, and dyslipidemia prevalence [21–23]. The prevalence of MS in these phenotypes are higher than in non-classic PCOS phenotypes (HA + PCOM or OA + PCOM) (odds ratio [OR] 2.1 in classic PCOS vs. 1.62 in non-classic phenotypes) [24, 25]. Additionally, an increased risk of MS is observed in obese (OR 1.75) and lean PCOS women (OR 1.45), when compared with body mass index (BMI)-matched control groups [24, 25]. On the other hand, the presence of HA, higher BMI, and ovulatory dysfunction are independent predictors of MS in PCOS patients [4, 5, 23].

Finally, reduction in BMI and adiposity are correlated with a recovery of cyclic menses with a parallel improvement of the MS [4, 26–28], suggesting that there is a relation between metabolic dysfunction and folliculogenesis disruption in PCOS.

7.2.1 Insulin Resistance and Hyperinsulinism in PCOS

Insulin resistance (IR) is a common feature in PCOS and metabolic syndrome. Insulin resistance is found in approximately 44–85% PCOS women, and it is higher in obese PCOS subjects (80–95%) [29–32]. Recent studies have shown that PCOS has heterogeneous pathophysiology characterized by an intimate interrelation of hyperandrogenism, IR, and compensatory hyperinsulinemia and its effects on different target tissues [27, 33, 34].

The pathogenesis of IR in PCOS is complex and incompletely dilucidated. Insulin resistance is traditionally defined as a decreased ability of insulin to mediate these metabolic actions (glucose uptake, glucose production, and lipolysis) while preserving its mitogenic and steroidogenic actions. The primary mechanism of IR (Fig. 7.1) is insulin receptor post-bind signaling defect in the peripheral organs [31, 35]. An increase in the phosphorylation rate on serine rather than tyrosine residue in the insulin receptor and IRS-1 has been frequently described [35]. The latter leads to a diminished translocation of glucose transporter 4 (GLUT-4) to the cytoplasmic membrane, which finally leads to compensatory hypersecretion of insulin to overcome this defect [34, 35].

Several studies have shown that adipose tissue of PCOS women has decreased insulin sensitivity. A lower level of GLUT-4 protein has been found in subcutaneous adipocytes of PCOS women compared to weight-match controls [36]. Similar findings are observed in obesity and type 2 diabetes mellitus (T2D) that can be improved by weight loss [35, 37, 38]. However, weight loss does not always improve insulin sensitivity in PCOS patients. The persistence of this metabolic defect in adipocytes is observed in the absence of obesity, T2D, or after weight loss; in lean PCOS phenotypes, suggests an intrinsic IR defect [35, 39, 40]. Moreover, recent studies have shown that insulin action on glucose metabolism in granulosa-lutein cell cultures is sharply diminished, similarly to what is observed in the muscle cell and adipocytes. These data suggest an impairment of insulin's metabolic pathway in reproductive and non-reproductive tissues in PCOS [41].

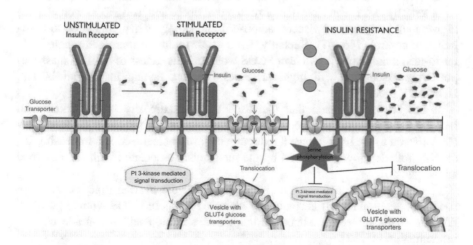

Fig. 7.1 Mechanism of insulin resistance in polycystic ovary syndrome. An excess of phosphorylation of serine rather than tyrosine residue in the insulin receptor and IRS-1 is found, leading to a diminished translocation of glucose transporter 4 (GLUT-4) to the cytoplasmic membrane. The latter leads to reduced glucose uptake by the cell, insulin resistance, and compensatory hypersecretion of insulin to overcome this defect. (adapted from [34])

As described above, the steroidogenic and mitotic functions of insulin signaling are preserved. Multiple studies have demonstrated that insulin and insulin-like growth factor-1 (IGF-1) receptors are expressed in theca and granulosa cells. Higher levels of circulating insulin bind to its receptor and IGF-1 receptor in theca cell, amplifying LH action. Compensatory hyperinsulinemia leads to an increase in CYP17 activity, rendering a higher androgen secretion [27, 31]. On the other hand, different studies have shown than insulin also induces theca cell hyperplasia [34, 35, 42]. Additionally, hyperinsulinemia has a negative effect over the liver, reducing the hepatic synthesis of SHBG, leading to increased free testosterone levels [34]. Thus, IR and compensatory hyperinsulinemia are responsible for or can aggravate hyper-androgenemia in PCOS.

7.2.2 Role of Adipose Tissue in Insulin Resistance in PCOS

In the last years, it has been found that adipose tissue plays a vital role in the development, improvement, or deterioration of IR and consequent follicle arrest in PCOS.

Adipose tissue is an endocrine organ that not only regulates glucose, lipid metabolism, and energy expenditure but also has an essential role in inflammation, immunity, and reproductive function. Obesity is defined as an abnormal accumulation of lipids in the adipose tissue. Obesity or abnormal fat body distribution is observed in PCOS women. Obesity and abdominal fat accumulation associate with a higher risk of ovulatory dysfunction, IR, and MS development in PCOS women [43, 44].

Obesity is observed in 44–88% of PCOS women [45]. Increased accumulation of abdominal adipose tissue has been found in PCOS patients. Body composition measurements by DXA scan have demonstrated that obese and lean PCOS women have higher total body fat and visceral adipose tissue storage when compared to BMI-matched controls [46, 47]. Recently, Ezeh et al. found an increased whole body fat-to-lean mass in obese and lean PCOS women. This excess of total fat mass was positively associated with higher free testosterone, fasting insulin levels, and HOMA-IR index [48].

It has been established that increased visceral adiposity is associated with increased catecholamine-induced lipolysis. The higher free fatty acid plasmatic levels delivered to the liver induce a reduction of insulin clearance and increasing IR, causing follicle growth impaired by the mechanism associated with IR described above [49, 50].

However, adipose can exert a direct effect over the ovarian function. Adipose tissue dysfunction (ATD) is frequently observed in obese PCOS women [45, 51]. ATD is characterized by abnormal adipokine secretion and low-grade chronic inflammation [45, 52].

Deregulation of adipokines secretion had been described in ATD associated with PCOS. Leptin and adiponectin are the most frequently studied since they play an essential role in ovarian function. Increased leptin levels are observed in obesity and PCOS [52]. In vitro studies have shown that higher leptin levels can inhibit follicle growth [27, 45, 51]. On the other hand, adiponectin levels are reduced in obesity and obese PCOS women [53, 54]. Lower adiponectin levels are associated with an increase in insulin resistance. Different studies have shown that lower adiponectin levels are related to increased LH secretion in the pituitary and lower estradiol secretion from granulosa cells [30, 54].

Low-grade chronic inflammation is characterized mainly by higher TNF-alfa and IL-6 levels [45]. TNF-alfa induces IR by inhibiting adiponectin secretion, increasing free fatty acid levels, and reducing GLUT-4 expression in peripheral tissues [55]. TNF-alfa exerts direct effects over the ovary. In vitro studies have shown that TNF-alfa stimulates proliferation and steroidogenesis in theca cells [43, 51]. It also facilitates insulin and IGF-1 action over theca cells. Recent studies have shown that TNF-alfa levels are strongly related to IR and HA in PCOS but not to BMI [44].

Higher levels of IL-6 and TNF-alfa levels are associated with the infiltration of monocyte-derived macrophages of the ovarian tissue. The local ovarian inflammatory reaction stimulates CYP17 activity, increasing ovarian androgen secretion [27, 45, 54].

7.2.3   Role of Androgen in Insulin Resistance

Hyperandrogenism is observed in at least 84.7% of PCOS patients, depending on the diagnostic criteria used [4, 5, 34]. Hyperandrogenic PCOS phenotypes (HA + OA + PCOM; HA + OA; HA + PCOM) have higher prevalence con IR, T2D, and dyslipidemia compared to non-hyperandrogenic PCOS phenotype (OA + PCOM) [23, 56]. Various studies have proposed that extremely low or high levels of androgens are associated with an increased risk of cardiovascular disease [57]. Daan et al. have shown that higher levels of androgens are associated with higher triglycerides and insulin, the prevalence of T2D and hypertension in different hyperandrogenic states in women, including PCOS [58].

Recent studies have shown a pleiotropic action of androgens over different organs that may lead to metabolic dysfunction in PCOS. Androgens play an essential role in body fat distribution, inducing android fat distribution. Obese and lean PCOS women have higher total body fat and visceral adipose tissue storage than BMI-matched controls [46, 47]. Moreover, under chronic flutamide treatment, PCOS women exhibit a decrease in abdominal fat depots [54]. In vitro studies have shown that androgens increase the size of adipocytes in subcutaneous adipose tissue [54, 59]. Hypertrophic adipocyte is more susceptible to local inflammation, macrophage infiltration that may impair insulin sensitivity, leading to ATD [49]. HA reduces the lipolytic rate of the adipose tissue, leading to an excessive depot of lipids in the cell. Excessive lipid accumulation causes lipotoxicity. This phenomenon is characterized by an impaired function of the endoplasmic reticulum and mitochondria, which finally increases insulin resistance on the cell [49]. Androgens also modulate adipokine secretion by the adipose tissue. Several studies have shown testosterone reduces adiponectin secretion, which is a crucial factor of insulin resistance development as stated earlier [49, 55].

HA also has adverse effects on skeletal muscle. Higher androgens levels are associated with reduced insulin-stimulated glucose uptake. Other studies have found that HA is associated with a diminished capillary density in the skeletal muscle, thereby hampering insulin access and insulin action in muscle cells [45, 54].

The high ovarian androgen production observed in PCOS is mainly due to increased androgen synthesis by ovarian theca cells. In vitro studies have shown that PCOS theca cells are more sensitive to insulin and LH-stimulated androgen secretion than those from healthy women [41]. The increased sensitivity is due to a higher expression of steroidogenic proteins and enzymes, such as StAR, 3-BHSD, cytochrome P450c17, that leads to HA [34, 39]. Additionally, an intrinsic cytochrome P450c17 hyperactivity even in the absence of LH or insulin stimuli [31].

7.3   Metabolic Syndrome, Hyperandrogenism, and Follicular Growth Arrest in PCOS

As described in previous sections of this chapter, PCOS has a complex pathophysiology that strongly links IR and HA.

The accumulated data suggest the presence of a common mechanism that leads to the development of the metabolic syndrome and follicular growth arrest in PCOS. Multiple studies have demonstrated that insulin and androgens receptors are also present in the hypothalamus and pituitary. Animal model studies have shown that insulin can increase LH pulse frequency and secretion. Euglycemic-hyperinsulinemic clamp studies have shown that hyperinsulinemia increases GnRH pulse frequency, LH pulse amplitude, and secretion in PCOS women [35]. A higher LH pulse frequency and amplitude of LH are also observed in lean PCOS, suggesting an inherent impaired pituitary function [35].

Ovarian HA causes a higher androgen influx to the adipocytes. HA increases aromatase activity leading to higher estradiol secretion from the adipose tissue [55]. Higher androgens and estradiol levels exert a negative feedback over FSH secretion, reducing FSH secretion [34]. These events lead to an increase in the LH:FSH ratio [10, 15, 27, 34]. Lower FSH levels are associated with lower aromatase activity in the granulosa. It has also been observed that under HA reduces granulosa cell proliferation and causing the resistance to FSH action [10]. According to the latter, granulosa cell dysfunction appears to contribute to theca cell overproduction of androgens.

These data suggest that IR and HA can lead to a higher LH/FSH ratio and a lower FSH sensitivity of granulosa cells, causing antral follicle growth impairment and follicular growth arrest in PCOS [15]. This way, a vicious circle in PCOS has been described, where hyperandrogenism favors abdominal fat accumulation and insulin resistance (Fig. 7.2). That reciprocally facilitates the hypersecretion of androgens in PCOS patients [27, 44, 60].

According to the mechanism described above, obesity has a binary effect over follicle arrest: (1) it could induce or worsen IR inducing increasing LH:FSH ratio and androgen secretion, and (2) a direct effect over the ovary leading to intraovarian hyperandrogenism and local inflammation.

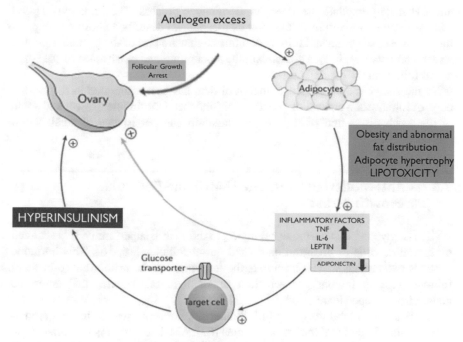

Fig. 7.2 Role of adipose tissue in insulin resistance and hyperandrogenemia. A vicious circle between abdominal fat accumulation and hyperandrogenism is observed in PCOS. Hyperandrogenism favors abdominal fat accumulation and insulin resistance. Adipose tissue excess facilitates the hypersecretion of androgens in PCOS patients by adipose tissue dysfunction. Deregulation of adipokine secretion, low-grade chronic inflammation, and lipotoxicity are observed. This phenomenon leads to hyperandrogenemia and follicle growth arrest, affecting the LH/FSH ratio and a direct effect on the ovary. (Adapted from [27])

These findings are strengthened by the fact that weight loss of abdominal fat reduction in PCOS women recovers regular menses, ovulation, and clinical pregnancy. These data suggest that weight loss could restore folliculogenesis in some PCOS phenotypes. Thus it has become one of the main recommendations for the management of PCOS to improve fertility and reduce long-term complications.

7.4   Intraovarian Mechanism of Follicular Growth Arrest in PCOS

Folliculogenesis is divided into two phases: a gonadotropin-independent period and a gonadotropin-dependent period. The gonadotropin-independent period comprehends the growth from primordial to the small antral follicle and is regulated mainly by local growth factors. On the other hand, the gonadotropin-dependent period comprehends the growth from small antral follicles to the Graafian follicle. FSH and LH mainly regulate the selection, dominance process. The impaired LH and FSH secretion observed in PCOS, and its mechanism described above can explain the absence of selection and follicle dominance that are part of the follicular growth arrest. Nevertheless, it does not explain the stockpiling and persistence of the small antral follicle in the ovarian cortex.

In the last years, a significant amount of data has been generated in the knowledge of intraovarian control of gonadotropin-independent follicle growth and some of the mechanisms underlying the accumulation and persistence of small antral follicles.

7.5   Anti-Müllerian Hormone (AMH) and Follicular Growth Arrest

AMH is a glycoprotein hormone belonging to the TGF-β superfamily. It is secreted by granulosa cells of preantral and small antral follicles [14, 16]. This hormone controls two critical stages: it inhibits the growth from the primordial-to-primary follicle stage. It inhibits the selection of small antral follicles that enter the gonadotropin-dependent period [61].

AMH plays an inhibitory role in follicular development, preventing the premature recruitment and maturation of follicles [62]. AMH secretion is maximal at the preantral and small antral stages in human follicles, and decreases in the large follicle PCOS ovaries have a higher number of pre-antral and antral follicles, indicating that follicular growth arrest occurs when AMH production is high [63]. Multiple studies have documented higher AMH levels in PCOS women than healthy women [64–67]. Moreover, other studies have suggested that AMH levels reflect the severity of PCOS [68]. MH levels are higher in anovulatory PCOS women compared with ovulatory PCOS women [69]. Hypersecretion of AMH by granulosa cells could impair follicular growth. AMH could increase FSH threshold small antral follicles, reducing granulosa cell sensitivity to FSH in the luteal-follicular phase transition causing follicle growth arrest [70]. AMH also blocks androgen conversion into estrogens by inhibiting aromatase activity, causing hyperandrogenism [71, 72]. Other authors found that follicular AMH levels are negatively correlated with FSH concentrations, indicating that AMH levels predict follicle responsiveness to FSH in ovulation induction cycles [17, 73].

Several studies suggested that androgens increase the secretion of AMH, which regulates the growth of primordial follicles. Androgen-induced AMH expression provides negative feedback inhibiting follicle growth because of HA [10, 61]. Finally, AMH influences transcription of genes in granulosa cells through Smad proteins and regulates gene expression to maintain primordial follicles in their arrested state [16].

The cause of AMH increased production is unknown. However, other factors related to PCOS pathophysiology such as LH, and androgen levels may be implicated. LH increases AMH expression in granulosa cells of anovulatory PCOS women, but not in ovulatory PCOS women or normal women, suggesting a role for

LH in AMH overexpression inducing follicular arrest [74, 75] However, AMH appears primarily related to androgen status, suggesting a direct and predominant role of androgens in the pathophysiology of reproductive dysfunction including follicular growth arrest [10].

Several studies have shown that women with classic PCOS also have higher AMH, androgens levels [4, 5]. These phenotypes are frequently associated with ovulatory dysfunction, expressed as PCOM or OA [1–4]. HA and higher AMH levels inhibit follicle growth that is clinically observed by the presence of PCOM, ovulatory dysfunction, and a higher FSH threshold [10, 71]. Several studies have shown that weight loss, reduction of abdominal fat, or improvement of IR leads to a decrease in androgens levels, FSH follicle threshold, restoring follicle growth, and ovulation. Interestingly, this metabolic and reproductive improvement is not associated with a decrease of AMH levels [26, 34]. The latter suggests the presence of additional mechanisms responsible for follicular growth arrest.

7.6   Dysregulation of Ovarian Angiogenesis and Estrogen Metabolites in the Follicular Growth Arrest

Regulation of the ovary angiogenesis is critical for follicular growth and ovulation and the subsequent development and regression of the corpus luteum [19, 76]. Follicular atresia is associated with inadequate development of the thecal vasculature [77]. On the other hand, abnormalities of ovarian angiogenesis in PCOS increase the risk of ovarian hyperstimulation syndrome during ovulation induction [78, 79].

The importance of vascular endothelial growth factor (VEGF) in ovarian function is well known [80, 81]. Previous studies have shown that the HIF-1α/VEGF signaling pathway plays a crucial role in both angiogenesis and tumor growth [82, 83]. HIF-1α is known to regulate cellular adaptation to hypoxic conditions. Stabilized HIF-1α translocates to the nucleus and binds to the hypoxia-response elements of several target genes (such as VEGF) that are involved in the modulation of angiogenesis [82–84]. Additionally, FSH induces angiogenesis by stimulating HIF-1α expression and VEGF secretion [85, 86]. Previously, Levin et al. found a strong correlation between VEGF levels in follicular fluid (FF), follicle growth, and the number of mature oocytes retrieved in IVF cycles [87]. The latter suggests that an impaired follicle vascularization has adverse effects on oocyte maturation. VEGF expression is low during preantral follicle growth and increases in granulosa cells and theca cells through dominant follicle development [77].

Järvela et al. studied follicular vascularization in the follicle of PCOS and non-PCOS women undergoing controlled ovarian hyperstimulation for IVF treatment, using three-dimensional power Doppler ultrasound. These authors found a reduced follicular vascularization in ovaries of PCOS women compared to normal women after GnRH treatment but not after gonadotropin stimulation [88].

The latter suggests that an impaired follicle vascularization has adverse effects on oocyte maturation. It seems plausible that abnormal angiogenesis can be involved in the follicular growth arrest and infertility in PCOS.

On the other hand, the secretion of estradiol throughout the ovarian cycle depends upon follicle recruitment and selection of a single dominant follicle followed by the LH/FSH surge, which ends the program of FSH-dependent steroidogenesis [89]. Estrogens can be metabolized in the ovary by alternative pathways to form estrogen metabolites with endogenous action (EMs). It has been established that other signaling pathways rather than the classical estradiol receptor pathway mediate EMs action [90, 91].

We have extensively studied the role of VEGF and EMs in ovarian angiogenesis, particularly in human corpus luteum function. We found that EMs such as 2-methoxyestradiol (2-ME2) and 2-methoxyestrone (2-ME1) have an anti-angiogenic effect. On the other hand, 16-ketoestradiol (16-kE2) and 4-hydroxyestrone (4-OHE1) have a pro-angiogenic effect, during the development and regression of corpus luteum [84, 92, 93]. Interestingly, these metabolites also participate in follicular development.

Data recently published by our group have demonstrated, for the first time, the importance of pro-angiogenic estrogen metabolites in healthy follicular development and follicular growth arrest in PCOS. In unstimulated ovarian cycles, we have found lower pro-angiogenic EMs and VEGF levels in the follicular fluid (FF) of small antral follicles of PCOS women compared to fertile women with regular menstrual cycles [[20], in press] (Table 7.1). On the other hand, in the IVF-stimulated cycles, the exogenous gonadotropin administration increases pro-angiogenic EMs and VEGF FF levels in PCOS and control women. Similar pro-angiogenic EMs and VEGF levels in FF were found in PCOS compared to control women in IVF treatment for male infertility at the time of oocyte pick up [[20], in press]. These data suggest that the administration of exogenous gonadotrophins during ovulation induction increases intrafollicular angiogenic factors and angiogenesis in PCOS, restoring follicular growth. The latest results are in agreement with previous publications that showed the presence of a pro-angiogenic intrafollicular environment in PCOS women undergoing IVF treatment [94]. These data strongly suggest the

Table 7.1 Intrafollicular levels of AMH, VEGF and estrogens metabolites (EMs) in follicle of women with spontaneous cycles and PCOS women with follicular arrest

	Ovulary (n = 10) (antral follicle)	PCOS (n = 10) (antral follicle)	Ovulatory (n = 10) (dominant follicle)
AMH (ng/mL)	213.2 ± 28.0	546 ± 16.7[a]	2.9 ± 0.09[b]
VEGF (pg/mL)	503.2 ± 101.40	33.1 ± 5.9[a]	6529.6 ± 514.3[b]
$\sum$EMs pro-angio/ $\sum$EMs anti-angio ratio	1.59	0.35[a]	1.15

Note: $\sum$ EMs = sum of estrogens metabolites
EMs pro-angio (2-OHE2, 16KE2, 4-OHE1). EMs anti-angio (2-ME2, 2-ME1)
[a]Comparing the difference between antral follicles of ovulatory and PCOS women (P < 0.05). Values are mean ± SEM
[b]Comparing the difference between antral and dominant follicles of ovulatory women (P < 0.05). Values are mean ± SEM

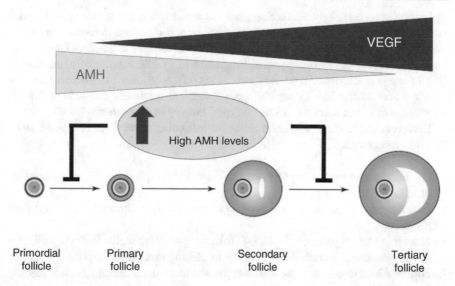

Fig. 7.3 Anti-müllerian hormone and follicle growth. AMH is secreted by granulosa cells of pre-antral and small antral follicles. It controls two critical stages in follicle growth. Higher AMH expression in PCOS follicle may impair follicular growth. The possible mechanisms involved are the inhibition of aromatase activity and estradiol secretion, an increase of the FSH threshold of small antral follicles leading to an FSH resistance, and diminished vascularization due to a decrease of proangiogenic EMs and VEGF intrafollicular levels

importance of angiogenesis in follicular growth, suggesting that an altered balance of pro- and anti-angiogenic factors could induce follicular arrest observed in PCOS.

As we mentioned earlier, AMH plays a crucial role in PCOS pathogenesis (Fig. 7.3). Previous publications have shown that AMH inhibits TGF beta signaling pathways, leading to decreased cell differentiation and angiogenesis [95]. In a recent study, we found high AMH levels and low VEGF and pro-angiogenic EMs levels in FF of arrested follicles of PCOS women in unstimulated cycles ([20], in press). In summary, high AMH levels present in PCOS reduce sensitivity to FSH and are detrimental to follicular angiogenesis, resulting in follicular growth arrest.

7.7   Conclusions

PCOS is one of the most frequent endocrine diseases in women. It was initially described as a reproductive disease. However, growing data have shown a strong association with metabolic dysfunction.

Ovulatory dysfunction and metabolic syndrome are more frequently found in severe PCOS phenotypes. Insulin resistance and hyperandrogenemia are critical factors in PCOS pathophysiology and are strongly interrelated. A vicious circle where hyperandrogenism favors abdominal fat accumulation and insulin resistance has been described in PCOS. Furthermore, IR reciprocally facilitates the hypersecretion of androgens in PCOS patients.

In the last years, several mechanisms responsible for follicular growth arrest have been described. Extraovarian mechanism of follicle arrest demonstrates a crucial role of inheriting or acquired insulin resistance, because abdominal fat accumulation can induce or worsen hyperandrogenism in PCOS. Hyperandrogenism and HI can cause an impairment of FSH and LH secretion, leading to follicle arrest. The improvement of the MS by weight loss or medical treatment can restore follicle growth ovulation in some PCOS phenotypes, but not in all of them.

Different intraovarian mechanisms of follicular growth arrest have been recently suggested:

- Hyperinsulinemia is associated with theca cell hyperplasia and higher secretion of androgens.
- Intraovarian hyperandrogenism is associated with diminished atresia of theca cells.
- Higher AMH expression in PCOS follicle granulosa cells impairs follicular development and estradiol secretion by inhibiting aromatase activity.
- Higher AMH levels increase the FSH threshold of small antral follicles, leading to an FSH resistance.
- Higher AMH levels in FF are associated with lower proangiogenic EMs and VEGF intrafollicular level.

These data suggest that PCOS has an altered intrafollicular environment characterized by impaired theca-granulosa communication and higher AMH levels that decrease follicle FSH sensitivity and reduce angiogenesis, leading to follicular growth arrest. This inherent ovarian condition can be deteriorated by an extraovarian factor such as insulin resistance secondary to abnormal fat distribution or obesity.

The latter exemplifies the complex endocrine and paracrine mechanism related to metabolic follicle syndrome and its relation to follicle growth arrest in PCOS.

The precise mechanism that causes hyperandrogenism and hyperinsulinism and follicle growth arrest in a specific PCOS phenotype is not fully understood. Until now, PCOS treatment is based on reducing IR by weight loss, insulin sensitizers, and ovarian gonadotropin stimulation to improve hyperandrogenemia, metabolic syndrome, and restore follicle growth.

Future studies necessary to design a tailored treatment to tackle the predominant mechanism in a specific PCOS phenotype are needed.

References

1. Zawadzki J, Dunaif A. Diagnostic criteria for polycystic ovary syndrome: towards a rationale approach. In: Dunaif A, J.R. G, F. H, G.R. M, editors. Polycystic Ovary Syndrome. Boston, Ma: Blackwell Scientific Publications; 1992. p. 377–84.
2. The Rotterdam ESHRE/ASRM-Sponsored PCOS Consensus Workshop Group. Revised 2003 consensus on diagnostic criteria and long-term health risks related to polycystic ovary syndrome. Fertil Steril. 2004;81(1):19–25.

3. Azziz R, Carmina E, Dewailly D, Diamanti-Kandarakis E, Escobar-Morreale HF, Futterweit W, et al. Positions statement: criteria for defining polycystic ovary syndrome as a predominantly hyperandrogenic syndrome: an androgen excess society guideline. J Clin Endocrinol Metab. 2006;91(11):4237–45.
4. Teede HJ, Misso ML, Costello MF, Dokras A, Laven J, Moran L, et al. Recommendations from the international evidence-based guideline for the assessment and management of polycystic ovary syndrome. Fertil Steril. 2018;110(3):364–79.
5. Lizneva D, Suturina L, Walker W, Brakta S, Gavrilova-Jordan L, Azziz R. Criteria, prevalence, and phenotypes of polycystic ovary syndrome. Fertil Steril. 2016;106(1):6–15.
6. Patil K, Yelamanchi S, Kumar M, Hinduja I, Prasad TSK, Gowda H, et al. Quantitative mass spectrometric analysis to unravel glycoproteomic signature of follicular fluid in women with polycystic ovary syndrome. PLoS One. 2019;14(4):e0214742.
7. Ambekar AS, Kelkar DS, Pinto SM, Sharma R, Hinduja I, Zaveri K, et al. Proteomics of follicular fluid from women with polycystic ovary syndrome suggests molecular defects in follicular development. J Clin Endocrinol Metab. 2015;100(2):744–53.
8. Maciel GAR, Baracat EC, Benda JA, Markham SM, Hensinger K, Chang RJ, et al. Stockpiling of transitional and classic primary follicles in ovaries of women with polycystic ovary syndrome. J Clin Endocrinol Metabol. 2004;89(11):5321–7.
9. Stubbs SA, Webber LJ, Stark J, Rice S, Margara R, Lavery S, et al. Role of insulin-like growth factors in initiation of follicle growth in Normal and polycystic human ovaries. J Clin Endocrinol Metabol. 2013;98(8):3298–305.
10. Dewailly D, Robin G, Peigne M, Decanter C, Pigny P, Catteau-Jonard S. Interactions between androgens, FSH, anti-Müllerian hormone and estradiol during folliculogenesis in the human normal and polycystic ovary. Hum Reprod Update. 2016;22(6):709–24.
11. Dilaver N, Pellatt L, Jameson E, Ogunjimi M, Bano G, Homburg R, et al. The regulation and signalling of anti-Müllerian hormone in human granulosa cells: relevance to polycystic ovary syndrome. Hum Reprod. 2019;34(12):2467–79.
12. Valkenburg O, Uitterlinden AG, Piersma D, Hofman A, Themmen AP, de Jong FH, et al. Genetic polymorphisms of GnRH and gonadotrophic hormone receptors affect the phenotype of polycystic ovary syndrome. Hum Reprod. 2009;24(8):2014–22.
13. Laven JSE. Follicle stimulating hormone receptor (FSHR) Polymorphisms and Polycystic Ovary Syndrome (PCOS). Front Endocrinol (Lausanne). 2019;10:23-.
14. Broekmans FJ, Visser JA, Laven JS, Broer SL, Themmen AP, Fauser BC. Anti-Mullerian hormone and ovarian dysfunction. Trends Endocrinol Metab. 2008;19(9):340–7.
15. Banaszewska B, Spaczynski RZ, Pelesz M, Pawelczyk L. Incidence of elevated LH/FSH ratio in polycystic ovary syndrome women with normo- and hyperinsulinemia. Rocz Akad Med Bialymst. 2003;48:131–4.
16. Durlinger AL, Visser JA, Themmen AP. Regulation of ovarian function: the role of anti-Mullerian hormone. Reproduction. 2002b;124(5):601–9.
17. Villarroel C, Merino PM, Lopez P, Eyzaguirre FC, Van Velzen A, Iniguez G, et al. Polycystic ovarian morphology in adolescents with regular menstrual cycles is associated with elevated anti-Mullerian hormone. Hum Reprod. 2011;26(10):2861–8.
18. Di Pietro M, Pascuali N, Parborell F, Abramovich D. Ovarian angiogenesis in polycystic ovary syndrome. Reproduction. 2018;155(5):R199–209.
19. Robinson RS, Woad KJ, Hammond AJ, Laird M, Hunter MG, Mann GE. Angiogenesis and vascular function in the ovary. Reproduction. 2009;138(6):869–81.
20. Henriquez S, Kohen P, Villarroel C, Muñoz A, Godoy A, Strauss JF, 3rd, et al. Significance of pro-angiogenic estrogen metabolites in normal follicular development and follicular growth arrest in Polycystic Ovary Syndrome (PCOS). Human Reproduction. 2020;(in press).
21. Jacewicz-Święcka M, Kowalska I. Polycystic ovary syndrome and the risk of cardiometabolic complications in longitudinal studies. Diabetes Metab Res Rev. 2018;34(8):e3054.
22. Carmina E, Lobo RA. Use of fasting blood to assess the prevalence of insulin resistance in women with polycystic ovary syndrome. Fertil Steril. 2004;82(3):661–5.

23. Behboudi-Gandevani S, Ramezani Tehrani F, Hosseinpanah F, Khalili D, Cheraghi L, Kazemijaliseh H, et al. Cardiometabolic risks in polycystic ovary syndrome: long-term population-based follow-up study. Fertil Steril. 2018;110(7):1377–86.
24. Zhu S, Zhang B, Jiang X, Li Z, Zhao S, Cui L, et al. Metabolic disturbances in non-obese women with polycystic ovary syndrome: a systematic review and meta-analysis. Fertil Steril. 2019;111(1):168–77.
25. Lim SS, Kakoly NS, Tan JWJ, Fitzgerald G, Bahri Khomami M, Joham AE, et al. Metabolic syndrome in polycystic ovary syndrome: a systematic review, meta-analysis and meta-regression. Obes Rev. 2019;20(2):339–52.
26. Christ JP, Falcone T. Bariatric surgery improves Hyperandrogenism, menstrual irregularities, and metabolic dysfunction among women with polycystic ovary syndrome (PCOS). Obes Surg. 2018;28(8):2171–7.
27. Escobar-Morreale HF. Polycystic ovary syndrome: definition, aetiology, diagnosis and treatment. Nat Rev Endocrinol. 2018;14(5):270–84.
28. Costello MF, Misso ML, Balen A, Boyle J, Devoto L, Garad RM, et al. Evidence summaries and recommendations from the international evidence-based guideline for the assessment and management of polycystic ovary syndrome: assessment and treatment of infertility. Hum Reprod Open. 2019;2019(1):hoy021-hoy.
29. Wild RA, Carmina E, Diamanti-Kandarakis E, Dokras A, Escobar-Morreale HF, Futterweit W, et al. Assessment of cardiovascular risk and prevention of cardiovascular disease in women with the polycystic ovary syndrome: a consensus statement by the androgen excess and polycystic ovary syndrome (AE-PCOS) society. J Clin Endocrinol Metabol. 2010;95(5):2038–49.
30. Jeanes YM, Reeves S. Metabolic consequences of obesity and insulin resistance in polycystic ovary syndrome: diagnostic and methodological challenges. Nutr Res Rev. 2017;30(1):97–105.
31. Escobar-Morreale HF, Luque-Ramirez M, San Millan JL. The molecular-genetic basis of functional hyperandrogenism and the polycystic ovary syndrome. Endocr Rev. 2005;26(2):251–82.
32. DeUgarte CM, Bartolucci AA, Azziz R. Prevalence of insulin resistance in the polycystic ovary syndrome using the homeostasis model assessment. Fertil Steril. 2005;83(5):1454–60.
33. Legro RS, Bentley-Lewis R, Driscoll D, Wang SC, Dunaif A. Insulin resistance in the sisters of women with polycystic ovary syndrome: association with hyperandrogenemia rather than menstrual irregularity. J Clin Endocrinol Metab. 2002;87(5):2128–33.
34. Azziz R. Polycystic Ovary Syndrome Obstetrics & Gynecology 2018;132(2).
35. Diamanti-Kandarakis E, Dunaif A. Insulin resistance and the polycystic ovary syndrome revisited: an update on mechanisms and implications. Endocr Rev. 2012;33(6):981–1030.
36. Seow KM, Juan CC, Hsu YP, Hwang JL, Huang LW, Ho LT. Amelioration of insulin resistance in women with PCOS via reduced insulin receptor substrate-1 Ser312 phosphorylation following laparoscopic ovarian electrocautery. Hum Reprod. 2007;22(4):1003–10.
37. Caro JF. Clinical review 26: insulin resistance in obese and nonobese man. J Clin Endocrinol Metab. 1991;73(4):691–5.
38. Freidenberg GR, Reichart D, Olefsky JM, Henry RR. Reversibility of defective adipocyte insulin receptor kinase activity in non-insulin-dependent diabetes mellitus. Effect of weight loss. J Clin Invest. 1988;82(4):1398–406.
39. Dunaif A. Insulin resistance and the polycystic ovary syndrome: mechanism and implications for pathogenesis. Endocr Rev. 1997;18(6):774–800.
40. Sorbara LR, Tang Z, Cama A, Xia J, Schenker E, Kohanski RA, et al. Absence of insulin receptor gene mutations in three insulin-resistant women with the polycystic ovary syndrome. Metabolism. 1994;43(12):1568–74.
41. Rice S, Christoforidis N, Gadd C, Nikolaou D, Seyani L, Donaldson A, et al. Impaired insulin-dependent glucose metabolism in granulosa-lutein cells from anovulatory women with polycystic ovaries. Hum Reprod. 2005;20(2):373–81.
42. Cardoso RC, Veiga-Lopez A, Moeller J, Beckett E, Pease A, Keller E, et al. Developmental programming: impact of gestational steroid and metabolic milieus on adiposity and insulin sensitivity in prenatal testosterone-treated female sheep. Endocrinology. 2016; 157(2):522–35.

43. Georgios KD, Ioannis K, Harpal SR. Polycystic ovary syndrome as a Proinflammatory state: the role of Adipokines. Curr Pharm Des. 2016;22(36):5535–46.
44. Escobar-Morreale HF, San Millan JL. Abdominal adiposity and the polycystic ovary syndrome. Trends Endocrinol Metab. 2007;18(7):266–72.
45. Poli Mara S, Sheila BL, Fabíola S, Debora MM. Adipose tissue dysfunction, adipokines, and low-grade chronic inflammation in polycystic ovary syndrome. Reproduction. 2015;149(5):R219–R27.
46. Satyaraddi A, Cherian KE, Kapoor N, Kunjummen AT, Kamath MS, Thomas N, et al. Body composition, metabolic characteristics, and insulin resistance in obese and nonobese women with polycystic ovary syndrome. J Hum Reprod Sci. 2019;12(2):78–84.
47. Polak AM, Adamska A, Krentowska A, Łebkowska A, Hryniewicka J, Adamski M, et al. Body composition, serum concentrations of androgens and insulin resistance in different polycystic ovary syndrome phenotypes. J Clin Med. 2020;9(3):732.
48. Ezeh U, Pall M, Mathur R, Azziz R. Association of fat to lean mass ratio with metabolic dysfunction in women with polycystic ovary syndrome. Hum Reprod. 2014;29(7): 1508–17.
49. Brennan KM, Kroener LL, Chazenbalk GD, Dumesic DA. Polycystic ovary syndrome: impact of lipotoxicity on metabolic and reproductive health. Obstet Gynecol Surv. 2019; 74(4):223–31.
50. Vazquez-Vela ME, Torres N, Tovar AR. White adipose tissue as endocrine organ and its role in obesity. Arch Med Res. 2008;39(8):715–28.
51. Delitala AP, Capobianco G, Delitala G, Cherchi PL, Dessole S. Polycystic ovary syndrome, adipose tissue and metabolic syndrome. Arch Gynecol Obstet. 2017;296(3):405–19.
52. Carmina E, Bucchieri S, Mansueto P, Rini G, Ferin M, Lobo RA. Circulating levels of adipose products and differences in fat distribution in the ovulatory and anovulatory phenotypes of polycystic ovary syndrome. Fertil Steril. 2009;91(4 Suppl):1332–5.
53. Toulis KA, Goulis DG, Farmakiotis D, Georgopoulos NA, Katsikis I, Tarlatzis BC, et al. Adiponectin levels in women with polycystic ovary syndrome: a systematic review and a meta-analysis. Hum Reprod Update. 2009;15(3):297–307.
54. Sanchez-Garrido MA, Tena-Sempere M. Metabolic dysfunction in polycystic ovary syndrome: pathogenic role of androgen excess and potential therapeutic strategies. Molecular Metabolism. 2020;35:100937.
55. Chazenbalk G, Trivax BS, Yildiz BO, Bertolotto C, Mathur R, Heneidi S, et al. Regulation of adiponectin secretion by adipocytes in the polycystic ovary syndrome: role of tumor necrosis factor-{alpha}. J Clin Endocrinol Metab. 2010;95(2):935–42.
56. Gunning MN, Sir Petermann T, Crisosto N, van Rijn BB, de Wilde MA, Christ JP, et al. Cardiometabolic health in offspring of women with PCOS compared to healthy controls: a systematic review and individual participant data meta-analysis. Hum Reprod Update. 2019;26(1):104–18.
57. Yucel A, Noyan V, Sagsoz N. The association of serum androgens and insulin resistance with fat distribution in polycystic ovary syndrome. Eur J Obstet Gynecol Reprod Biol. 2006;126(1):81–6.
58. Daan NMP, Jaspers L, Koster MPH, Broekmans FJM, de Rijke YB, Franco OH, et al. Androgen levels in women with various forms of ovarian dysfunction: associations with cardiometabolic features. Hum Reprod. 2015;30(10):2376–86.
59. Echiburú B, Pérez-Bravo F, Galgani JE, Sandoval D, Saldías C, Crisosto N, et al. Enlarged adipocytes in subcutaneous adipose tissue associated to hyperandrogenism and visceral adipose tissue volume in women with polycystic ovary syndrome. Steroids. 2018;130:15–21.
60. Kawwass JF, Sanders KM, Loucks TL, Rohan LC, Berga SL. Increased cerebrospinal fluid levels of GABA, testosterone and estradiol in women with polycystic ovary syndrome. Hum Reprod. 2017;32(7):1450–6.
61. Baba T, Ting AY, Tkachenko O, Xu J, Stouffer RL. Direct actions of androgen, estrogen and anti-Müllerian hormone on primate secondary follicle development in the absence of FSH in vitro. Hum Reprod. 2017;32(12):2456–64.

62. Weenen C, Laven JSE, von Bergh ARM, Cranfield M, Groome NP, Visser JA, et al. Anti-Müllerian hormone expression pattern in the human ovary: potential implications for initial and cyclic follicle recruitment. Mol Hum Reprod. 2004;10(2):77–83.
63. Pellatt L, Hanna L, Brincat M, Galea R, Brain H, Whitehead S, et al. Granulosa cell production of anti-Müllerian hormone is increased in polycystic ovaries. J Clin Endocrinol Metabol. 2007;92(1):240–5.
64. Laven JSE, Mulders AGMGJ, Visser JA, Themmen AP, de Jong FH, Fauser BCJM. Anti-Müllerian hormone serum concentrations in Normoovulatory and Anovulatory women of reproductive age. J Clin Endocrinol Metabol. 2004;89(1):318–23.
65. Villarroel C, López P, Merino PM, Iñiguez G, Sir-Petermann T, Codner E. Hirsutism and oligomenorrhea are appropriate screening criteria for polycystic ovary syndrome in adolescents. Gynecol Endocrinol. 2015;31(8):625–9.
66. Codner E. Iñíguez Gn, Villarroel C, Lopez P, Soto ns, Sir-Petermann T, et al. hormonal profile in women with polycystic ovarian syndrome with or without type 1 diabetes mellitus. J Clin Endocrinol Metabol. 2007;92(12):4742–6.
67. Codner E, Iñiguez G, Hernández IM, Lopez P, Rhumie HK, Villarroel C, et al. Elevated anti-Müllerian hormone (AMH) and inhibin B levels in prepubertal girls with type 1 diabetes mellitus. Clin Endocrinol. 2011;74(1):73–8.
68. Jacob SL, Field HP, Calder N, Picton HM, Balen AH, Barth JH. Anti-Müllerian hormone reflects the severity of polycystic ovary syndrome. Clin Endocrinol. 2017;86(3):395–400.
69. Das M, Gillott DJ, Saridogan E, Djahanbakhch O. Anti-Mullerian hormone is increased in follicular fluid from unstimulated ovaries in women with polycystic ovary syndrome. Hum Reprod. 2008;23(9):2122–6.
70. Hsueh AJW, Kawamura K, Cheng Y, Fauser BCJM. Intraovarian control of early Folliculogenesis. Endocr Rev. 2015;36(1):1–24.
71. Eldar-Geva T, Margalioth EJ, Gal M, Ben-Chetrit A, Algur N, Zylber-Haran E, et al. Serum anti-Mullerian hormone levels during controlled ovarian hyperstimulation in women with polycystic ovaries with and without hyperandrogenism. Hum Reprod. 2005;20(7):1814–9.
72. Piouka A, Farmakiotis D, Katsikis I, Macut D, Gerou S, Panidis D. Anti-Müllerian hormone levels reflect severity of PCOS but are negatively influenced by obesity: relationship with increased luteinizing hormone levels. Am J Physiol Endocrinol Metab. 2009;296(2):E238–E43.
73. Dumesic DA, Lesnick TG, Stassart JP, Ball GD, Wong A, Abbott DH. Intrafollicular antimüllerian hormone levels predict follicle responsiveness to follicle-stimulating hormone (FSH) in normoandrogenic ovulatory women undergoing gonadotropin releasing-hormone analog/recombinant human FSH therapy for in vitro fertilization and embryo transfer. Fertil Steril 2009;92(1):217–221.
74. Pierre A, Peigne M, Grynberg M, Arouche N, Taieb J, Hesters L, et al. Loss of LH-induced down-regulation of anti-Mullerian hormone receptor expression may contribute to anovulation in women with polycystic ovary syndrome. Hum Reprod. 2013;28(3):762–9.
75. Chun S. Serum luteinizing hormone level and luteinizing hormone/follicle-stimulating hormone ratio but not serum anti-Mullerian hormone level is related to ovarian volume in Korean women with polycystic ovary syndrome. Clin Exp Reprod Med. 2014;41(2):86–91.
76. Tamanini C, De Ambrogi M. Angiogenesis in developing follicle and Corpus luteum. Reprod Domest Anim. 2004;39(4):206–16.
77. Wulff C, Wilson H, Wiegand SJ, Rudge JS, Fraser HM. Prevention of thecal angiogenesis, antral follicular growth, and ovulation in the primate by treatment with vascular endothelial growth factor trap R1R2. Endocrinology. 2002;143(7):2797–807.
78. Pau E, Alonso-Muriel I, Gomez R, Novella E, Ruiz A, Garcia-Velasco JA, et al. Plasma levels of soluble vascular endothelial growth factor receptor-1 may determine the onset of early and late ovarian hyperstimulation syndrome. Hum Reprod. 2006;21(6):1453–60.
79. Pellicer A, Albert C, Mercader A, Bonilla-Musoles F, Remohi J, Simon C. The pathogenesis of ovarian hyperstimulation syndrome: in vivo studies investigating the role of interleukin-1beta, interleukin-6, and vascular endothelial growth factor. Fertil Steril. 1999;71(3):482–9.

80. LeCouter J, Kowalski J, Foster J, Hass P, Zhang Z, Dillard-Telm L, et al. Identification of an angiogenic mitogen selective for endocrine gland endothelium. Nature. 2001;412(6850):877–84.
81. Kamat BR, Brown LF, Manseau EJ, Senger DR, Dvorak HF. Expression of vascular permeability factor/vascular endothelial growth factor by human granulosa and theca lutein cells. Role in corpus luteum development. Am J Pathol. 1995;146(1):157–65.
82. Jang Y, Han J, Kim SJ, Kim J, Lee MJ, Jeong S, et al. Suppression of mitochondrial respiration with auraptene inhibits the progression of renal cell carcinoma: involvement of HIF-1α degradation. Oncotarget. 2015;6(35):38127–38.
83. Wan J, Chai H, Yu Z, Ge W, Kang N, Xia W, et al. HIF-1α effects on angiogenic potential in human small cell lung carcinoma. J Exp Clin Cancer Res. 2011;30(1):77-.
84. Devoto L, Henriquez S, Kohen P, Strauss JF 3rd. The significance of estradiol metabolites in human corpus luteum physiology. Steroids. 2017;123:50–4.
85. Kuo SW, Ke FC, Chang GD, Lee MT, Hwang JJ. Potential role of follicle-stimulating hormone (FSH) and transforming growth factor (TGFbeta1) in the regulation of ovarian angiogenesis. J Cell Physiol. 2011;226(6):1608–19.
86. Stilley JA, Guan R, Duffy DM, Segaloff DL. Signaling through FSH receptors on human umbilical vein endothelial cells promotes angiogenesis. J Clin Endocrinol Metab. 2014;99(5):E813–20.
87. Levin ER, Rosen GF, Cassidenti DL, Yee B, Meldrum D, Wisot A, et al. Role of vascular endothelial cell growth factor in ovarian Hyperstimulation syndrome. J Clin Invest. 1998;102(11):1978–85.
88. Jarvela IY, Sladkevicius P, Kelly S, Ojha K, Campbell S, Nargund G. Comparison of follicular vascularization in normal versus polycystic ovaries during in vitro fertilization as measured using 3-dimensional power Doppler ultrasonography. Fertil Steril. 2004;82(5):1358–63.
89. Hillier SG. Current concepts of the roles of follicle stimulating hormone and luteinizing hormone in folliculogenesis. Hum Reprod. 1994;9(2):188–91.
90. Rosenfeld CS, Wagner JS, Roberts RM, Lubahn DB. Intraovarian actions of oestrogen. Reproduction. 2001;122(2):215–26.
91. Zhu BT, Conney AH. Is 2-Methoxyestradiol an endogenous estrogen metabolite that inhibits mammary carcinogenesis? Cancer Res. 1998;58(11):2269
92. Kohen P, Henriquez S, Rojas C, Gerk PM, Palomino WA, Strauss JF 3rd, et al. 2-Methoxyestradiol in the human corpus luteum throughout the luteal phase and its influence on lutein cell steroidogenesis and angiogenic activity. Fertil Steril. 2013;100(5):1397–404.
93. Henriquez S, Kohen P, Xu X, Veenstra TD, Munoz A, Palomino WA, et al. Estrogen metabolites in human corpus luteum physiology: differential effects on angiogenic activity. Fertil Steril. 2016;106(1):230–7. e1
94. Tal R, Seifer DB, Arici A. The emerging role of angiogenic factor dysregulation in the pathogenesis of polycystic ovarian syndrome. Semin Reprod Med. 2015;33(3):195–207.
95. Nilsson E, Rogers N, Skinner MK. Actions of anti-Mullerian hormone on the ovarian transcriptome to inhibit primordial to primary follicle transition. Reproduction. 2007;134(2):209–21.

Quality of Life and Sexual Health

8

Lara Tiranini, Giulia Stincardini, Alessandra Righi,
Laura Cucinella, Manuela Piccinino, Roberta Rossini,
and Rossella E. Nappi

8.1 Quality of Life

According to the World Health Organization (WHO), quality of life (QoL) is the "individual perception of human beings of their position in life in the context of the culture and value systems in which they live and in relation to their goals." In this setting, health-related quality of life (HRQoL) is a multidimensional concept that examines the impact of a specific disease or its treatment on physical, mental, emotional, and social aspects and provides information on the benefits of medical therapies from the patient's perspective.

Polycystic ovarian syndrome (PCOS) is a major cause of psychological morbidity. Several systematic reviews have shown that PCOS has an overall negative impact on HRQoL [1–3]. It is not clear which aspects of PCOS have the strongest influence on HRQoL in affected women. Different traditions, religions, cultural-gender identity, and ethnicity are likely to influence the impact of PCOS on HRQoL in various societies. In a study by Benetti-Pinto et al. [4], Brazilian PCOS patients had worse self-perception regarding their general health with a negative correlation between weight and the physical domain. PCOS occurring in South Asian women adversely affected psychological well-being, especially due to the presence of hirsutism rather than obesity [5]; however, their HRQoL resulted not poorer than Caucasian women with PCOS [6]. In Iranian women, hirsutism has the strongest

L. Tiranini · G. Stincardini · A. Righi · L. Cucinella · R. E. Nappi (✉)
Research Center for Reproductive Medicine, Gynecological Endocrinology and Menopause,
IRCCS San Matteo Foundation, Pavia, Italy

Department of Clinical, Surgical, Diagnostic and Pediatric Sciences, University of Pavia,
Pavia, Italy

M. Piccinino · R. Rossini
Research Center for Reproductive Medicine, Gynecological Endocrinology and Menopause,
IRCCS San Matteo Foundation, Pavia, Italy

© International Society of Gynecological Endocrinology 2021
A. R. Genazzani et al. (eds.), *Impact of Polycystic Ovary, Metabolic Syndrome and Obesity on Women Health*, ISGE Series,
https://doi.org/10.1007/978-3-030-63650-0_8

93

impact on HRQoL, followed by infertility and menstrual irregularity [7]. Thus, the subjectively perceived impact of PCOS symptoms on women's lives, as well as cultural considerations or women's expectations, provides a basis for a better understanding of this large variability in QoL.

The polycystic ovary syndrome health-related quality of life questionnaire (PCOSQ) is the only specific validated instrument to measure QoL in these women population. It includes 26 items categorized into five domains, i.e., hirsutism, emotions, body weight, infertility, and menstruation [8]. Subsequently, the PCOSQ was modified by adding four questions to evaluate issues associated with acne [9]. Even generic questionnaires, validated for chronic diseases, have been used to assess HRQoL in PCOS women.

8.1.1 Hirsutism and Acne

Symptoms affecting appearance and body image, as hair and skin problems, reduce self-confidence and self-esteem causing marked psychological distress. The symptom of acne was reported in very few studies, probably because it is not included as a domain in the PCOSQ. Hirsutism, together with menstruation, is the most affected domain of HRQoL in PCOS women [3], but QoL may vary through different populations according to differences in cultural heritage, value systems, and family structure. In a German PCOS population, an elevated Ferriman-Gallwey score for hirsutism was associated with a low SF-36 scale including bodily pain, general health and physical domains, as well as decreased sexual satisfaction, but no correlation was detected between hirsutism and psychological or emotional distress [10]. On the other hand, a UK study involving PCOS women with self-reported facial hair showed an elevated incidence of depression and anxiety; the subsequent randomization to a laser treatment revealed a positive impact upon HRQoL with reduction in self-reported severity of hirsutism, time spent on hair removal, and depression and anxiety scores [11]. Thus, as demonstrated in a sample of adolescent girls with PCOS [12], self-perceived severity of illness such as hirsutism might correlate more directly with HRQoL than clinical assessment, further supporting the importance of measuring HRQoL from the patient's perspective. The pathogenesis of skin issues (hirsutism and acne) includes both hyperandrogenemia and insulin-resistance; therefore, it was demonstrated that both combined hormonal contraceptives and lifestyle changes have a positive effect on QoL [13].

8.1.2 Body Weight

PCOS is associated with higher rates of obesity and metabolic syndrome, leading to an increased prevalence of cardiovascular risk factors, such as insulin resistance, dyslipidemia, and diabetes. Weight gain appears to exert the greatest negative influence upon HRQoL in women with PCOS, and many of them report frustration with inability to lose weight, low self-esteem, and consequently a poor body image [8]. Cultural influences are likely involved in body image distress, as the android fat pattern commonly associated with PCOS is considered unattractive in many context. Moreover, social expectations of thinness in Western countries may also play a role. However, the role of body mass index (BMI) in self-reported QoL of women with PCOS appears to be complex. Some studies have shown that reductions in HRQoL are associated with an elevated BMI [10, 14], not only in the adult population but also in PCOS adolescents [15]. Other studies do not suggest a relationship between BMI status and HRQoL in PCOS women. For example, Hashimoto et al. [16] found similar HRQoL weight scores comparing two ethnicities (Austrian and Brazilian women) with significant differences in BMI (Austrian women were leaner than Brazilians); the weight domain resulted the worst area of HRQoL in both populations. These findings indicate that all women with PCOS have weight concerns regardless of their BMI; therefore, relying on this clinical measurement alone as an indicator of poor QoL would overlook the difficulties experienced by PCOS women who have a "normal" weight. One potential explanation of the reduction in HRQoL may be that PCOS women with normal BMI struggle to maintain their weight at this level. There is also the need to look beyond BMI and measure waist circumference which is more directly proportional to total body fat and to metabolically active visceral fat, a more accurate measure of metabolic risk. In any case, a reduction in weight appears to improve HRQoL significantly. A combined treatment with lifestyle interventions and hormonal contraceptives was associated with improvement in all domains of HRQoL in overweight/obese PCOS women [13], confirming some findings previously obtained in obese adolescents with or without the addiction of metformin [17]. Even if changes in insulin sensitivity did not correlate with changes in HRQoL [13], Hahn et al. [18] showed that treatment with metformin induces an improvement in SF-36 HRQoL scores significantly correlated with a reduction in weight. In women with multiple comorbidities, such as depression, even cognitive-behavioral therapy added to an intensive lifestyle intervention showed a positive impact on PCOSQ scores [19]. Therefore, efforts to identify appropriate long-term weight loss programs and treatments would be beneficial to these women, and physicians must provide early interventions because young, obese adolescents with PCOS have a high prevalence of early endocrine, metabolic, and cardiovascular characteristics.

8.1.3 Menstruation

Menstrual irregularity (oligomenorrhea and amenorrhea) is one the most distressing symptoms in PCOS women determining a reduced feeling of femininity and a significant concern about fertility [9]. In a US sample, menstrual cycle disorders were the second most important factor after obesity in reducing QoL in women with PCOS [14], whereas by comparing Asian and Caucasian PCOS women, menstrual problems were found to be of least concern for Asians [6]. Indeed, different studies display a variability in the distribution and frequency of PCOSQ sub-scale domains, which is probably determined not only by ethnicity and culture but also by the enrollment of women with different phenotypes of PCOS [20].

8.1.4 Infertility

PCOS is the most common endocrine disorder causing female anovulatory infertility regardless of ethnicity. Infertility has been reported as the worse domain of HRQoL in some studies [21], but selection bias must be considered as women could have been referred to clinic due to infertility problems. Several factors modulate the emotional consequences of infertility, including duration of infertility, previous treatment failure, age, and socio-cultural background. Reproductive history predicted scores in the infertility domain of the PCOSQ: women with PCOS who had given birth to at least one viable infant exhibited better functioning in this domain in comparison to women without children. Moreover, women who experienced spontaneous abortions reported the lowest scores in the infertility domain, exceeding those of women who had been unsuccessful in establishing pregnancy [14]. Infertility is not only a concern of women trying to conceive since it has been shown that even adolescent girls with PCOS are worried about their future ability to become pregnant with an impact on their QoL [22].

8.1.5 Psychological Distress (Depression and Anxiety)

Women with PCOS have higher levels of emotional distress with excessive weight, hirsutism, and infertility having a strong influence on the psychological experience of women because they evoke negative emotions of low self-esteem, frustration, and anxiety [23]. A recent meta-analysis showed that PCOS women have over three times the risk of depressive symptoms and over five times the risk of anxiety symptoms if compared to controls [24]. The association remained significant also restricting the analysis to moderate and severe depressive and anxiety scores [24]. Other psychiatric disorders have been found to correlate with PCOS, with increased odds of personality disorder, schizoaffective disorder, withholding anger, obsessive compulsive disorder, panic disorder, and attention deficit disorder [25]. Disordered eating behaviors, as bulimia and binge eating disorder, are also more prevalent in adult women with PCOS.

The exact mechanism underlying the increased prevalence of depressive and anxiety symptoms in women with PCOS is unclear, but many potential factors may play a role. In the general population, some meta-analyses have shown association between depression and factors such as obesity, insulin resistance, and diabetes [26]. In PCOS, although weight concerns are common and are associated with low QoL scores, a meta-analysis showed only a modest impact of weight on depression and anxiety scores [27]; in addition, women maintained higher odds of psychological disturbances after matching for BMI, suggesting an independent relationship. Insulin resistance, common in both obese and lean PCOS women, showed a bidirectional relationship with depression, but not with anxiety [28]. Infertility does not seem to correlate with an increased risk of depression or anxiety. The relationship between androgens and mood in women is controversial. Biochemical hyperandrogenemia, in particular higher free testosterone, was observed in PCOS women with anxiety compared to PCOS women without anxiety [29], whereas no association was seen between testosterone and depression [24]. Clinical hyperandrogenism was associated with elevated depression and anxiety scores, when the Ferriman-Gallwey scale is self-administered. By contrast, when the clinician filled-in the same scale of hirsutism, there was no correlation with depression, indicating the importance of the subjective experience of hirsutism. Stress and increased activity of hypothalamic-pituitary-adrenal axis have been implicated as a possible mechanism contributing to depression both in the general population and in PCOS patients ([30]), but very few studies are available.

Depression and anxiety, as well as other psychiatric disturbances, should be routinely screened in PCOS patients. Indeed, some of PCOS specific treatments have shown favorable emotional effects, but there are no studies evaluating anti-depressant or anti-anxiety medications specifically in the PCOS population. Lifestyle interventions (i.e., dietary, exercise) have been shown to decrease weight, testosterone, and hirsutism, potentially improving depressive and anxiety symptoms. The addition of hormonal contraception regulating the menstrual cycle and reducing hyperandrogenism showed a better efficacy [13]. On the other hand, hormonal contraceptives given to lean PCOS women showed no improvement in psychological domains [17]. Other potential treatments are laser hair removal, which improved psychological aspects related to hirsutism without changes in androgen levels [11], and pioglitazone, an insulin sensitizer which determined a greater decrease in depression scores if compared to metformin, probably because of its anti-inflammatory properties (in the general obese population, dysregulation of inflammatory pathways is associated to depression). Finally, cognitive behavioral therapy is one of the first-line treatments for patients with depression, with data confirming an improvement in weight loss and stress responsiveness and a small improvement in depression and anxiety scores [19].

Body image distress (BID) is an important mediator and predictor of depression and anxiety, and, in PCOS women, skin problems and obesity are the main determinants of body dissatisfaction. BID is defined as a distortion of perception, behavior, or cognition related to body weight or shape. The Multidimensional Body Self Relations-Appearance Subscales (MBSRQ-AS) (a 34-item questionnaire) and the Stunkard Figure Rating Scale (an image of multiple female silhouettes increasing in size) are validated instruments to measure body image distress. The most recent and larger controlled study by Alur-Gupta [31] confirmed a worse body image score on all subscales of MBSRQ-AS in PCOS patients, and this result is maintained even after adjustment for BMI and other confounders. Moreover, PCOS women expressed greater differences between ideal and perceived images of their own body, also indicative of BID. These results point to the need for screening and counseling women with PCOS regarding the higher predisposition for BID and the associated depressive and anxiety symptoms which may jeopardize motivation and compliance to treatments. Management of BID includes cognitive behavioral therapy, stress management training, and psychoeducation, associated with specific therapies for PCOS. Thus, a strict collaboration with nutritionists, endocrinologists, and behavioral health specialists is essential to provide a comprehensive care, and early intervention decreases psychological disturbances by improving QoL.

8.2   Sexual Health

In PCOS women, body image issues (i.e., obesity, hirsutism, and acne), irregular menstrual bleeding, and infertility may influence the feminine identity with consequent frustration, unhappiness, and psychological distress. In addition, the perceived unattractiveness may induce alteration of sexual behavior and loss of self-esteem with effects on both intimate and social relationships. Sexual function depends on the integration of physical, emotional, cognitive, and socio-cultural aspects. Female sexual dysfunction (FSD) may affect any phase of the sexual response cycle preventing the individual or the couple from experiencing satisfactory sexual behavior. The Female Sexual Function Index (FSFI) is the most used self-reporting instrument to assess six domains of sexual function (desire, arousal, lubrication, orgasm, satisfaction, pain) and has been largely used even in PCOS.

Current opinions about sexual function in women with PCOS are controversial; contrasting results observed in different studies might be explained by the multifactorial nature of women's sexual function, different phenotypes, and characteristics of study populations, as well as the spectrum of PCOS severity.

8.2.1   Impact of PCOS Traits on Sexual Function

Changes in appearance might impair feminine identity and compromise sexual satisfaction. In the general population, it has been shown that obesity affected several aspects of sexual function (except desire and pain) in women with FSD, whereas no correlation was demonstrated between BMI and FSFI in women without FSD. This finding indicates that obesity might be an important factor once sexual dysfunction is already manifested [32]. In PCOS women, some studies reported a weak correlation between BMI and FSD. For example, increasing BMI resulted in diminished FSFI scores on desire and sexual satisfaction domains [33]. In another study, high BMI had only a minor effect on sexual function, determining a lower satisfaction with sexual life [34]. Whereas obese healthy women had low FSFI score, PCOS women yielded borderline FSFI scores regardless of their obesity status [35]. On the other hand, Elsenbruch et al. [23] concluded that in PCOS women BMI had no impact on sexual satisfaction and no effect on the frequency of sexual intercourse or sexual thought and fantasies. The same results were found in Brazilian [4] and in North American PCOS women with a lack of correlation between BMI and sexual function, apart a mild association with orgasmic dysfunction [36].

As already mentioned, hirsutism is another important trait of PCOS able to alter body image and affect one's perception of sexual attractiveness. In an Iranian sample of infertile PCOS women, Eftekhar et al. [33] found significantly lower scores in all FSFI domains using the Ferriman-Gallwey score, while in other studies [10, 23] PCOS women believed more than controls that their excessive body hair negatively affected their sexuality and caused difficulty in making social contacts due to appearance. Instead, Stovall et al. [36] did not find an association between hirsutism and sexual dysfunction in PCOS. Hashemi et al. [37] reported a lower but not significant score of sexual function in hirsute women with PCOS, while alopecia, another distressful characteristic of PCOS, correlated to sexual dysfunction. In a study including lean PCOS and control women, those with clinical hyperandrogenism showed higher scores in the Visual/Proximity domain of the Cues of Sexual Desire Scale in respect with those with biochemical hyperandrogenism [38].

Concerning infertility, in an Iranian sample of married PCOS women a 10% wider prevalence of FSD in the infertile group compared to fertile counterpart was reported [37]. On the other hand, another study concluded that having children or not was not associated with sexual function in women with PCOS [34]. That being so, the wide variability in the perception of PCOS symptoms according to sociocultural factors may explain such controversial results.

Finally, sexual debut and behavior have been also investigated in adolescent with PCOS. These girls were less likely to be sexually active than their healthy peers, but the mean ages of initiation of sexual activity were not significantly different [22].

8.2.2   General Impact of PCOS on Sexual Function

We have stated that several studies have reported a possible association between PCOS and sexual dysfunction. However, a recent meta-analysis by Zhao et al. [39] concluded that PCOS did not significantly impair sexual functioning and the prevalence rate of FSD was similar in PCOS women and in healthy controls (34.6% and 33.5%, respectively). These results confirm the findings of a pilot study including PCOS women and controls with normal weight in order to avoid the bias of obesity on psychological distress and sexual function [40]. The incidence of FSD was similar in PCOS and control women even in the context of partnership (i.e., partner's sexual health and feelings, relationship) [40]. Other studies reported that women with PCOS felt less sexually attractive, were less satisfied with their sex life, and thought their partners were less satisfied too, even if they did not differ in the frequency of sexual intercourses and sexual thoughts and fantasies when compared to controls [10, 23]. Treatment with metformin increased the frequency of sexual intercourses, improved the satisfaction with sexual life, reduced pain during sexual intercourses, and diminished the self-reported impact of hirsutism on sexuality [18].

According to Zhang et al. [39], even if the total FSFI score did not differ between the PCOS group and the control group, women with PCOS had significantly lower values in the arousal and lubrication domains. A possible explanation is the relationship between arousal disorder and physical appearance (i.e., obesity, hirsutism) and between vaginal lubrication and psychological inhibition during sexual intercourse.

8.2.3 Androgens and Sexual Function in PCOS

Hyperandrogenemia is the hallmark of PCOS, and it is associated with a reduction of sexual hormone binding globulin (SHBG) levels that increase free circulating androgens. Androgens seem deeply involved in the modulation of sexual function by positively acting on sexual desire (thoughts and fantasies); however, the exact role of androgens in sexual response remains controversial and not completely understood because normal sexual function has been documented even in women with low androgen levels across the menstrual cycle [41]. Several studies have found that hyperandrogenemia had a negative effect on sexual function, probably because of the clinical signs of hyperandrogenism (hirsutism, acne, alopecia) which impair body image. On the contrary, some investigators suggested that hyperandrogenemia might act as a protecting factor for sexual function: Stovall et al. [36] reported that PCOS women with the lowest total serum testosterone levels tended to have the lowest sexual function scores, while higher testosterone levels were associated with greater desire/frequency. Discrepancies in linking androgen circulating levels and sexual function are well known and may be due to a variety of mechanisms, including intracrinology, bioavailability, and enzymatic and receptor activity [42]. Indeed, high testosterone levels in PCOS women did not produce any beneficial effects on their sexual function [35]; similarly, higher circulating androgen levels in PCOS women did not influence sexual function nor modify clitoral body volume if compared to women without PCOS showing normal androgen levels [40]. Consistent with this, Rellini et al. [38] demonstrated that clinical signs of hyperandrogenism, rather than biochemical signs of hyperandrogenemia, were associated with specific cues of sexual desire levels, implying that the link between androgens and sexual desire relies on individual androgen sensitivity.

8.3 Conclusions

The multifaceted aspects of PCOS coupled to the multidimensional nature of QoL and sexual function offer a complex view to the readers, fully opened to further research. It is likely that genetic and epigenetic mechanisms play a crucial role in setting different phenotypes of PCOS women giving origin to a multitude of behavioral patterns.

References

1. Jones GL, Hall JM, Balen AH, Ledger WL. Health-related quality of life measurement in women with polycystic ovary syndrome: a systematic review. Hum Reprod Update. 2008;14:15–25.
2. Veltman-Verhulst SM, Boivin J, Eijkemans MJ, Fauser BJ. Emotional distress is a common risk in women with polycystic ovary syndrome: a systematic review and meta-analysis of 28 studies. Hum Reprod Update. 2012;18:638–51.

3. Bazarganipour F, Taghavi SA, Montazeri A, Ahmadi F, Chaman R, Khosravi A. The impact of polycystic ovary syndrome on health-related quality of life: a systematic review and meta-analysis. Iran J Reprod Med. 2015;13:61–70.
4. Benetti-Pinto CL, Ferreira SR, Antunes A, Yela DA. The influence of body weight on sexual function and quality of life in women with polycystic ovary syndrome. Arch Gynecol Obstet. 2015;291:451–5.
5. Kumarapeli V, Seneviratne R, Wijeyaratne C. Health-related quality of life and psychological distress in polycystic ovary syndrome: a hidden facet in south Asian women. BJOG. 2011;118:319–28.
6. Jones GL, Palep-Singh M, Ledger WL, Balen AH, Jenkinson C, Campbell MJ, Lashen H. Do south Asian women with PCOS have poorer health-related quality of life than Caucasian women with PCOS? A comparative cross-sectional study Health and Quality of Life Outcomes. 2010;8:149.
7. Moghadam ZB, Fereidooni B, Saffari M, Montazeri A. Polycystic ovary syndome and its impact on Iranian women's quality of life: a population-based study. BMC Womens Health. 2018;18:164.
8. Cronin L, Guyatt G, Griffith L, Wong E, Azziz R, Futterweit W, et al. Development of a health-related quality of life questionnaire (PCOSQ) for women with polycystic ovary syndrome (PCOS). J Clin Endocrinol Metab. 1998;83:1976–87.
9. Barnard L, Ferriday D, Guenther N, Strauss B, Balen AH, Dye L. Quality of life and psychological Well-being in polycystic ovary syndrome. J Obstet Gynecol Neonatal Nurs. 2005;34:12–20.
10. Hahn S, Janssen OE, Tan S, Pleger K, Mann K, Schedlowski M, Kimming R, Benson S, Balamitsa E, Elsenbruch S. Clinical and psychological correlates of quality-of life in polycystic ovary syndrome. Eur J Endocrinol. 2005;153:853–60.
11. Clayton WJ, Lipton M, Elford J, Rustin M, Sherr L. A randomized controlled trial of laser treatment among hirsute women with polycystic ovary syndrome. Br J Dermatol. 2005;152:986–92.
12. Trent ME, Rich M, Austin SB, Gordon CM. Quality of life in adolescent girls with polycystic ovary syndrome. Arch Pediatr Adolesc Med. 2002;156:556–60.
13. Dokras A, Sarwer DB, Allison KC, Milman L, Kris-Etherton PM, Kunselman AR, Stetter CM, Williams NI, Gnatuk CL, Estes SJ, Fleming J, Coutifaris C, Legro RS. Weight loss and lowering androgens predict improvements in health-related quality of life in women with PCOS. J Clin Endocrinol Metab. 2016;101:2966–74.
14. McCook JC, Reame NE, Thatcher SS. Health-related quality of life issues in women with polycystic ovary syndrome. J Obstet Gynecol Neonatal Nurs. 2005;34:12–20.
15. Trent ME, Austin SB, Rich M, Gordon CM. Overweight status of adolescent girls with polycystic ovary syndrome: body mass index as mediator of quality of life. Ambul Pediatr. 2005;5:107–11.
16. Hashimoto DM, SchmidJ MFM, Fonseca AM, Andrade LH, Kirchengast S, Eggers S. The impact of the weight status on subjective symptomatology of the polycystic ovary syndrome: a cross-cultural comparison between Brazilian and Austrian women. Anthropol Anz. 2003;61:297–310.
17. Harris-Glocker M, Davidson K, Kochman L, Guzik D, Hoeger K. Improvement in quality-of-life questionnaire measures in obese adolescent females with polycystic ovary syndrome treated with lifestyle changes and oral contraceptives, with or without metformin. Fertil Steril. 2010;93:1016–9.
18. Hahn S, Benson S, Elsenbruch S, Pleger K, Tan S, Mann K, Schedlowski M, Bering van Halteren W, Kimmig R, Janssen OE. Metformin treatment of polycystic ovary syndrome improves health-related quality-of-life, emotional distress and sexuality. Hum Reprod. 2006;21:1925–34.
19. Cooney LG, Milman LW, Hantsoo L, Kornfield S, Sammel MD, Allison KC, Epperson N, Dokras A. Cognitive-behavioral therapy improves weight loss and quality of life in women with polycystic ovary syndrome. Fertil Steril. 2010;110:161–71.

20. Bazarganipour F, Ziaei S, Montazeri A, Foroozanfard F, Kazemnejad A, Faghihzadeh S. Predictive factors of health-related quality of life in patients with polycystic ovary syndrome: a structural equation modelling approach. Fertil Steril. 2013;100:1390–6. e3
21. Schmid J, Kirchengast S, Vytiska-Binstorfer E, Huber J. Infertility caused by PCOS – health-related quality of life among Austrian and Moslem immigrant women in Austria. Hum Reprod. 2004;19:2251–7.
22. Trent ME, Rich M, Austin SB, Gordon CM. Fertility concerns and sexual behavior in adolescent girls with polycystic ovary syndrome: implications for quality of life. J Pediatr Adolesc Gynecol. 2003;16:33–7.
23. Elsenbruch S, Hahn S, Kowalsky D, Offner AH, Schedlowski M, Mann K, Janssen OE. Quality of life, psychosocial Well-being, and sexual satisfaction in women with polycystic ovary syndrome. J Clin Endocrinol Metab. 2003;88:5801–7.
24. Cooney LG, Lee I, Sammel MD, Dokras A. High prevalence of moderate and severe depressive and anxiety symptoms in polycystic ovary syndrome: a systematic review and meta-analysis. Hum Reprod. 2017;32:1091–2017.
25. Cesta CE, Mansson M, Palm C, Lichtenstein P, Thadou AN, Landen M. Polycystic ovary syndrome and psychiatric disorders: comorbidity and heritability in a nationwide Swedish cohort. Psychoneuroendocrinology. 2016;73:196–203.
26. Luppino FS, de Wit LM, Bouvy PF, Stijnen T, Cuijpers P, Pennix BW, Zitman FG. Overweight, obesity, and depression: a systematic review and meta-analysis of longitudinal studies. Arch Gen Psychiatry. 2010;67:220–9.
27. Barry JA, Kuczmierczky AR, Hardiman PJ. Anxiety and depression in polycystic ovary syndrome: a systematic review and meta-analysis. Hum Reprod. 2011;26:2442–51.
28. Greenwood EA, Pasch LA, Shinkai K, Cedars MI, Huddleston HG. Putative role for insulin resistance in depression risk in polycystic ovary syndrome. Fertil Steril. 2015;104:707–14. e1
29. Weiner CL, Primeau M, Ehrmann DA. Androgens and mood dysfunction in women: comparison of women with polycystic ovarian syndrome to healthy controls. Psychosom Med. 2004;66:356–62.
30. Benson S, Hahn S, Tan S, Mann K, Janssen OE, Schedlowski M, Elsenbruch S. Prevalence and implications of anxiety in polycystic ovary syndrome: results of an internet-based survey in Germany. Hum Reprod. 2009;24:1446–51.
31. Alur-Gupta S, Chemerinski A, Liu C, Lipson J, Allison K, Sammel MD, Dokras A. Body image distress is increased in women with polycystic ovary syndrome and mediates depression and anxiety. Fertil Steril. 2019;112:930–8. e1
32. Esposito K, Ciotola M, Giugliano G, Bisogni C, Schisano B, Autorino R, Cobellis L, De Sio M, Colacurci N, Giugliano D. Association of body weight with sexual function in women. Int J Impot Res. 2007;19:353–7.
33. Eftekhar T, Sohrabvand F, Zabandan N, Shariat M, Haghollahi F, Ghahghaei-Nezamabadi A. Sexual dysfunction in patients with polycystic ovary syndrome and its affected domains. Iran J Reprod Med. 2014;8:539–46.
34. Mansson M, Norstrom K, Holte J, Landin-Wilhelmsen K, Dahlgren E, Landen M. Sexuality and psychological wellbeing in women with polycystic ovary syndrome compared with healthy controls. Eur J Obstet Gynecol Reprod Biol. 2011;2:161–5.
35. Ferraresi SR, Lara LA, Reis RM, Rosa ESA. Changes in sexual function among women with polycystic ovary syndrome. Eur J Endocrinol. 2005;6:853–60.
36. Stovall DW, Scriver JL, Clayton AH, Williams CD, Pastore LM. Sexual function in women with polycystic ovary syndrome. J Sex Med. 2012;1:224–30.
37. Hashemi S, Ramezani TF, Farahmand M, Bahri KM. Association of PCOS and its clinical signs with sexual function among Iranian women affected by PCOS. J Sex Med. 2014;10:2508–14.
38. Rellini AH, Stratton N, Tonani S, Santamaria V, Brambilla E, Nappi RE. Differences in sexual desire between women with clinical versus biochemical signs of hyperandrogenism in polycystic ovarian syndrome. Hormones Behavior. 2013;63:65–71.

39. Zhao S, Wang J, Xie Q, Luo L, Zhu Z, Liu Y, Zhao Z. Is polycystic ovary syndrome associated with risk of female sexual dysfunction? A systematic review and meta-analysis. Reprod Biomed Online. 2019;38:979–89.
40. Battaglia C, Nappi RE, Mancini F, Cianciosi A, Persico N, Busacchi P, Facchinetti F, Sisti G. PCOS, sexuality, and clitoral vascularisation: a pilot study. J Sex Med. 2008;12:2886–94.
41. Nappi RE. To be or not to be in sexual desire: the androgen dilemma. Climacteric. 2015 Oct;18:672–4.
42. Salonia A, Pontillo M, Nappi RE, Zanni G, Fabbri F, Scavini M, Daverio R, Gallina A, Rigatti P, Bosi E, Bonini PA, Montorsi F. Menstrual cycle-related changes in circulating androgens in healthy women with self-reported normal sexual function. J Sex Med. 2008;5:854–63.

Infertility Management in Lean Versus Obese PCOS

9

Duru Shah and Madhuri Patil

9.1 Introduction

Polycystic ovary syndrome (PCOS) is a common polygenic endocrinopathy in women of reproductive age. PCOS is associated with menstrual irregularities, hyperandrogenism, polycystic ovarian morphology and fertility issues. It is the cause of anovulatory infertility in almost 70% of women in the reproductive age group [1]. PCOS also has a high prevalence of metabolic disorders, obesity, increased anxiety and depression which can have a negative impact on women's health. Insulin resistance and hyperinsulinemia are common and are responsible for hormonal and metabolic dysfunction. The presentation can be heterogeneous as the diagnosis of PCOS is based on the Rotterdam criteria, which include two of the three findings – polycystic ovarian morphology (PCOM), chronic anovulation (CA) and hyperandrogenism (HA). Other features, which have been associated with PCOS, include insulin resistance (IR) and metabolic syndrome (MS). Different PCOS phenotypes differ significantly in their metabolic risk due to insulin resistance and dyslipidaemia which worsens with the severity of androgen excess. PCOS can significantly affect a woman's ability to conceive and her quality of life. There are two types of PCOS patients, one obese and other non-obese or lean. The two groups differ in their clinical, metabolic and hormonal parameters and also respond differently to treatment. Although a majority of cases with PCOS are obese/overweight, a small but significant proportion of patients present with normal or low body mass index (BMI; ≤ 25 kg/M^2).

D. Shah (✉)
Gynaecworld, The Center for Women's Health and Fertility, Mumbai, India

M. Patil
Patil's Fertility and Endoscopy Clinic, Bangalore, India

© International Society of Gynecological Endocrinology 2021
A. R. Genazzani et al. (eds.), *Impact of Polycystic Ovary, Metabolic Syndrome and Obesity on Women Health*, ISGE Series,
https://doi.org/10.1007/978-3-030-63650-0_9

9.2   Pathophysiology of PCOS

The pathophysiology is complex and is thought to be a result of interactions between genetics, epigenetics, ovarian dysfunction and endocrine, neuroendocrine and metabolic alterations. Due to the possibility of there being various combinations of polycystic ovarian morphology, anovulatory cycles and hyperandrogenism, PCOS women have been assigned various phenotypes such as Phenotype A, B, C and D as seen in Fig. 9.1.

9.2.1   Insulin Resistance and Hyperandrogenaemia

Insulin resistance (IR) is thought to be responsible for PCOS both in obese and lean women, the latter being a much less common presentation of the syndrome. It is still controversial whether hyperandrogenaemia (HA) or hyperinsulinemia is the primary defect. Hyperinsulinemia, the consequence of insulin resistance, stimulates androgen secretion both from ovarian (mainly) and adrenal gland. It also suppresses sex hormone-binding globulin (SHBG) synthesis from the liver, thereby resulting in a further increase in free, biologically active androgens. Thus, IR contributes to hyperandrogenism through insulin-induced increased ovarian androgen production, both directly and synergistically with luteinizing hormone [2], and by reduction of hepatic sex hormone-binding globulin production [3] thus contributing to both reproductive and metabolic disturbances. Figure 9.1 A depicts why insulin resistance could be the primary defect. Foetal and/or prepubertal androgen excess

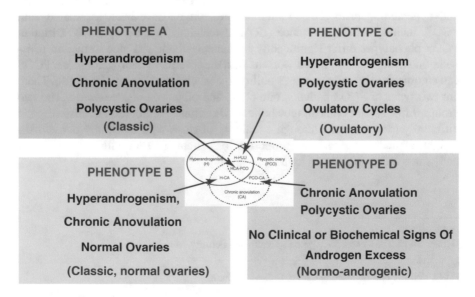

Fig. 9.1 Phenotypes of PCOS based on Rotterdam criteria

'programmes' the hypothalamic–pituitary control of LH and enhances visceral fat distribution and predisposes to insulin resistance (IR) and anovulation. Genetic and environmental factors like diet may interact with this underlying linear process and modify the final phenotype to produce the heterogeneous nature of the syndrome. Figure 9.1 B depicts how hyperandrogenaemia could be the primary defect (Fig. 9.2).

In PCOS, extra and intra-ovarian factors may have an impact on granulosa cell (GC) oocyte interaction, oocyte maturation and embryonic developmental competence. The extra-ovarian factors identified include gonadotrophins, hyperandrogenaemia and hyperinsulinemia, whilst the intra-ovarian factors include members of the epidermal, fibroblast, insulin-like and neurotrophin families of growth factors, as well as cytokines [4]. These abnormalities are possibly linked to abnormal endocrine/paracrine factors, metabolic dysfunction and alterations in the intrafollicular microenvironment during folliculogenesis and follicle maturation [4]. The paracrine/endocrine factors include several diverse proteins of the TGFβ

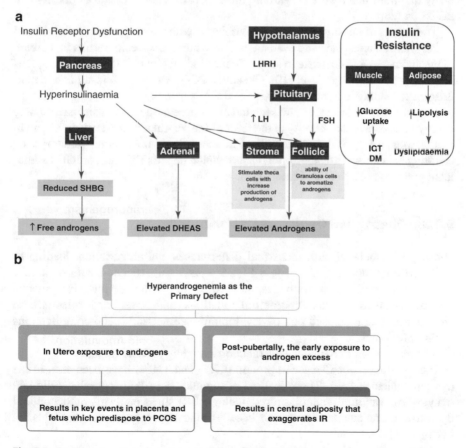

Fig. 9.2 (**a**) Hyperinsulinemia as primary defect. (**b**) Hyperandrogenaemia as primary defect

superfamily – TGFβ, anti-Mullerian hormone (AMH), inhibin, activins, bone mor-
phogenetic protein 15 (BMP15) and growth differentiation factor 9 (GDF9) [5].
Deficiency of FSH, hypersecretion of LH, hyperandrogenaemia, hyperinsulinemia,
and altered growth factors and cytokines can influence follicular growth and oocyte
meiotic maturation processes [6].

9.2.2   Obesity and Fertility

Obesity in PCOS women is one of the most important factors influencing various
phenotypes. Hence the problems of obesity add on to the prominent pathologies
noted in every phenotype of PCOS. Both lean and obese PCOS can affect the infertility treatment outcome, poorer outcomes being higher in obese women [7]. Obesity
influences outcomes of fertility treatment by affecting oocyte quality [8] and endometrial receptivity [9]. There exists a controversy on the various ways obesity exerts
its effect on oocytes, both fresh and vitrified, and the endometrium. There remain
many questions unanswered regarding the effects of a combination of obesity and
PCOS on fertility.

The impact of obesity on PCOS is significant, with a high prevalence of visceral
obesity, insulin resistance and even metabolic syndrome. Obesity results in increase
in the androgens and decrease in sex hormone binding globulin (SHBG) levels, thus
increasing free androgen level [10]. Obesity in PCOS women can result in hyperandrogenism leading to hyperinsulinemia and vice versa.

Leptin, which is produced and secreted by adipose tissue, has a role in regulating
energy homeostasis and obesity at the level of the central nervous system. Leptin in
PCOS women is raised and centrally stimulates the hypothalamic–pituitary axis
resulting in increased gonadotropin release, which impairs FSH and/or IGF-I stimulated granulosa cell steroidogenesis [11].

9.2.3   Obesity and Ovulatory Dysfunction

Obesity is associated with menstrual disturbances and anovulation, leading to
poor fertility outcomes. Obesity in PCOS women is associated with ovulatory
dysfunction, reduced ovarian responsiveness to ovulation inducing agents,
altered oocyte as well as endometrial functions, and lower birth rates. Obese
women are at an increased risk of developing maternal and foetal complications
during pregnancy.

The mechanism of ovulatory dysfunction is highlighted in Fig. 9.3.

Increased levels of C-reactive protein (CRP) and TNF-a have been seen in the
ovarian follicular fluid. There is lipid accumulation in both cumulus cells and
oocytes. Activation of endoplasmic reticulum (ER) stress pathway, mitochondrial
dysfunction, and increased apoptosis in cells of the developing ovarian follicles has
been noted [12].

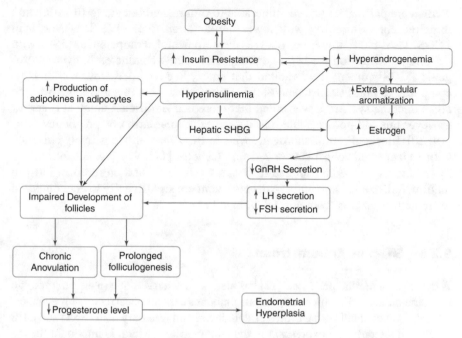

Fig. 9.3 Mechanism of ovulatory dysfunction in obese PCOS

9.2.4 Lean Phenotype and Fertility

A small but significant proportion (20–30%) of women with PCOS have a normal or low BMI and may or may not have symptoms such as irregular menstrual cycles, hirsutism and acne [13]. The clinical manifestations in lean and overweight women with PCOS are comparable [14] with similar prevalence of IR, menstrual dysfunction, PCOM at ultrasound, hirsutism, acanthosis nigricans and endometrial hyperplasia. Hormonal profiles are similar in both obese and lean PCOS, though the severity is much more in the obese PCOS [14]. Lean PCOS have higher LH to FSH ratio and DHEAS levels than classical PCOS [14]. Lean PCOS has higher ovulatory cycles and pregnancy rates with lower requirement of gonadotropin dose and also a lower miscarriage rate.

9.2.5 Effect on Oocytes and Embryos

The hyperandrogenaemia and IR in PCOS patients results in abnormal oocyte developmental competence [15], which in turn result in decreased fertilization rates and impaired embryogenesis [16]. Preovulatory follicles in PCOS are hyperandrogenic in women undergoing COS and contain metaphase II oocytes with distinctly abnormal gene expression profiles [4]. Overweight PCOS women are particularly more vulnerable to diminished oocyte fertilization and impaired embryo quality with lower implantation rates [17]. However, lean PCOS also have impaired oocyte developmental competence [58], with impaired fertilization [6, 18]. In a prospective study conducted in hyperandrogenic PCOS women, it was found that embryos developed slower after ICSI compared to non-PCOS women [19]. Delay in early embryo kinetics in time lapse imaging system, it was noted that there is a significant delay at t_2 and t_3; however this did not translate into decreased implantation or pregnancy rates [19, 20]. Elevated serum androgen levels in PCOS patients positively correlate with an increased cohort size of 2–5 mm follicles [14]. When small follicles in PCOS are aspirated and immature oocytes recovered and cultured in vitro to mature, fertilization and embryo development are significantly lower compared to immature oocytes from normal women [21].

9.2.6   Effect on Endometrium

A decrease in uterine perfusion [22] has also been observed due to an embryotoxic cytokine milieu [23], which may impair implantation and occurrence of pregnancy. Obesity is associated with elevated circulating serum free fatty acid (FFA) and CRP levels and altered gene expression in the endometrium, which is important for the activation of the immune system and inflammation. The above factors result in compromised decidualization and excessive inflammation, which may impair implantation and predispose to endometrial cancer [24].

9.3   Management of Infertility

In obese PCOS, targeting obesity improves fertility outcome in PCOS women [25, 26]. (Table 9.1).

Table 9.1 Effect of weight loss on fertility

Effect of weight loss
• reduction in insulin and LH concentration
• increased insulin sensitivity
• increased concentration of SHBG resulting in reciprocal decrease in free testosterone
• reduced hirsutism and acne
• improvement in reproductive function – Restores menstrual function and ovulation resulting in spontaneous conceptions
• increase in the number of embryos available for transfer with higher clinical pregnancy rate (CPR) and livebirth rate (LBR)
• reduction in miscarriage rates
• reduces the risk of IGT, type 2 diabetes mellitus and GDM

9.3.1 Lifestyle Modification in Obese PCOS

Weight loss can be achieved through diet, exercise and behavioural modification, which improve both metabolic and reproductive abnormalities. However, the optimal diet composition and type of exercise remains unknown. Health benefits of postponing pregnancy to achieve weight loss must be balanced against the risk of declining fertility with advancing age [27]. Therefore, in obese PCOS women who have poor ovarian reserve or are of advanced reproductive age (ARA), it is not advisable to wait for weight loss prior to IVF as it may compromise the IVF outcome [25, 26].

Lifestyle management for weight loss, for fertility enhancement and also for general health benefits should be recommended in PCOS (Level B evidence) and should include both dietary and exercise interventions as first-line therapy (Level C evidence) [14]. Healthy food choices, irrespective of diet composition, should be used for weight loss or maintenance in conjunction with behavioural change techniques (Level C/D evidence) [14]. Exercise participation of ≥150 min/week (≥90 min mod-high intensity aerobic activity 60–90% maximum heart rate) should be recommended to all women (especially overweight) with PCOS (Level D evidence) [14].

There is emerging evidence from RCTs that apart from diet, physical activity (PA) may improve pregnancy rates in women with reproductive health problems [26]. Whilst the type, intensity, frequency and duration of optimal PA intervention and the role of PA independent of weight loss remain unclear [26], these preliminary findings suggest that PA may be an affordable and feasible alternative or complementary therapy to fertility treatments [26].

9.3.2 Lifestyle Modification in Lean PCOS

Lean PCOS women should aim to maintain their weight. Lifestyle modifications by dietary interventions and regular physical activity, especially resistance exercises to build muscles, have demonstrated improved insulin resistance and ameliorated hyperandrogenism [28]. Lean PCOS must be encouraged to consume vegetables, fruits and proteins and restrict carbohydrates and fats. It is also very important to curb stress with mindfulness, sleep, yoga and meditation [29].

9.3.3 Bariatric Surgery

Bariatric surgery should be considered if BMI is ≥35 kg/m2 and lifestyle modification therapy has failed to achieve sufficient weight loss. Obese patients undergoing bariatric surgery have been able to conceive spontaneously [25]. According to the 2018 international guidelines on PCOS, bariatric surgery should be considered an experimental therapy in women with PCOS, for the purpose of having a healthy baby. Currently, risk to benefit ratio is too uncertain to advocate this as fertility therapy [14].

If bariatric surgery is to be prescribed, the following needs to be considered [14]:
- Comparative cost.
- The need for a structured weight management program involving diet, physical activity and interventions to improve psychological, musculoskeletal and cardiovascular health to continue post-operatively.
- Perinatal risks such as small for gestational age, premature delivery and possibly increased infant mortality.

9.3.4 Anti-Obesity Drugs

In a recent review, anti-obesity drugs were evaluated [30]. It was found that Orlistat played a role in reducing IR and androgen levels. It also helped in reducing blood pressure and correcting the lipid profile. It appears to be equally effective when used with metformin in reducing weight, IR and testosterone levels [30]. Anti-obesity drugs are not recommended, when attempting pregnancy and during pregnancy. More studies are needed to evaluate the effect of other agents like liraglutide and naltrexone/bupropion.

9.4 Oral Contraceptive Pills (OCP) [31]

OCPs supress FSH, LH and oestrogen levels and therefore could be used in those patients who have high day 2 LH and in those patients who have asynchronous development of follicles in an GnRH antagonist cycle. Outcome of ART after OCP pre-treatment depends on pill-free interval prior to a treatment cycle and duration of pill administration. A 5-day washout period after OCP discontinuation is optimal before the initiation of COS. Duration of pill administration may also have an impact on the reproductive hormones and endometrium. More than 16 days of pill administration results in a greater suppression of pituitary–ovarian axis, which is then associated with a longer duration and higher consumption of gonadotropins.

Higher serum leptin levels in PCOS patients may be reduced with short-term OC treatment. Suppression of ovarian function and reduction of luteinizing hormone (LH) and/or insulin level may be the likely mechanisms in decreasing leptin concentration. Hence OC pills may be used to abolish the untoward effect of leptin on granulosa cells [27].

9.5 Ovulation Induction

Abnormalities in circulating hormones due to elevated testosterone and LH levels can result in failure to ovulate and compromised maturation of oocyte or endometrium or both.

9.5.1 Oral Ovulation Inducing Agents

Letrozole should be considered as the first-line pharmacological treatment for ovulation induction in women with PCOS and anovulatory infertility, to improve ovulation, pregnancy and live birth rates. Aromatase inhibitors inhibit oestrogen synthesis, resulting in enhanced GnRH pulses with consequent FSH and inhibin secretion. It also stimulates ovarian follicular development by augmenting follicular FSH receptor expression in the ovary, the result of increased local androgen concentration. It also results in induction of high intrafollicular IGF-I concentrations, which synergize with FSH action and increase follicular growth.

Advantages of letrozole over clomiphene citrate are as follows:
- No adverse antioestrogenic effect on the endometrium or cervical mucus.

- Absence of oestrogen receptor depletion.
- Associated with significantly lower serum and intrafollicular concentration of E2 at midcycle per mature follicle.
- Rapid elimination from the body (half-life of 45 hours).
- Better uterine blood flow.
- Limited number of mature follicles.
- Associated with decreased incidence of OHSS and multiple pregnancy.

Letrozole is used in the dose of 2.5 to 5 mg per day from day 3 to 7 of the menstrual cycle. Where letrozole is not available or its use is not permitted in certain countries, or the cost is prohibitive, then health professionals can use other ovulation induction agents like Clomiphene Citrate (CC) and Tamoxifen.

Clomiphene citrate (CC) could be used alone or in combination with metformin in women with PCOS with anovulatory infertility. Combined therapy of CC with metformin is beneficial in PCOS women who are CC-resistant. Improvement is noted both in the ovulation and pregnancy rates. CC resulted in improvement in CPR and ovulation as compared to Metformin alone in obese women with PCOS. CC should be discontinued if 6 ovulatory cycles fail to yield a pregnancy or when there is no ovulation with 150 mg of CC per day or the endometrial growth is less than 7 mm at ovulation.

Reasons for CC failure are as follows:

(a) Failure to ovulate due to raised BMI, free androgen index, LH and insulin.
(b) Ovulation, but no conception.
- Antioestrogenic effects on cervical mucus and endometrium.
- High LH.
(c) Antioestrogenic effect on endometrium resulting in endometrial thinning due to:
- Oestrogen receptor downregulation and depletion.
- Suppression of pinopode formation.

The risk of multiple pregnancy is increased with CC use and therefore monitoring needs to be considered. Letrozole as compared to CC appears to improve ovulation rate, CPR and LBR, with a shorter time-to-pregnancy in sub-fertile women with anovulatory PCOS. The quality of this evidence is low [32]. No difference was noted in effectiveness between letrozole and laparoscopic ovarian drilling, and occurrence of OHSS was very rare [32].

Tamoxifen in a dose of 20–40 mg from day 2 to 6 is a promising alternative to CC for ovarian stimulation in the subgroup of patients who fail to develop an adequate endometrial thickness in a previous OI cycle.

Infertile women who fail to conceive following CC or aromatase inhibitors (AIs) require an alternative, second-line approach which includes gonadotropins (GT) and/or laparoscopic ovarian drilling. It is also an indication to expand diagnostic evaluation to exclude other infertility factors if not done earlier.

9.5.2 Gonadotropins

Gonadotropins could be used alone or in combination with CC/Letrozole/Tamoxifen.

CC/Letrozole/Tamoxifen stimulate recruitment of a number of small follicles, and gonadotropins sustain the growth of recruited follicles (Fig. 9.4).

Homburg et al. examined the feasibility of low-dose FSH as first-line treatment. Pregnancies and live births were achieved faster with low-dose FSH than with CC. As gonadotropins are expensive and injectable drugs, their use should be balanced by convenience and cost in favour of CC. FSH may be an appropriate first-line treatment for some women with PCOS and anovulatory infertility [33].

Increased BMI and IR render the management of the PCOS patient difficult. Increased BMI increases GT requirements; the dose and response is unpredictable and can result in explosive ovarian response. Therefore, choosing the right gonadotropin and dose is important, and it is safer to use low-dose step-up protocol or chronic low-dose protocol (Fig. 9.5).

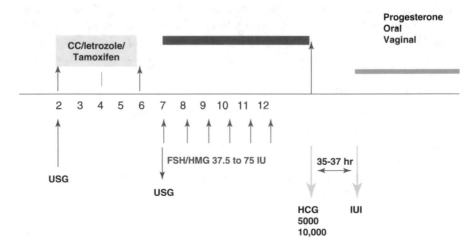

Fig. 9.4 Combined oral ovulogen and gonadotropin protocol

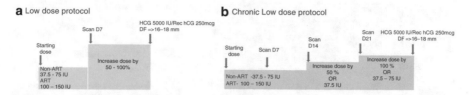

Fig. 9.5   (**a**) Low-dose and (**b**) chronic low-dose protocol

When the ovarian response has been documented in a previous cycle, the threshold dose can be initiated from the start in the next cycle. There is no difference in the CPR and LBR whether Rec follicle stimulating hormone (FSH)/urinary FSH/human menopausal gonadotropin (hMG) or HP-hMG has been used [34]. Thus, urinary or recombinant FSH can be used in women with PCOS undergoing COS for IVF ± ICSI, with insufficient evidence to recommend any specific FSH preparation [14].

When using gonadotropins for ovulation induction in PCOS, it is important to:

1. Increase safety and effectiveness.
2. Optimize response and outcome to increase the LBR with decreased birth defects, imprinting and epigenetic disorders.
3. Minimize the risks of Ovarian Hyperstimulation Syndrome (OHSS) and multiple pregnancies.

This can be achieved by adopting different strategies for an optimal outcome and maximizing success rates by individualized stimulation. Most individualized controlled ovarian stimulation (iCOS) protocols are based on age, AMH and AFC and are amended further for BMI of women. In PCOS, due to the large number of follicles, there are higher chances of complications. Hence we need to individualize COS and substitute the earlier outcome parameters like follicle number, oocyte number, embryo number, implantation rate and pregnancy rate per cycle with healthy LBR, decreased patient discomfort, cost, risks and complications (Fig. 9.6).

The selection of a dominant follicle occurs in the early follicular phase, and therefore ovulation induction drugs should be initiated within 3 days of the start of menstrual cycle, when the follicular size is less than 10 mm, there is absence of ovarian cysts and endometrial thickness is less than 6 mm. In an ART cycle the oestradiol should be less than 50 pg/ml and progesterone less than 1.0 ng/ml to initiate GT therapy. GT dose can then be adjusted depending on the follicular growth and oestradiol levels.

9.5.3   GnRH Analogues

A gonadotrophin releasing hormone (GnRH) antagonist protocol is preferred in women with PCOS undergoing an IVF ± ICSI cycle, over a GnRH agonist long protocol. This is to reduce the duration of stimulation, total gonadotrophin dose administered and incidence of OHSS [14]. The GnRH agonist protocols increase the

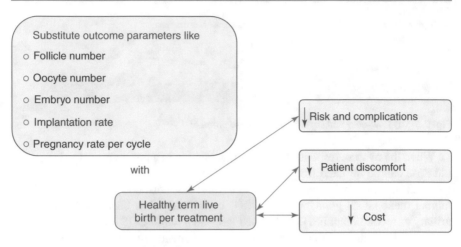

Fig. 9.6 Principles of individualized COS

number of retrieved oocytes, pregnancy rate and decrease the number of cycle cancelations, but increase the risk of OHSS [35]. Hence use on GnRH antagonist protocol is recommended in PCOS women, mainly due to a reduction of complications.

9.6   Laparoscopic Ovarian Drilling (LOD)

Laparoscopic ovarian surgery could be the second-line therapy for women with PCOS, women who are CC resistant, have anovulatory infertility and no other infertility factor. Laparoscopic ovarian surgery could potentially be offered as first-line treatment if laparoscopy is indicated for another reason in women with PCOS. When laparoscopic ovarian surgery is recommended, it is important to consider comparative cost, expertise required and intra-operative and post-operative risks, which are higher in women who are overweight and obese [36]. There is no evidence of a significant difference in rates of clinical pregnancy, live birth or miscarriage in women with clomiphene-resistant PCOS undergoing LOD compared to other medical treatments [36], except that it is a one-time event with its effect lasting for at least a year. On the contrary there is an increased risk of associated lower ovarian reserve, probable loss of ovarian function and peri-adnexal adhesion formation due to the surgery. This information needs to be shared with all women with PCOS considering laparoscopic ovarian surgery.

9.7   Assisted Reproductive Technologies (ART)

ART is not the first line of treatment in PCOS associated infertility. It is generally the last option unless there is another reason to use ART to treat infertility in PCOS women. In the absence of an absolute indication for IVF ± ICSI, women with PCOS and anovulatory infertility could be offered IVF as third-line therapy where first- or second-line ovulation induction therapies have failed.

Ovulatory dysfunction can be overcome by ovulation induction and ART. The outcome following these treatment modalities may still not be optimum due to the impact of obesity on oocytes, embryos and endometrium. BMI appears to have a marked effect on in vitro fertilization (IVF) outcomes. Oocyte maturation, quality and fertilization are reduced in obese PCOS patients with a better fertilization rate in lean PCOS as compared with overweight counterparts (BMI ≥25 kg/M²) [37].

Implantation, clinical pregnancy, miscarriage and live birth rates progressively worsen with increasing BMI [27]. The deleterious effect of obesity on assisted reproduction outcome reduces the probability of achieving and maintaining pregnancy (Table 9.2) [38]. Weight loss in these patients has been found to improve the outcome of ART in obese women [27].

In women with anovulatory PCOS, the use of IVF is effective, and multiple pregnancies can be minimized when elective single embryo transfer is used. Women with PCOS undergoing IVF ± ICSI therapy therefore need to be counselled prior to starting treatment, on cost, convenience, increased risk of ovarian hyperstimulation syndrome (OHSS) and about options to reduce the risk of OHSS. PCOS women tend to be more hypersensitive to gonadotropins and therefore have a higher risk of OHSS and multiple pregnancies. Ovarian stimulation should be initiated with low doses of gonadotropins (100 to 150 IU), and use of GnRH antagonist protocol is recommended with regard to improved safety and efficacy. In the lean PCOS pregnancy rates are higher with ovarian stimulation using mid-luteal long GnRH agonist suppressive regimens. This may be because lean PCOS women are associated with high LH levels that are reduced with the mid-luteal long GnRH agonist protocol, improving the implantation potential [39]. Both recombinant hCG and urinary hCG can be used for triggering final oocyte maturation. A reduced dose of urinary hCG (5000 IU instead of 10,000 IU) is recommended in a GnRH agonist protocol to improve safety [14]. A GnRH agonist trigger is recommended for final oocyte maturation in women at risk of OHSS, when GnRH antagonist is used for downregulation [14]. We also need to avoid elevation of progesterone in the late follicular phase, by preventing early rise in LH levels. Progesterone elevation (PE) suggests a high ovarian response and usually occurs with an administration of a greater dose of FSH [40]. To avoid progesterone rise, it is helpful to use the modified natural cycle, mild stimulation protocols or individualized COS protocol with low dose of FSH and use of hMG for COS as LH activity offsets the rise of P4 induced by FSH [40]. It can also be achieved by early initiation of GnRH antagonist which will prevent early rise in LH levels. In cycles where elevated pre-ovulatory progesterone does occur, the probabilities of implantation rate, CPR and LBR can be increased if all embryos are cryopreserved and subsequently thawed and transferred in a natural or HRT cycle [40]. Luteal phase support is best given by using progesterone and avoiding hCG. The clinical pregnancy and implantation rates in PCOS women are 30–35% and 10–15%, respectively [41]. Despite a higher oocyte yield in all age groups, women with PCOS over 40 years of age have similar CPR and LBR when compared to women with tubal factor infertility at the same age. The reproductive window thus may not be extended

Table 9.2 Effect of obesity on ART outcome

Deleterious effects of obesity on ovarian stimulation and IVF laboratory parameters	Obesity and pregnancy outcome following ART
• higher gonadotrophin requirement	• altered endometrial receptivity due to elevated circulating serum FFA and CRP levels, altered gene expression in endometrium
• longer period of ovarian stimulation	• lower implantation rates
• higher cancellation rates	• lower pregnancy rates
• higher incidence of follicular asynchrony	• higher preclinical miscarriage rates (biochemical pregnancies)
• decreased periovulatory intrafollicular hCG concentrations	• higher clinical miscarriage rates
• lower peak of serum oestradiol	• increased risk of foetal defects
• premature granulosa cell (GC) luteinizsation	• increased complications in second and third trimesters of pregnancy (for mother and foetus)
• defective oocyte meiotic resumption	• lower live birth rates
• reduced oocyte retrieval	• morbid obesity is strongly associated with GDM, hypertension, preeclampsia, preterm delivery, stillbirth, increased caesarean or instrumental delivery, shoulder dystocia, foetal distress, early neonatal death; and small- as well as large-for-gestational age infants
• less mature follicles	
• altered cumulus/corona mass–oocyte interaction	
• poorer oocyte quality	
• mitochondrial abnormalities	
• dysregulated meiotic/mitotic spindle dynamics	
• lower fertilization rates	
• poorer embryo quality	
• smaller size of blastocyst due to increased triglycerides and decreased glucose consumption with altered amino acid metabolism	
• lower incidence of embryo transfer	
• lower mean number of transferred embryos	

in PCOS, and hence PCOS patients with infertility should be treated in a timely manner despite indicators of high ovarian reserve [41].

Adjuvant Therapy The aim of treatment in PCOS is to achieve optimal outcome for which certain adjuvants may be used.

9.8   Insulin Sensitizers

9.8.1   Metformin

90% of obese women with PCOS have IR, which exacerbates ovulatory dysfunction [42, 43]. Mechanism of action and side effects of metformin in PCOS are highlighted in Table 9.3.

Metformin can be used in a dose of 1000 mg to 2550 mg daily and stopped when the pregnancy test is positive or menstruation occurs, unless the metformin therapy is otherwise indicated. Combined therapy of metformin and CC versus CC alone results in improved ovulation rate and CPR [44]. Recent updated Cochrane review suggests that metformin may be beneficial over placebo for live birth, but women do experience gastrointestinal side effects. This beneficial effect was uncertain when used alone or in combination with CC as compared to CC alone [45].

A Cochrane review in 2017 concluded that metformin may increase the LBR among women undergoing ovulation induction with gonadotropins in a timed intercourse and intrauterine insemination (IUI) cycle [44].

As per the latest international guidelines on PCOS, adjunct metformin therapy could be used before and/or during ovulation induction with gonadotropins in women undergoing IVF /ICSI therapy with a GnRH agonist protocol, to improve the clinical pregnancy rate and reduce the risk of OHSS [14]. Several lean PCOS

Table 9.3 Mechanism of action and side effects of metformin

Action	Side effects
• ↑ glucose tolerance	• gastrointestinal disturbance in 1/3 of patients
• ↑ insulin sensitivity and insulin related signalling mechanisms	• generalized feeling of unwellness
• ↓ blood lipid levels	• decreased absorption of vitamin B-12
• ↑ weight loss or stabilization	• lactic acid buildup
• improved fat distribution	
• ↓ blood pressure	
• ↓ androgen levels	
• improves ovarian environment with restoration of regular menses due to its effect on ovarian steroidogenesis and intraovarian IR	
Postponement of diabetes	

women are able to achieve regular menstrual cycles and ovulation with metformin therapy [46]. Significant reductions in fasting glucose, testosterone and insulin resistance were seen with the use of metformin in lean PCOS [47].

9.8.2   Inositols

Inositol, a member of the B-complex family of vitamins, is found to be deficient in women with PCOS. Myo-inositol is an insulin sensitizer which has beneficial effects on ovarian function and response to ART in women with PCOS. Though it induces nuclear and cytoplasmic oocyte maturation and promotes embryo development, till date there is no data on its effects on pregnancy and live birth rate. Further research on larger patient populations is needed to determine whether inositol supplementation, possibly in combination with other drugs, could improve CPR and LBRs in PCOS women undergoing ART [48]. Due to small sample size, use of D-chiro-inositol (2 studies), rosiglitazone (1 study) or pioglitazone has limited evidence [14].

The international guidelines on PCOS also recommend that Inositol (in any form) should currently be considered as an experimental therapy in PCOS, with emerging evidence on efficacy highlighting the need for further research [14]. Myo-inositol in the dose of 3 grams per day has shown to have a positive effect even on lean PCOS women. It has shown to reduce luteinizing hormone (LH), androgen levels and 'high-sensitivity C-reactive protein' with improved insulin resistance [49]. Agarwal A et al. evaluated the benefit of combined use of Metformin plus Myo-inositol versus Metformin alone in infertile PCOS women undergoing ovulation induction [50]. This study concluded that there were significantly higher live birth rates in women receiving the combination therapy as compared to metformin alone [50].

There is still not much evidence for use of newer insulin-sensitizing agents like glucagon-like peptide 1 (GLP-1) analogues (exenatide and liraglutide) in women attempting pregnancy [14].

9.8.3   Other Adjuvants

Table 9.4 gives the list of other adjuvants that are used.

Most of these adjuvants used are off-label prescriptions for the treatment of infertility associated with PCOS. Therefore, one needs to balance the benefits with the evidence, when using adjuvants in PCOS.

9.9   Psychological Intervention

Behavioural problems, damaged self-confidence, increased levels of anxiety and depression benefit with psychological counselling, both individually and as group therapy to improve infertility treatment outcome.

Table 9.4 Adjuvant therapy in PCOS

Androgen Excess	Others - May improve ovulation	Reduce risk of OHSS
Prednisone	N acetyl cysteine	Cabergoline
Methyl prednisolone	Melatonin	Calcium
Dexamethasone	Vitamin D	Prophylactic albumin
Hyper Insulinemia/ Insulin Resistance	Chromium polynicotinate	Hydroxyl starch
Metformin	L Methyl folate	Immunoglobulin
Inositol	Phytoestrogens	Metformin
		Aspirin
		GnR Hantagonist

9.9.1 Difference in Results between Obese and Lean PCOS

Most studies which evaluated the association between BMI and outcome of ART are small and retrospective. Lean patients have less retrieved oocytes than obese. Though the dose of gonadotropins required is less, the implantation, CPR and LBR does not differ among both groups [51]. Patients with PCOS with higher BMI require higher doses of gonadotropin and have fewer oocytes retrieved with significantly lower CPR and LBR compared with those with lower BMI [52]. The incidence of ovarian hyperstimulation syndrome (OHSS) was higher in lean PCOS as compared to obese PCOS [39]. There was one study which reported lower fertilization rates in obese PCOS with BMI > 25 kg/m^2 than those with a BMI of $\leq$25 kg/m^2 [51]. In the experience of the author (unpublished data), number of retrieved and mature oocytes and fertilization and cleavage rates were significantly lower in the obese group (p value <0.05). The pregnancy rate (p value = 0.0005) and LBR (p value = 0.002) was statistically lower in the obese patients. There was no difference in the incidence of OHSS and missed abortion.

9.10 Preventing Complications

OHSS is a serious, detrimental and unintended consequence of COS due to excessive ovarian stimulation and excessive ovarian response to COS when HCG is used for triggering ovulation. We need to increase the safety of infertility treatment in PCOS by minimizing the risk of OHSS, and therefore prevention is of utmost importance.

(a) Prevention of OHSS – the strategies to prevent OHSS have been enumerated in Table 9.5.

In the past apart from cancellation, none of the approaches were totally efficient, although they decreased the incidence of OHSS in patients at high risk. But today with the option of GnRH agonist trigger in a GnRH antagonist cycle along with an elective decision to freeze-all the embryos with transfer in a subsequent cycle, it can minimize the occurrence of OHSS.

Table 9.5 Strategies to minimize risk of OHSS

Before initiation of treatment	• Identification of risk factors to individualize COS.
	• Correct adoption of stimulation protocols.
	• Monitoring COS using USG and E2 assays constitutes the 'gold standard'.
	• Use of GnRh antagonist protocol.
During treatment	• Limit the dose or concentration of hCG.
	• Use rec LH/GnRH agonist to trigger ovulation.
	• IVM.
	• Prophylactic albumin at oocyte retrieval in high-risk patients.
	• Transfer of single embryo to prevent multiple pregnancy.
After oocyte retrieval	• Using only progesterone for luteal phase support.
	• Dopamine agonist – Cabergoline 0.5 mg daily for 7–10 days.
	• Cryopreservation of all embryos for transfer in subsequent cycle.
	• Use of antagonist after cryofreezing all embryos.

Freeze-all Strategy: Elective frozen embryo transfer (eFET) is preferred in PCOS women who are at an increased risk of OHSS and develop progesterone elevation more than 1.5 ng/ml on the day of trigger. Personalized ET based on receptivity profile (ERA) in women with recurrent implantation failure is recommended. Elective frozen embryo transfer is also recommended, when pre-implantation genetic testing for aneuploidy is used as an embryo selection technique. Improved pregnancy rates have been reported after eFET by employing strategies to improve embryo implantation such as increasing the endometrial receptivity (ER) [53]. Decreased ER in PCOS women is related to endometrial advancement as a result of COS [54], and altered genes that are crucial for the endometrium-embryo interaction [55]. Elective FET is associated with a decreased incidence of ectopic pregnancy, as it does not involve COS, which is associated with an increase in uterine contractility and embryo-endometrium asynchrony [56]. Altered trophoblast expansion and invasion due to COS is also responsible to some extent for obstetric and perinatal complications [57], such as pre-term birth [58], and small for gestational age babies [59]. Few studies have even reported a lower risk of low birth weight [58]. Elective FET cycles are associated with increased time to pregnancy, higher incidence of large for gestational age and higher risk of placenta accreta [58].

A study looked at the effect of BMI on pregnancy outcomes with the freeze-all strategy [59]. In this study 3079 women with PCOS underwent 1168 elective frozen embryo transfer cycles and were categorized into three groups based on their BMI [59]. Implantation rate, clinical pregnancy rate, early miscarriage and live birth rate (LBR) were evaluated in all three groups. Obesity remained a risk factor for reduced rates of implantation and LBR, with an increased risk of early abortion with the freeze-all strategy [59]. Hence advising weight loss even prior to a freeze-all cycle should be considered.

(b) Prevention of multiple pregnancies.

Preventing multiple pregnancies is of utmost importance. Multiple pregnancies are associated with higher maternal and neonatal morbidity and mortality and shift

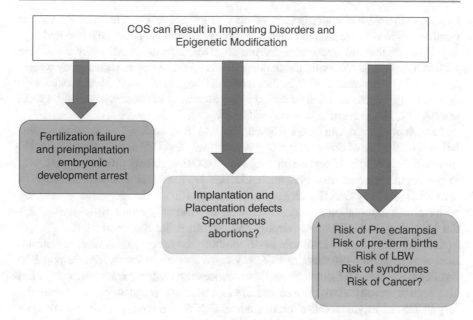

Fig. 9.7 Effects of imprinting disorders and epigenetic modification

results of infertility treatment from success to complications. In an ovulation induction cycle, either with timed intercourse or intrauterine insemination, multiple pregnancy can be prevented by using oral ovulogens and low-dose gonadotropin protocols. In case three or more dominant follicles develop, the cycle should be cancelled or converted into an ART cycle. In an ART cycle, multiple pregnancies can be prevented by limiting the number of embryos transferred to one embryo in women less than 36 years and two embryos in women 37 years or more and in those women who have had at least two previous failed IVF cycles.

(c) Prevention of imprinting disorders and epigenetic modification.

Imprinting disorders and epigenetic modification may contribute to aneuploidy and recurrent implantation failure of euploid embryos [60]. Fig. 9.7 highlights the other effects of imprinting disorders and epigenetic modification.

This can be prevented by adopting mild stimulation protocols, improving in vitro culture systems, lifestyle changes and with supplementation of adequate folate.

9.11 Conclusion

Metabolic, hormonal and clinical derangements exist in both lean and obese PCOS. Insulin resistance and hyperinsulinemia are inherent in PCOS women regardless of BMI and should be managed accordingly. This makes it mandatory to extend early screening and intervention to women with both lean and obese phenotype. Determinants of success of infertility treatment are obesity, degree of hyperinsulinemia and concentration of circulatory LH levels. The primary goal of treatment is to manage insulin resistance and hyperandrogenaemia, the two underlying disorders that are responsible for the negative sequelae in infertility associated with PCOS. Key to successful treatment depends on the ability to reduce body weight by lifestyle modifications such as diet modification, exercise and psychosocial support. Dietary intervention and increased physical activity in obese women with PCOS improve IR, HA, menstrual function and fertility.

In both obese and lean PCOS women, lifestyle modifications, restoration of ovulation with the use of oral ovulogens/gonadotropins and IVF in refractory cases will increase the chances of successful pregnancy. COH regimens offer an opportunity to correct in vivo abnormal systemic endocrine environment with normalization of serum LH levels by GnRH analogues during late follicular development. Modifying conventional stimulation protocols according to patients' characteristics and on initial screening makes it patient-friendly and optimizes the chance of LBR.

Obesity plays a significant role in determining the severity of clinical manifestations and metabolic disorders of PCOS. Weight loss improves ovarian response to fertility drugs and ART outcome and also reduces the obstetric complications. It has also been observed that weight loss increases spontaneous pregnancy rates in anovulatory PCOS. Lifestyle modification in the lean PCOS also results in a better outcome after treatment. OI protocols should be safe and efficacious which result in a pregnancy with low risk of OHSS and multiple pregnancies, with better neonatal outcomes.

Individualizing OI protocols based on patient characteristics such as BMI, LH and AMH levels, AFC, gonadotropin type and dose, in association with GnRH analogue, increases the likelihood of pregnancy.

Women with PCOS have more favourable ART outcome if they have a lower BMI though the CPR and LBR may not significantly differ. It is still not very clear, whether weight loss improves the outcome in an ART cycle. When lifestyle management is advised, it is very important to weigh the benefits of weight loss against postponing pregnancy, especially in those with advanced age and decreased ovarian reserve. However, obese patients must still be made aware of their increased obstetric risks of preeclampsia, gestational diabetes and caesarean section and should be encouraged to lose weight before attempting conception. Individualized COS, freeze-all strategy and elective single embryo transfer could help in increasing the success of ART and decreasing stress, anxiety and complications in PCOS women undergoing fertility treatment.

References

1. Brassard, M., AinMelk, Y., and Baillargeon, J.P. Basic infertility including polycystic ovary syndrome. (xi). Med Clin North Am. 2008; 92: 1163–1192.
2. Barbieri RL, Makris A, Randall RW, Daniels G, Kistner RW, Ryan KJ. Insulin stimulates androgen accumulation in incubations of ovarian stroma obtained from women with hyperandrogenism. J Clin Endocrinol Metab. 1986;62:904–10.
3. Plymate SR, Matej LA, Jones RE, Friedl KE. Inhibition of sex hormone-binding globulin production in the human hepatoma (Hep G2) cell line by insulin and prolactin. J Clin Endocrinol Metab. 1988;67:460–4.

4. Wood JR, Dumesic DA, Abbott DH, et al. Molecular abnormalities in oocytes from women with polycystic ovary syndrome revealed by microarray analysis. J Clin Endocrinol Metab. 2007;92:705–13.
5. Knight PG, Glister C. Local roles of TGF- β superfamily members in the control of ovarian follicle development. Anim Reprod Sci. 2003;78:165–83.
6. Qiao J, Feng HL. Extra-and intra-ovarian factors in polycystic ovary syndrome: impact on oocyte maturation and embryo developmental competence. Hum Reprod Update. 2010;17(1):17–33.
7. Fedorcsak P, Dale PO, Storeng R, Ertzeid G, Bjercke S, Oldereid N, et al. Impact of overweight and underweight on assisted eproduction treatment. Hum Reprod. 2004;19:2523–8.
8. Zhang JJ, Feret M, Chang L, Yang M, Merhi Z. Obesity adversely impacts the number and maturity of oocytes in conventional IVF not in minimal stimulation IVF. Gynecol Endocrinol. 2015;31:409–13.
9. Bellver J, Pellicer A, Garcia-Velasco JA, Ballesteros A, Remohi J, Meseguer M. Obesity reduces uterine receptivity: clinical experience from 9,587 first cycles of ovum donation with normal weight donors. Fertil Steril. 2013;100:1050–8.
10. Yuan C, Liu X, Mao Y, Diao F, Cui Y, Liu J. Polycystic ovary syndrome patients with high BMI tend to have functional disorders of androgen excess: a prospective study. J Biomed Res. 2016;30:197–202.
11. Koyuncu FM, Kuscu NK, Var A, Onur E. Leptin levels in patients with polycystic ovary syndrome in response to two different oral contraceptive treatments. Acta Obstet Gynecol Scand. 2003;82(8):767–8.
12. Wu LL, Norman RJ, Robker RL. The impact of obesity on oocytes: evidence for lipotoxicity mechanisms. Reprod Fertil Dev. 2011;24(1):29–34.
13. Williams RM, Ong KK, Dunger DB. Polycystic ovarian syndrome during puberty and adolescence. Mol Cell Endocrinol. 2013;373:61–7.
14. Teede HJ, Misso ML, Costello MF, Dokras A, Laven J, Moran L, Piltonen T, Norman RJ. Recommendations from the international evidence-based guideline for the assessment and management of polycystic ovary syndrome. Hum Reprod. 2018;33(9):1602–18.
15. Heijnen EMEW, Eijkemans MJC, Hughes EG, et al. A meta-analysis of outcomes of conventional IVF in women with polycstic ovary syndrome. Human Reprod Update. 2006; 12:13–21.
16. Schramm RD, Bavister BD. A macaque model for studying mechanisms controlling oocyte development and maturation in human and nonhuman primates. Hum Reprod. 1999;14:2544–55.
17. Cano F, Garcia-Velasco JA, Millet A. Oocyte quality in polycystic ovaries revisited: identification of a particular subgroup of women. J Assist Reprod Genet. 1997;14:254–60.
18. Hwang JL, Seow KM, Lin YH, et al. IVF versus ICSI in sibling oocytes from patients with polycystic ovarian syndrome: a randomized controlled trial. Hum Reprod. 2005; 20:1261–5.
19. Wissing ML, Bjerge MR, Olesen AI, Hoest T, Mikkelsen AL. Impact of PCOS on early embryo cleavage kinetics. Reprod Biomed Online. 2014;28(4):508–14.
20. Bellver J, Mifsud A, Grau N, Privitera L, Meseguer M. Similar morphokinetic patterns in embryos derived from obese and normoweight infertile women: a time-lapse study. Hum Reprod. 2013;28:794–800.
21. Barnes FL, Kausche A, Tiglias J, et al. Production of embryos from in vitro-matured primary human oocytes. Fertil Steril. 1996;65:1151–6.
22. Chekir C, Nakatsuka M, Kamada Y, Noguchi S, Sasaki A, Hiramatsu Y. Impaired uterine perfusion associated with metabolic disorders in women with polycystic ovary syndrome. Acta Obstet Gynecol Scand. 2005;84:189–95.
23. Ledee-Bataille N, Lapree-Delage G, Taupin JL, Dubanchet S, Taieb J, Moreau JF, et al. Follicular fluid concentration of leukaemia inhibitory factor is decreased among women with polycystic ovarian syndrome during assisted reproduction cycles. Hum Reprod. 2001;16:2073–8.
24. Broughton DE, Moley KH. Obesity and female infertility: potential mediators of obesity's impact. Fertil Steril. 2017 Apr 1;107(4):840–7.

25. Tziomalos K, Dinas K. Obesity and outcome of assisted reproduction in patients with polycystic ovary syndrome. Front Endocrinol. 2018 Apr 4;9:149.
26. Mena GP, Mielke GI, Brown WJ. The effect of physical activity on reproductive health outcomes in young women: a systematic review and meta-analysis. Hum Reprod Update. 2019;25(5):542–64.
27. Practice Committee of the American Society for Reproductive Medicine. Obesity and reproduction: a committee opinion. Fertil Steril. 2015;104(5):1116–26.
28. Goyal M, Dawood AS. Debates regarding lean patients with poly- cystic ovary syndrome: a narrative review. J Hum Reprod Sci. 2017;10:154–61.
29. Pascoe MC, Thompson DR, Ski CF. Yoga, mindfulness-based stress reduction and stress-related physiological measures: a meta-analysis. Psychoneuroendocrinology. 2017 Dec 1;86:152–68.
30. Chatzis P, Tziomalos K, Pratilas GC, Makris V, Sotiriadis A, Dinas K. The role of Antiobesity agents in the Management of Polycystic Ovary Syndrome. Folia Med. 2018 Dec 1;60(4):512–20.
31. Shah D. Madhuri Patil on behalf of the national PCOS working group, consensus statement on the use of oral contraceptive pills in polycystic ovarian syndrome women in India. J Hum Reprod Sci. 2018;11(2):96.
32. Amer SA, Smith J, Mahran A, Fox P, Fakis A. Double-blind randomized controlled trial of letrozole versus clomiphene citrate in subfertile women with polycystic ovarian syndrome. Hum Reprod. 2017;32(8):1631–8.
33. Homburg R, Hendriks ML, König TE, Anderson RA, Balen AH, Brincat M, Child T, Davies M, D'Hooghe T, Martinez A, Rajkhowa M. Clomifene citrate or low-dose FSH for the first-line treatment of infertile women with anovulation associated with polycystic ovary syndrome: a prospective randomized multinational study. Hum Reprod. 2012;27(2):468–73.
34. Weiss NS, Nahuis M, Bayram N, Mol BW, Van der Veen F, van Wely M. Gonadotrophins for ovulation induction in women with polycystic ovarian syndrome. Cochrane Database Syst Rev. 2015;9
35. Lambalk CB, Banga FR, Huirne JA, Toftager M, Pinborg A, Homburg R, et al. GnRH antagonist versus long agonist protocols in IVF: a systematic review and meta-analysis accounting for patient type. Hum Reprod Update. 2017;23:560–79.
36. Farquhar C, Brown J, Marjoribanks J. Laparoscopic drilling by diathermy or laser for ovulation induction in anovulatory polycystic ovary syndrome. Cochrane Database Syst Rev. 2012;6
37. Kar S. Anthropometric, clinical, and metabolic comparisons of the four Rotterdam PCOS phenotypes: a prospective study of PCOS women. J Hum Reprod Sci. 2013;6:194–200.
38. Bellver J, Busso C, Pellicer A, Remohí J, Simón C. Obesity and assisted reproductive technology outcomes. Reprod Biomed Online. 2006;12(5):562–8.
39. Orvieto R, Nahum R, Meltcer S, Homburg R, Rabinson J, Anteby EY, et al. Ovarian stimulation in polycystic ovary syndrome pa- tients: the role of body mass index. Reprod Biomed Online. 2009;18:333–6.
40. Fleming R, Jenkins J. The source and implications of progesterone rise during the follicular phase of assisted reproduction cycles. Reprod Biomed Online. 2010;21(4):446–9.
41. Kalra SK, Ratcliffe SJ, Dokras A. Is the fertile window extended in women with polycystic ovary syndrome? Utilizing the Society for Assisted Reproductive Technology registry to assess the impact of reproductive aging on live-birth rate. Fertil Steril. 2013 Jul 1;100(1):208–13.
42. Practice Committee of the American Society for Reproductive Medicine. Role of metformin for ovulation induction in infertile patients with polycystic ovary syndrome (PCOS): a guideline. Fertil Steril. 2017;108(3):426–41.
43. Palomba S, Falbo A, La Sala GB. Metformin and gonadotropins for ovulation induction in patients with polycystic ovary syndrome: a systematic review with meta-analysis of randomized controlled trials. Reprod Biol Endocrinol. 2014;12(1):3.
44. Rocha AL, Oliveira FR, Azevedo RC, Silva VA, Peres TM, Candido AL, Gomes KB, Reis FM. Recent advances in the understanding and management of polycystic ovary syndrome. F1000Research. 2019;8.

45. Sharpe A, Morley LC, Tang T, Norman RJ, Balen AH. Metformin for ovulation induction (excluding gonadotrophins) in women with polycystic ovary syndrome. Cochrane Database Syst Rev. 2019;12
46. Anastasiou OE, Canbay A, Fuhrer D, Reger-Tan S. Metabolic and androgen profile in underweight women with polycystic ovary syndrome. Arch Gynecol Obstet. 2017;296:363–71.
47. Popova P, Ivanova L, Karonova T, Grineva E. Ovulation induction by metformin in lean and obese women with polycystic ovary syndrome. Endocr Abstr 2011;26(P90).
48. Garg D, Tal R. Inositol treatment and ART outcomes in women with PCOS. Int J Endocrinol. 2016;2016
49. Genazzani AD, Santagni S, Ricchieri F, Campedelli A, Rattighieri E, Chierchia E, et al. Myo-inositol modulates insulin and luteinizing hormone secretion in normal weight patients with polycystic ovary syndrome. J Obstet Gynaecol Res. 2014;40:1353–60.
50. Agrawal A, Mahey R, Kachhawa G, Khadgawat R, Vanamail P, Kriplani A. Comparison of metformin plus myoinositol vs metformin alone in PCOS women undergoing ovulation induction cycles: randomized controlled trial. Gynecol Endocrinol. 2019;35(6):511–4.
51. McCormick B, Thomas M, Maxwell R, Williams D, Aubuchon M. Effects of polycystic ovarian syndrome on in vitro fertilization-embryo transfer outcomes are influenced by body mass index. Fertil Steril. 2008;90:2304–9.
52. Bailey AP, Hawkins LK, Missmer SA, Correia KF, Yanushpolsky EH. Effect of body mass index on in vitro fertilization outcomes in women with poly- cystic ovary syndrome. Am J Obstet Gynecol. 2014;211:e1–6.
53. Roque M, Valle M, Kostolias A, Sampaio M, Geber S. Freeze-all cycle in reproductive medicine: current perspectives. JBRA Assist Reprod. 2017;21(1):49.
54. Kolibianakis E, Bourgain C, Albano C, Osmanagaoglu K, Smitz J, Van Steirteghem A, Devroey P. Effect of ovarian stimulation with recombinant follicle-stimulating hormone, gonadotropin releasing hormone antagonists, and human chorionic gonadotropin on endometrial maturation on the day of oocyte pick-up. Fertil Steril. 2002;78(5):1025–9.
55. Labarta E, Martínez-Conejero fnameJA, Alamá P, Horcajadas JA, Pellicer A, Simón C, Bosch E Endometrial receptivity is affected in women with high circulating progesterone levels at the end of follicular phase: a functional genomics analysis Hum Reprod 2011;26:1813–5.
56. Londra L, Moreau C, Strobino D, Garcia J, Zacur H, Zhao Y. Ectopic pregnancy after in vitro fertilization: differences between fresh and frozen-thawed cycles. Fertil Steril. 2015;104:110–8.
57. Mainigi MA, Olalere D, Burd I, Sapienza C, Bartolomei M, Coutifaris C. Peri-implantation hormonal milieu: elucidating mechanisms of abnormal placentation and fetal growth. Biol Reprod. 2014;90:26.
58. Ishihara O, Araki R, Kuwahara A, Itakura A, Saito H, Adamson GD. Impact of frozen-thawed single-blastocyst transfer on maternal and neonatal outcome: an analysis of 277,042 single-embryo transfer cycles from 2008 to 2010 in Japan. Fertil Steril. 2014;101:128–33.
59. Qiu M, Tao Y, Kuang Y, Wang Y. Effect of body mass index on pregnancy outcomes with the freeze-all strategy in women with polycystic ovarian syndrome. Fertil Steril. 2019 Dec 1;112(6):1172–9.
60. Osman E, Franasiak J, Scott R. Oocyte and embryo manipulation and epigenetics. InSeminars in reproductive medicine 2018 may (Vol. 36, no. 03/04, pp. e1-e9). Thieme Medical Publishers.

Polycystic Ovary Syndrome: Fertility Treatment Options

10

Gesthimani Mintziori, Dimitrios G. Goulis, and Basil C. Tarlatzis

10.1 Introduction

Polycystic ovary syndrome (PCOS) is one of the most prevalent causes of infertility, as it comprises the most common endocrine disorder in premenopausal women. The main pathophysiological mechanism, anovulation, results in an increased time-to-conception.

During the second international symposium, held in Thessaloniki in 2007, and adopted by the European Society of Human Reproduction and Embryology (ESHRE) and the American Society for Reproductive Medicine (ASRM), all the therapeutic options regarding fertility for women with PCOS were discussed [1]. Recently, the International Evidence-Based Guideline for the Assessment and Management of PCOS addressed all fertility treatment options and critically appraised the available evidence [2].

10.2 Fertility Treatment Options

10.2.1 Lifestyle Change for Weight Loss

Lifestyle interventions include diet, physical exercise and behavioral management techniques. Lifestyle changes to induce weight loss are considered the first-line treatment for infertility in women with PCOS, with parallel overall health, metabolic, and psychological benefits. It has been suggested that lifestyle modifications should be advised and implemented in obese women with PCOS before the ovulation induction, mainly to avoid obesity-related pregnancy complications;

G. Mintziori · D. G. Goulis · B. C. Tarlatzis (✉)
Unit of Reproductive Endocrinology, 1st Department of Obstetrics and Gynecology, Medical School, Aristotle University of Thessaloniki, Thessaloniki, Greece

© International Society of Gynecological Endocrinology 2021
A. R. Genazzani et al. (eds.), *Impact of Polycystic Ovary, Metabolic Syndrome and Obesity on Women Health*, ISGE Series,
https://doi.org/10.1007/978-3-030-63650-0_10

nevertheless, it is unclear if this approach increases the cumulative pregnancy or live birth rates. A recent Cochrane review on lifestyle changes in women with PCOS, which synthesized 15 studies with 498 participants, showed that lifestyle interventions could have a positive impact on the free androgen index (FAI) [mean difference (MD) -1.11, 95% confidence interval (CI) -1.96 to −0.26, 6 randomized controlled trials (RCTs), $n = 204$, I^2 71%]. Unfortunately, no studies were found reporting data on miscarriage, pregnancy or live birth rates [3]. In any case, obesity constitutes an independent risk factor for anovulation, failed or delayed response to treatment [e.g., clomiphene citrate (CC), gonadotropins], first trimester miscarriages, and third trimester complications. Thus, weight loss is recommended as a first-line treatment for obese women with PCOS desiring fertility. No type of diet seems to be more beneficial compared with the others [4]. A moderate reduction in body weight (5–10%) in overweight women can restore menstruation and fertility.

10.2.2 Pharmacological and Surgical Ovulation Induction

Letrozole and CC are the treatment of choice for ovulation induction in women with PCOS. CC has traditionally been used as an ovulation induction agent for over 40 years. Nevertheless, according to recent data, letrozole is more effective compared with CC in anovulatory women with PCOS, with the likelihood of a live birth increasing by 40–60% with letrozole compared to CC [5].

10.2.2.1   Letrozole

Letrozole is the most common aromatase inhibitor (AI) used for ovulation induction. AIs inhibit the aromatase action, the enzyme that converts androgens to estrogens and increase the secretion of follicle-stimulating hormone (FSH) needed to stimulate the development and maturation of the ovarian follicle. A 2019 individual patient data (IPD) meta-analysis assessing letrozole vs. CC showed that letrozole leads to higher ovulation [relative risk (RR) 1.13, 95% CI 1.07–1.2], clinical pregnancy (RR 1.45, 95% CI 1.23–1.70, I^2), and live birth rates (RR 1.43, 95% CI 1.17–1.75) compared with CC [6]. Similarly, letrozole decreased the time-to-pregnancy [(hazard ratio [HR] 1.72, 95% CI 1.38–2.15)] [6]. These observations are more evident in women with high baseline serum concentrations of total testosterone. According to the 2018 International Evidence-Based Guideline for the Assessment and Management of PCOS, letrozole comprises a first-line pharmacological treatment for ovulation induction in women with PCOS [2]. Despite this evidence as well as its affordable cost, the use of letrozole remains off-label, and women have to provide informed consent.

10.2.2.2   Clomiphene Citrate

CC is a selective estrogen-receptor modulator (SERM) traditionally used as an ovulation induction agent for over 40 years. Compared with placebo or no treatment, CC leads to higher clinical pregnancy rates. Its primary indication is infertility due to oligoovulation or anovulation. CC is administered at a starting dose of 50 mg/day and is taken orally for 5 days. It is a cheap and safe drug, as it does not require frequent ultrasound monitoring. It is taken orally and has relatively few adverse effects. Multiple pregnancy rates with CC administration range from 0.3% (triplets) to 5–7% (twin pregnancies), and the risk for developing ovarian hyperstimulation syndrome (OHSS) is <1% [7].

10.2.2.3 Metformin

Metformin is a simple, low-cost, and safe treatment option for obese women with PCOS. Metformin is an insulin-sensitizing drug, taken orally twice daily. Although it is commonly associated with gastrointestinal disorders, there are no other serious adverse effects. A recent Cochrane meta-analysis, which included 41 studies and 4552 women, showed that metformin increases ovulation [odds ratio (OR) 2.64, 95% CI 1. –3.75; I^2 61%; 13 studies, 684 women), clinical pregnancy (OR 1.98, 95% CI 1.47–2.65; I^2 30%; 11 studies, 1213 women), and live birth rates (OR 1.59, 95% CI 1.00–2.51; 4 studies, 435 women) compared to placebo [8].

In obese women with PCOS, CC could be used in combination with metformin to improve the reproductive outcomes (ovulation, pregnancy, and live birth rates) [2]. The addition of metformin to CC may also decrease the time-to-pregnancy, especially in specific PCOS subgroups (e.g., obese and CC-resistant women). When metformin and CC are compared, in terms of their efficacy on the reproductive outcomes, the baseline body mass index (BMI) seems to play a role: normal-weight women benefit more from metformin. In contrast, obese women with PCOS have better reproductive outcomes (clinical pregnancy and live birth rates) after ovulation induction with CC [8].

10.2.2.4 Gonadotropins

Gonadotropins are used as a second-line treatment for ovulation induction in women with PCOS. This strategy is mainly due to their cost, availability, as well as the need for expertise and intensive ultrasound monitoring. In addition, the risk of multiple pregnancies is increased. The clinical efficacy of the different gonadotrophin preparations seems comparable. As women with PCOS receiving exogenous gonadotropins are at an increased risk for developing OHSS, a low-dose, step-up ovarian stimulation protocol has been suggested.

10.2.2.5 Assisted Reproduction Technology

About one-fifth of women undergoing assisted reproduction technology (ART) have been diagnosed with PCOS. However, in vitro fertilization (IVF) should only be used in the event of failure of other treatments in women with PCOS, due to the lack of consistency in stimulating the ovaries in a controlled manner, or if there are specific indications for IVF, e.g., tubal or male factor infertility. Although there is no agreement on the optimal stimulation protocol, most studies indicate that the use of GnRH-antagonists per se can significantly reduce the risk of developing OHSS compared to other protocols [9]. Moreover, in an antagonist protocol, it is possible to induce final oocyte maturation with GnRH-agonist triggering instead of hCG, which, associated with freezing of all embryos and subsequent frozen embryo transfer (FET), maintains high pregnancy rates and almost eliminates the risk for OHSS [10]. Additionally, IVF is a reasonable treatment strategy, since multiple pregnancy rate can be minimized by single embryo transfer (SET), which is not the case with ovulation induction and especially gonadotrophin administration. It is important to note that with IVF, women with PCOS have similar pregnancy rates compared with women without PCOS.

10.2.2.6 Ovarian Drilling

There is insufficient evidence that laparoscopic ovarian diathermy ("drilling") in CC-resistant women is associated with increased rates of clinical pregnancies and live births compared with other treatments [5]. However, a reduction in the incidence of multiple pregnancies has been observed in women undergoing laparoscopic ovarian drilling [11]. The main concerns for its use are related to the long-term effects on the ovarian function and the development of intra-abdominal adhesions.

10.2.3 Other Treatment Options to Enhance Fertility

Alternative assisted reproduction options in women with PCOS include in vitro maturation (IVM) of eggs collected from unstimulated ovaries [12]; as the method requires considerable expertise, it is not available widely. Given the current evidence, the use of anti-obesity medications aiming at improving fertility is not justified [5].

According to an overview of systematic reviews of non-pharmacological interventions in women with PCOS, N-acetyl-cysteine and inositol could induce ovulation, though the evidence is not strong [13]. Regarding alternative medicine, Chinese herbals and acupuncture on top of pharmacological therapies for ovulation induction in women with PCOS may improve clinical pregnancy rates compared with pharmacological therapies alone [13].

10.3 Selecting the Optimal Fertility Treatment Option

A meta-analysis of 57 RCTs, which studied 8082 women who were treated with CC, metformin (or their combination), tamoxifen, FSH, or laparoscopic ovarian drilling, demonstrated that all pharmacological treatments result in a higher pregnancy rate compared with placebo or no treatment [14]. Letrozole and the combination of CC with metformin resulted in higher pregnancy rates compared to CC, tamoxifen, or metformin alone [14]. An IPD meta-analysis demonstrated that letrozole improved time-to-pregnancy (HR 1.72, 95% CI 1.38–2.15), clinical pregnancy rates (RR 1.45, 95% CI 1.23–1.70), and live birth rates (RR 1.43, 95% CI 1.17–1.75) compared with CC [6].

10.4 Conclusions

Women with PCOS and infertility should be reassured that many treatment options are available. A moderate reduction in body weight (5–10%) in overweight women can restore fertility, without taking any other measure. First-line treatments include lifestyle modifications and CC/letrozole, while second-line treatments include medications that increase insulin sensitivity, exogenous gonadotropins, and laparoscopic ovarian drilling. The choice of treatment should be the result of a joint decision after an informed discussion between the infertile couple and the medical team, based on a woman's special characteristics and the couple's wishes and choices.

References

1. Thessaloniki ESHRE/ASRM-Sponsored PCOS Consensus Workshop Group. Consensus on infertility treatment related to polycystic ovary syndrome. Hum Reprod. 2008;23(3):462–77.
2. Teede HJ, Misso ML, Costello MF, et al. Recommendations from the international evidence-based guideline for the assessment and management of polycystic ovary syndrome. Hum Reprod. 2018;33(9):1602–18.
3. Lim SS, Hutchison SK, Van Ryswyk E, Norman RJ, Teede HJ, Moran LJ. Lifestyle changes in women with polycystic ovary syndrome. Cochrane Database Syst Rev. 2019;3:CD007506.
4. Moran LJ, Tassone EC, Boyle J, et al. Evidence summaries and recommendations from the international evidence-based guideline for the assessment and management of polycystic ovary syndrome: lifestyle management. Obes Rev. 2020;
5. Costello MF, Misso ML, Balen A, et al. Evidence summaries and recommendations from the international evidence-based guideline for the assessment and management of polycystic ovary syndrome: assessment and treatment of infertility. Hum Reprod Open. 2019;2019(1):hoy021.
6. Wang R, Li W, Bordewijk EM, et al. First-line ovulation induction for polycystic ovary syndrome: an individual participant data meta-analysis. Hum Reprod Update. 2019;25(6):717–32.
7. Kafy S, Tulandi T. New advances in ovulation induction. Curr Opin Obstet Gynecol. 2007;19(3):248–52.
8. Sharpe A, Morley LC, Tang T, Norman RJ, Balen AH. Metformin for ovulation induction (excluding gonadotrophins) in women with polycystic ovary syndrome. Cochrane Database Syst Rev. 2019;12:CD013505.
9. Luo S, Li S, Li X, Bai Y, Jin S. Effect of gonadotropin-releasing hormone antagonists on intrauterine insemination cycles in women with polycystic ovary syndrome: a meta-analysis. Gynecol Endocrinol. 2014;30(4):255–9.
10. Youssef MA, Van der Veen F, Al-Inany HG, et al. Gonadotropin-releasing hormone agonist versus HCG for oocyte triggering in antagonist-assisted reproductive technology. Cochrane Database Syst Rev. 2014;10:CD008046.
11. Farquhar C, Brown J, Marjoribanks J. Laparoscopic drilling by diathermy or laser for ovulation induction in anovulatory polycystic ovary syndrome. Cochrane Database Syst Rev. 2012;6:CD001122.
12. Walls ML, Hunter T, Ryan JP, Keelan JA, Nathan E, Hart RJ. In vitro maturation as an alternative to standard in vitro fertilization for patients diagnosed with polycystic ovaries: a comparative analysis of fresh, frozen and cumulative cycle outcomes. Hum Reprod. 2015;30(1):88–96.
13. Pundir J, Charles D, Sabatini L, et al. Overview of systematic reviews of non-pharmacological interventions in women with polycystic ovary syndrome. Hum Reprod Update. 2019;25(2):243–56.
14. Wang R, Kim BV, van Wely M, et al. Treatment strategies for women with WHO group II anovulation: systematic review and network meta-analysis. BMJ. 2017;356:j138.

Management of PCOS Women Preparing Pregnancy

Xiangyan Ruan and Alfred O. Mueck

11.1 Introduction

As well known, infertility is a prevalent presenting feature of PCOS with ~75% of these women suffering infertility due to anovulation, making PCOS the most common cause of anovulatory infertility. Women with PCOS often have many concerns about childbearing including whether they could become pregnant and what they should do before they try to become pregnant. Polycystic ovary syndrome (PCOS) is a common female reproductive endocrine disease. The prevalence in premenopausal women ranges from 6 to 20%, possibly making this syndrome as the most common endocrine and metabolic disorder in women of reproductive age [1–3]. According to the reports in specialized departments of China like in our "Department of Gynecological Endocrinology," it stands as the most important disease – in our daily clinic from more than 500 outpatients, at least 50% are diagnosed with PCOS, and more than 50,000 per year of our PCOS patients get treatment as described in this chapter. The disease can begin in early adolescence, the etiology is not yet clear, the pathogenesis is complex, and it is related to environmental (especially nutrition) factors. Particularly, genetical factors may also play an important role in the development of the disease and differences in type and outcome [4]. Changes of endocrine and metabolic markers are often associated with PCOS although are not decisive for the diagnosis. In 2003, the "European Society for Human Reproduction and Embryology (ESHRE)" and the "American Society of Reproductive Medicine (ASRM)" revised the diagnostic criteria for PCOS at the Rotterdam meeting [5]: (1) rare ovulation or anovulation; (2) abnormal clinical manifestations and/or

X. Ruan (✉) · A. O. Mueck
Department of Gynecological Endocrinology, Beijing Obstetrics and Gynecology Hospital, Capital Medical University, Beijing, People's Republic of China

Research Centre for Women's Health and University Women's Hospital of Tuebingen, University of Tuebingen, Tuebingen, Germany

© International Society of Gynecological Endocrinology 2021
A. R. Genazzani et al. (eds.), *Impact of Polycystic Ovary, Metabolic Syndrome and Obesity on Women Health*, ISGE Series,
https://doi.org/10.1007/978-3-030-63650-0_11

biochemical indicators of hyperandrogenism; and (3) polycystic ovarian morphology (PCOM): follicle number of 2–9 mm in diameter in one or both ovaries ≥12 and/or ovarian volume >10 cm³. In 2018 the cut-off for follicle number was raised to 20 or more in either ovary [2]. If at least two of the three abovementioned criteria are met, "PCOS" can be diagnosed, whereby diseases such as thyroid dysfunction, Cushing's syndrome, androgen-secreting tumors, hyper-prolactinemia, pituitary gland diseases, and premature ovarian failure must be excluded.

Currently there is controversial discussion about the value of the assessment of anti-Müllerian hormone (AMH) in context with the diagnosis of PCOS. However, according to our own and other recent research, we conclude that AMH may be a useful parameter to assess the severity and prognosis of PCOS and may help to differentiate the main phenotypes of the disease, being higher in PCOS patients compared to controls especially in non-obese women [6–8]. However, the mechanisms resulting in increased AMH in PCOS are poorly understood and have been attributed to obesity, insulin resistance (IR), hyperandrogenism, complex interactions with gonadotrophins, etc. [9].

PCOS is characterized by biochemical and clinical hyperandrogenic features and menstrual and ovulation disorders. Related metabolic disorders include IR, abnormal glucose, and abnormal lipid metabolism, which can increase the risk of cardiovascular disease [10]. Primary disease characteristics of PCOS, mainly hyperandrogenism and impaired glucose tolerance, also predict suboptimal obstetric and neonatal outcomes. Increased rates of gestational diabetes mellitus, pregnancy induced hypertension, preeclampsia, caesarean section delivery, and preterm birth have been reported among pregnant women with PCOS.

It is very important to strengthen the need of the individualized long-term management of PCOS patients. Thus, this article will elaborate preferably on the long-term complications of PCOS and new developments in long-term management.

11.2 Pathophysiology of PCOS

The pathophysiology of PCOS is complex and not fully understood [11–14]. Women with PCOS experience an increase in frequency of hypothalamic gonadotropin-releasing hormone (GnRH) pulses which, in turn, results in an increase in the luteinizing hormone (LH)/follicle stimulating hormone (FSH) ratio. The dominance of LH over FSH increases ovarian androgen production and decreases follicular maturation. This leads to an increase in the level of biologically active testosterone and contributes to the clinical consequences of hyperandrogenemia in PCOS [15]. Abnormalities in both androgen metabolism and the control of androgen production, when accompanied by anovulation, increase the likelihood of metabolic dysfunction [16]. The majority of women with PCOS have insulin resistance and/or are obese [16]. Their elevated insulin levels increase GnRH pulse frequency and either contribute to or cause the abnormalities seen in the hypothalamic–pituitary–ovarian axis that lead to PCOS [15]. Normal patterns of gonadotropin secretion are essential for reproduction, and any imbalance may contribute to decreased fertility and pregnancy problems [17]. The pathological imbalance of LH and FSH, present in women with PCOS, explains the rationale for pretreatment with combined hormonal contraceptives to increase fertility and improve pregnancy outcomes; however, more studies are needed regarding this important topic.

11.3 Long-Term Consequences of PCOS

Studies show a link between hyperandrogenic PCOS and disturbances in metabolic parameters which could lead to an increased risk of cardiovascular disease (CVD) [12, 16]. Obesity, impaired glucose tolerance, and type 2 diabetes are all more prevalent in women with PCOS when compared with the general population [18]. Although conventional cardiovascular risk calculators such as the Framingham Index have not been validated within this patient population and there is no real proof of an increased risk of CVD as main endpoint in studies, there is clear evidence of higher incidence of hypertension, impaired lipid and glucose metabolism, and increased risk of developing gestational diabetes and type 2 diabetes, which indeed all can increase the risk of CVD [12, 16]. In addition, polycystic ovary syndrome is associated with poorer pregnancy outcomes, for example, an increase in risk of pre-term delivery and preeclampsia. Decreased quality of life, including an increased risk of depression and anxiety, is also an important risk in untreated PCOS patients [11].

11.4 Treatment Targets

11.4.1 Lifestyle

Lifestyle modification involving a healthy diet and exercise and achievement of optimal BMI is important for all women affected by PCOS. Evidence from observational studies shows that moderate weight loss (5–10%) in women with PCOS can improve insulin resistance as well as androgenic and reproductive outcomes.

11.4.2 Hyperandrogenism

Pharmacological treatment of PCOS is aimed to reduce the level of circulating androgens and to control their effect at tissue level in order to ameliorate symptoms such as hirsutism and acne and reduce the risk of long-term metabolic consequences. Combinations of ethinyl-estradiol (EE) and progestogens, especially those containing antiandrogenic progestogens such as cyproterone acetate (CPA), chlormadinone acetate (CMA), and drospirenone (DRSP), have traditionally been the first choice for management of PCOS [19]. Almost all combined oral contraceptives (COCs) and other estrogen/progestogen combinations like vaginal rings and contraceptive patches contain EE as the estrogenic component. Reason for this is the good cyclical stability because of the long half-life of EE which can stabilize the endometrial situation during the use of those combined contraceptives. Only two newer COCs available in many Western countries contain estradiol instead of EE, in combination with newer special progestogens, dienogest (DNG) or nomegestrol acetate (NOMAC), respectively, which due to their strong endometrial efficacy can avoid breakthrough bleedings in contrast to other combinations with estradiol (E2) which have been tested for their potential use in contraception.

The antiandrogenic effect of the estrogen/progestogen combinations is achieved via a number of different mechanisms, which mainly are (1) increase in hepatic SHBG production with all estrogens in a dose-dependent manner; however, the effect is much stronger using EE compared with E2; (2) suppression of LH secretion and thereby ovarian androgen production, achieved with all progestogens (including androgenic progestogens such as levonorgestrel [LNG]) if used in ovulatory inhibition dosages; (3) competition at the 5-alpha-reductase and androgen receptors by progestogens, effect strongest when using CPA; (4) competition at the androgen-receptor with antiandrogenic progestogens like CPA, CMA, DNG, and DRSP can block the action of testosterone; (5) in addition the ovarian androgen production can be blocked directly, especially when using EE/CPA combinations.

11.4.3 Identifying Treatment Priorities in PCOS

The management of PCOS should be tailored to each woman's specific goals, reproductive interests, and particular symptomatic presentation. The presenting primary complaint may vary depending on age or ethnic variation. Treatment may primarily focus on the symptom generating the greatest level of distress, such as hirsutism or infertility, and often require a multidisciplinary approach. When discussing long-term management of PCOS, women should be advised regarding the risks and benefits of treatment and the elements of lifestyle management to reduce the metabolic and cardiovascular consequences of the syndrome. Recognition of the symptoms of venous thromboembolism (VTE) and knowledge how to respond are also important.

11.4.4 Obesity

Obesity is a common problem in patients with PCOS. In the United States, 80% of women with PCOS suffer from obesity. According to a recent meta-analysis [20], women with PCOS had an increased prevalence of overweight [RR (95% CI): 1.95 (1.52, 2.50)], obesity [2.77 (1.88, 4.10)], and central obesity [1.73 (1.31, 2.30)] compared with women without PCOS; Caucasian women with PCOS had a greater increase in obesity prevalence than Asian women with PCOS compared with women without PCOS [10.79 (5.36, 21.70) versus 2.31 (1.33, 4.00), P < 0.001]. Numerous studies have shown that centripetal obesity and visceral hypertrophy are associated with PCOS. High insulin levels due to hyperandrogenism and IR in PCOS can lead to centripetal fat distribution, mainly manifested as an increase in the ratio of waist circumference to hip circumference [21, 22]. Moreover, non-targeted and targeted studies suggest that the genomic, transcriptomic, and proteomic profiles of visceral adipose tissue from women with PCOS are quite different from those of healthy women and resemble those of men, indicating that androgen excess contributes to their adipose tissue dysfunction.

In addition to reducing ovulation, obesity is also associated with endometrial changes associated with IR, which reduces the rate of implantation and increases the rate of abortion and is closely related to complications in the third trimester of pregnancy, leading to low fertility. At the same time, obesity is likely to aggravate the hyperandrogenism of PCOS and menstrual disorders to form a vicious circle. It can also lead to psychological complications of women with PCOS, such as anxiety and depression. The accumulation of abdominal fat can induce IR and hyperinsulinemia, and insulin can stimulate the production of ovarian androgens, further aggravating hyperandrogenism. Overweight and obesity are prone to increase the risk of type 2 diabetes (T2DM) [23]. Some studies have shown that for every 1% increase in body mass index (BMI), the risk of T2DM can increase by 2%. The amount of visceral fat and abdominal fat is positively correlated with the risk of IR, inflammation, T2DM, dyslipidemia, metabolic syndrome (MetS), and cardiovascular disease, but metabolic disorders can also be seen in some nonobese PCOS women [24].

Weight management is crucial for treatment of PCOS patients. Weight loss is beneficial for improving the menstrual cycle and restoring ovulation. In a randomized trial of PCOS female infertility, it was found that both COC or separate lifestyle changes aiming for weight loss significantly improved ovulation rates compared with immediate clomiphene citrate treatment, i.e., live birth rates increased more [25].

We found that letrozole combined with low-dose highly purified human menopausal gonadotrophin (HMG) may be an effective and safe choice for reducing hyperstimulation and can increase the pregnancy rate by ovulation induction of clomiphene-resistant women with PCOS [26]. However, a recent randomized trial found that weight loss even is superior to oral contraceptive pretreatment in improving induced ovulation in overweight and obese PCOS women, providing additional evidence for the importance of weight loss to improve the reproductive function of PCOS [27]. As "COC" in China mostly EE plus CPA is used, although according to the new labeling the indication now only is "for treatment of biochemical and clinical signs of hyperandrogenism." Indeed in our department thousands of PCOS patients every year are treated with EE/CPA, and only since recently we use more EE/DRSP in obese patients, mostly together with lifestyle changes. Within a large cohort study using EE/CPA together with standardized lifestyle change, we observed significant improvement in physical aspects like weight loss associated with increased quality of life and a decrease of depressive symptoms and anxiety [28]. Weight loss is also beneficial for improving metabolism [29]. Lifestyle improvement can be achieved with diet, exercise adjustment, etc. Existing dietary and reproductive physiological data suggest that specific dietary improvements may help to counteract the chronic low-grade inflammatory process in the disease. The reproductive outcome of these patients is improved [30]. It was recommended that for overweight PCOS patients the diet should be controlled keeping it at 1200 ~ 1500 kcal/day, and moderate-intensity exercise for more than 5 days per week during at least 30 minutes should be performed. A specific recommendation is to increase whole grain intake and avoid refined carbohydrates, including oats, brown rice, and quinoa. Encouragingly, it was found that women who received in vitro fertilization and had a nutrition with higher content of grains had higher live birth rates. Within a large prospective cohort study including more than 5000 women, it was demonstrated that for obese women any form of exercise is beneficial to improve the fertility [31]. Recent studies have shown that weight loss in the first 2 months is a good predictor of prognosis after 1 year of lifestyle intervention. Therefore, early identifying if individuals will have unsuccessful or successful weight loss may be a promising solution providing tailored treatments for long-term weight loss. For women with obesity who are not able or not really willing to change their lifestyle, as medical treatment the widely used insulin sensitizer metformin may be considered for patients with pre-diabetes or diabetes mellitus. In most countries (like also in China), metformin is labelled only for patients with diabetes mellitus, and if used as "off-label," the patients must be informed. The newest recommendations from the "International evidence-based guideline for the assessment and management of PCOS" suggest that metformin in addition to lifestyle changes could be recommended in adult women with PCOS to treat overweight, hormonal, and metabolic disorders [2]. Metformin may offer especially benefit in high metabolic risk groups including those with risk factors for diabetes or impaired glucose tolerance, whereby with respect to symptoms and treatment effect there could be genetical differences. For the use of metformin, it needs to be considered that adverse effects, including gastrointestinal side effects, are generally dose-dependent, and it is recommended to start with low dose, i.e., with 500 mg increments 1–2 weekly.

We found that the use of EE/CPA can restore the regularity of menstrual cycles and does not deteriorate the glucose and lipid metabolism [32]. To investigate also the new treatment options, we compared metformin, EE/CPA with orlistat, which has the indication to help getting weight loss in obese patients [32, 33]. Within a prospective randomized placebo-controlled four-arm study comparing (a) orlistat combined with EE/CPA vs. (b) metformin plus EE/CPA vs. (c) orlistat plus metformin plus EE/CPA vs. (d) EE/CPA, we found that the combination EE/CPA plus orlistat has been the best choice in reducing weight, reducing androgen levels, improving glucose metabolism, and reducing systemic fat content, with less adverse reactions [33]. According to the newest guideline for the diagnosis and treatment of polycystic ovary syndrome in China, orlistat is recommended in obese women to improve weight loss [3]. However, the first advice always must be to inform the patients about the need of dietary restrictions and "healthy diet," respectively. Moreover, the benefit of orlistat observed in our studies may be dependent on genetical factors, so more research is still needed.

Some studies suggested glucagon-like peptide-1 analogue liraglutide in combination with metformin and lifestyle interventions resulted in significant reduction in body weight in overweight and obese women with PCOS, which indicates that also liraglutide may be an effective alternative for getting weight loss in such patients. Compared with metformin, short-term exenatide treatment had better efficacy in reducing body weight, improving IR, and reducing inflammation.

However, large and long-term clinical trials are needed to assess efficacy and safety. Patients with difficulty to get weight loss can also consider bariatric surgery, which can effectively alleviate PCOS and its clinical symptoms, including hirsutism and irregular menstruation in severely obese women [34]. A meta-analysis published in 2017 indicated that surgically induced weight loss in women with severe obesity and PCOS resulted in significant decreases in serum levels of total and free testosterone and improvement of hirsutism and menstrual dysfunction in as many as 53% and 96% of the patients, respectively [34].

11.5   Insulin Resistance and Diabetes Mellitus

IR is closely associated with increased risk of pre-diabetes and T2DM in PCOS, with IR in approximately 60–80% of PCOS patients and 95% in obese patients. In a large study of 11,035 patients with PCOS [35], the prevalence of T2DM was 2.5 times that of the age-matched control group. Using a meta-analysis it was calculated that the odds ratio (OR) of Impaired Glucose Tolerance (IGT), T2DM, and MetS in PCOS is 2.48 (95% CI 1.63, 3.77), 4.43 (95% CI 4.06, 4.82), and 2.88 (95% CI 2.40, 3.45), respectively. Subgroup analyses of studies with BMI-matched populations reveal the same risks. The OR for IGT in lean PCOS women has been estimated to be 3.22 (95% CI 1.26, 8.24), whereby the IR of patients with PCOS worsens with increasing age. IR certainly is a key player in the metabolic manifestations in PCOS patients and seems to be partially independent of obesity. Investigations in adolescents found that the frequency of IGT were equal between obese and non-obese PCOS patients. However, there is general agreement that obese women with PCOS have a higher risk to be insulin resistant, and some groups of lean affected PCOS women may have normal insulin sensitivity. A meta-analysis indicates that women with PCOS have a higher risk of IR and glucose intolerance than women of similar age and weight who do not have PCOS [36].

The pathogenesis of IR in patients with PCOS is multifactorial. Investigations on possible mechanisms suggest that there is a post-binding defect in receptor signaling likely due to increased receptor and insulin receptor substrate-1 serine phosphorylation that selectively affects metabolic but not mitogenic pathways in classic insulin target tissues and in the ovary [17]. Consecutive activation of serine kinases in the MAPK-ERK pathway may contribute to resistance in terms of insulin's metabolic actions in skeletal muscles. Insulin functions as a co-gonadotropin through its cognate receptor which can modulate ovarian steroidogenesis. Genetic disruption of insulin signaling in the brain has indicated that this pathway is important for ovulation and body weight regulation [17]. These insights have been directly translated into the novel therapy of PCOS with insulin-sensitizing drugs. Furthermore, androgens contribute to the development of IR in PCOS. IR not only predisposes patients to metabolic dysfunction and increased risk of type 2 diabetes mellitus but also is important within the pathophysiology of PCOS. High testosterone and SHBG concentrations (indicating a high fraction of the biological active free testosterone) are independently associated with IR, so there is a direct interactive relationship between hyperandrogenemia and IR, i.e., IR may induce an increased androgen action, and vice versa androgens may induce IR, respectively [17]. Androgen exposure at critical periods or intrauterine growth restriction may also have a causal relationship to the development of PCOS [17].

As already described above, lifestyle changes, including diet, exercise, and behavioral changes, are the first-line treatment for all overweight and obese patients with PCOS. In context with changes in glucose metabolism, it has been shown that changes in the diet can improve IR in patients with PCOS. In addition also exercise can improve IR and metabolic profiles and reduce visceral fat in women with PCOS [37]. Such lifestyle changes reduce the risk of IGT progression to T2DM in healthy women and in PCOS patients [37].

For PCOS patients diagnosed with T2DM, there are no specific recommendations for the various available anti-diabetic treatment options. However, metformin and lifestyle changes are suggested as the treatment of choice, and any antidiabetic drug (i.e., sulfonylureas, pioglitazone, dipeptidyl peptidase 4 inhibitors, glucagon-like peptide-1 receptor agonists, sodium-glucose cotransporter 2 inhibitors, or basal insulin) can be added to patients who are still unable to achieve their glycemic goals with metformin. Among the available alternative options, pioglitazone appears to improve insulin sensitivity to a similar extent like metformin, and both have synergistic effects on IR in patients with PCOS [38]. However, safety issues, including weight gain and the risk of edema, limit the use of pioglitazone in this population. Limited data also indicate that glucagon-like peptide 1 analogs combined with metformin are more effective in reducing IR and reducing body weight than metformin monotherapy. It is worth noting that only insulin, metformin, and glibenclamide can be safely used in pregnancy. Therefore, patients receiving other antidiabetic drugs should take appropriate contraceptive measures.

11.5.1 Decreased Fertility, Adverse Pregnancy Outcomes

Important long-term consequences of untreated PCOS are decreased fertility and adverse pregnancy outcomes [39, 40]. Infertility in PCOS is due to infrequent or absent ovulation, and no clear evidence exists that factors other than oligo-ovulation or anovulation contribute to reduced fertility. About 75% of women with PCOS have infertility, and PCOS accounts for the vast majority of cases of oligo-ovulation or anovulation requiring fertility treatment [2]. At the same time, women with PCOS are at increased risk of adverse pregnancy and neonatal complications; this information may be vital in clinical practice for the management of pregnancy in women with PCOS. According to various data, the risk of miscarriage in PCOS women is three times higher than the risk of miscarriage in healthy women [40]. Unfortunately, the risk of most frequent pregnancy pathologies is also higher for

PCOS patients, as gestational diabetes mellitus (GDM), pregnancy-induced hypertension and preeclampsia, and for gestational age (GA) children. IGT and GDM in pregnant PCOS patients occur more frequently than in healthy women. A quadruple increase in the risk of pregnancy-induced hypertension linked to arterial wall stiffness has also been observed in PCOS patients [40]. The risk of pre-eclampsia, the most severe of all complications, is also up to four times higher in those suffering from PCOS [40]. A meta-analysis in women with PCOS including 27 studies, analyzing 4982 women with PCOS and 119,692 controls [41], showed a significantly higher risk of developing GDM (OR 3.43; 95% CI: 2.49–4.74), pregnancy-induced hypertension (PIH) (OR 3.43; 95% CI:2.49–4.74), preeclampsia (OR 2.17; 95% CI: 1.91–2.46), preterm birth (OR 1.93; 95%CI: 1.45–2.57), and caesarean section (OR 1.74; 95% CI: 1.38–2.11) compared to controls. Women with PCOS had an increased risk of preterm delivery compared with the background population. The increased risk was confined to hyperandrogenic women with PCOS who had a two-fold increased risk of pre-term delivery and preeclampsia [42]. Our team found that follicular and embryo development and changes in endometrial receptivity in patients with PCOS were associated with adverse pregnancy outcomes [43]. As we always have stressed in our research and publications, based on the literature and our own experience treating during recent years thousands of PCOS patients, individualized comprehensive treatment combining lifestyle changes with pharmacological interventions has a positive effect on pregnancy outcomes in patients with PCOS [28, 33]. These women should be given notice of the additional risks their pregnancies may have, stronger surveillance and attention should be provided, as well as screening for these complications during pregnancy and parturition. According to a meta-analysis evaluating obstetric complications in women with PCOS [41], during pregnancy particularly close checks on a regular basis of glucose metabolism and hormonal status should be performed besides control of lifestyle modification and medical therapy. To reduce pregnancy-related complications, very recently our team found that the use of COC may not be valuable only in patients who want or need contraception but also as pretreatment in PCOS patients who want pregnancy: We evaluated the prevalence of adverse pregnancy outcomes in 6000 healthy Chinese women, selected from 24,566 pregnant women by randomized sampling, and investigated whether these outcomes could be decreased in patients with PCOS by pretreatment with EE/CPA. The result was that patients with PCOS are more likely to develop GDM, PIH, and premature delivery, and 3-monthly pretreatment with the COC was associated with a lower risk of GDM, PIH, and premature delivery [43]. Since this treatment concept has been already proven to be most successful in many of our patients, it is now included in our own routine management for treatment of PCOS patients who want pregnancy, together with individualized lifestyle interventions.

PCOS is a very frequent endocrine disorder. Figure 11.1 summarizes the long-term complications and management of this disease, with symptoms, complications, and risks dependent on the age of the patients. Because of the different symptoms and risks and the broad spectrum of possible symptomatic treatment options, often a multidisciplinary approach is needed. *Obesity* is one of the most

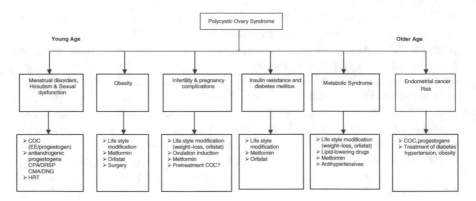

Fig. 11.1 Long-term complications and management of polycystic ovary syndrome; *COC* combined oral contraceptives, *EE* ethinyl-estradiol, *CPA* cyproterone acetate, *DRSP* drospirenone, *CMA* chlormadinone acetate, *DNG* dienogest, *HRT* hormone replacement therapy

common findings in PCOS, and is itself an independent risk factor for many of the symptoms and negative long-term consequences that have been attributed to PCOS. Patients with PCOS are at increased risk of *endometrial cancer*, whereas an association with other types of gynecological cancers like ovarian and breast cancer are controversial or have not been found, respectively. Untreated PCOS patients clearly have an increased long-term risk to develop *diabetes mellitus* and *metabolic syndrome*. In patients who are overweight or obese, lifestyle interventions, principally in terms of diet and exercise, are thought to be the most effective management. If proven to be unsuccessful, metformin is an effective pharmacological treatment and can prevent conversion of IGT to T2DM. At least in Chinese women orlistat combined with COC can help to reduce weight and can lower androgens, blood fat, and glucose, but more research is needed, especially if genetical factors may play a role. PCOS patients may have a *decreased fertility* and/or *adverse pregnancy outcomes*. According own research pretreatment with COC containing an antiandrogenic progestogen can be recommended to increase the fertility and decrease adverse pregnancy outcomes. The most important consideration of management is to tailor treatment choices to the specific needs of the patient.

11.6 Conclusion

Polycystic ovary syndrome (PCOS) is a frequent female reproductive endocrine disease. It has been associated with a number of severe reproductive complications. However, there are still open questions especially regarding the *Management of PCOS women preparing pregnancy*. We summarized the literature focused on the symptoms and negative long-term consequences of untreated PCOS and the existing options for the treatment. We reviewed the Pubmed and China National Knowledge Infrastructure databases and the relevant literature for the last 20 years, including new results of own (published) research and own experience from treating daily more than 200 PCOS patients. Obesity is one of the most common findings. It can cause abnormal ovulations which can lead to infertility. Important long-term consequences can be adverse pregnancy outcomes. Insulin resistance, important within the pathophysiology of PCOS, predisposes patients to metabolic dysfunction and increased risk of type 2 diabetes mellitus. Lifestyle modifications including dietary changes, exercise and weight loss are first-line interventions for many patients. Well known drug treatments such as metformin, oral contraceptives, etc. should be selected according to the individual situation and patients' needs. Regarding newer methods in the long-term management of PCOS, we found that orlistat may help to achieve weight loss and to improve lipid and glucose metabolism. In addition to pharmacological interventions, long-term standardized individualized management of PCOS patients is needed to achieve fertility and to reduce the risk of metabolic related diseases.

Acknowledgments Supported by Beijing Municipal Administration of Hospitals' Ascent Plan (DFL20181401), Beijing Municipal Administration of Hospitals Clinical Medicine Development of Special Funding Support (XMLX201710).

References

1. Escobar-Morreale HF. Polycystic ovary syndrome: definition, aetiology, diagnosis and treatment. Nat Rev Endocrinol. 2018;14:270–84.
2. Teede HJ, Misso ML, Costello MF, et al. Recommendations from the international evidence-based guideline for the assessment and management of polycystic ovary syndrome. Hum Reprod. 2018;33:1602–18.
3. Chen Z, Tian Q, Qiao J, et al. Guidelines for the diagnosis and treatment of polycystic ovary syndrome in China. Chinese J Obst Gynecol. 2018;53(1):2–6.
4. Conway G, Dewailly D, Diamanti-Kandarakis E, et al. The polycystic ovary syndrome: a position statement from the European Society of Endocrinology. Eur J Endocrinol. 2014;171:P1–29.
5. EA-SPcwg R (2004) Revised 2003 consensus on diagnostic criteria and long-term health risks related to polycystic ovary syndrome. Fertil Steril 81:19–25.
6. Tian X, Ruan X, Mueck AO, et al. Anti-Mullerian hormone levels in women with polycystic ovarian syndrome compared with normal women of reproductive age in China. Gynecol Endocrinol. 2014;30:126–9.
7. Tian X, Ruan X, Mueck AO, et al. Serum anti-Mullerian hormone and insulin resistance in the main phenotypes of non-obese polycystic ovarian syndrome women in China. Gynecol Endocrinol. 2014;30:836–9.
8. Jin J, Ruan X, Hua L, et al. Prevalence of diminished ovarian reserve in Chinese women with polycystic ovary syndrome and sensitive diagnostic parameters. Gynecol Endocrinol. 2017;33:694–7.
9. Cassar S, Teede HJ, Moran LJ, et al. Polycystic ovary syndrome and anti-Mullerian hormone: role of insulin resistance, androgens, obesity and gonadotrophins. Clin Endocrinol. 2014;81:899–906.
10. Ruan X, Kubba A, Aguilar A, et al. Use of cyproterone acetate/ethinylestradiol in polycystic ovary syndrome: rationale and practical aspects. Eur J Contracept Reprod Health Care. 2017;22(3):183–90.
11. Sirmans SM, Pate KA. Epidemiology, diagnosis, and management of polycystic ovary syndrome. Clin Epidemiol. 2014;6:1–13.

12. Fauser BCJM, Tarlatzis BC, Rebar RW, et al. Consensus on women's health aspects of poly-cystic ovary syndrome (PCOS): the Amsterdam ESHRE/ASRM-sponsored 3rd PCOS consensus workshop group. Fertil Steril. 2012;97:28–38.
13. Badawy AS, Elnashar A. Treatment options for polycystic ovary syndrome. Int J Women's Health. 2011;3:25–35.
14. Poretsky L, Piper B. Insulin resistance, hypersensitivity of LH, and dual defect hypothesis for the pathogenesis of polycystic ovary syndrome. Obstet Gynecol. 1994;84:613–21.
15. McCartney CR, Eagleson CR, Marshall JC. Regulation of gonadotropin secretion: implications for polycystic ovary syndrome. Semin Reprod Med. 2002;20:317–36.
16. Lizneva D, Suturina L, Walker W, et al. Criteria, prevalence, and phenotypes of polycystic ovary syndrome. Fertil Steril. 2016;106:6–15.
17. Diamanti-Kandarakis E, Dunaif A. Insulin resistance and the polycystic ovary syndrome revisited: an update on mechanisms and implications. Endocr Rev. 2012;33:981–1030.
18. Norman RJ, Dewailly D, Legro RS, et al. Polycystic ovary syndrome. Lancet. 2007;370:685–97.
19. Ruan X, Mueck AO. Oral contraception for women of middle age. Maturitas. 2015;82:266–70.
20. Lim SS, Davies MJ, Norman RJ, et al. Overweight, obesity and central obesity in women with polycystic ovary syndrome: a systematic review and meta-analysis. Hum Reprod Update. 2012;18:618–37.
21. Dumesic DA, Akopians AL, Madrigal VK, et al. Hyperandrogenism accompanies increased intra-abdominal fat storage in Normal weight polycystic ovary syndrome women. J Clin Endocrinol Metab. 2016;101:4178–88.
22. Arpaci D, Gurkan Tocoglu A, et al. The relationship between epicardial fat tissue thickness and visceral adipose tissue in lean patients with polycystic ovary syndrome. J Ovarian Res. 2015;8:71.
23. Ollila MM, West S, Keinanen-Kiukaaniemi S, et al. Overweight and obese but not normal weight women with PCOS are at increased risk of type 2 diabetes mellitus-a prospective population-based cohort study. Hum Reprod. 2017;32:968.
24. Delitala AP, Capobianco G, Delitala G, et al. Polycystic ovary syndrome, adipose tissue and metabolic syndrome. Arch Gynecol Obstet. 2017;296:405–19.
25. Legro RS, Dodson WC, Kunselman AR, et al. Benefit of delayed fertility therapy with preconception weight loss over immediate therapy in obese women with PCOS. J Clin Endocrinol Metab. 2016;101:2658–66.
26. Zhao Y, Ruan X, Mueck AO. Letrozole combined with low dose highly purified HMG for ovulation induction in clomiphene citrate-resistant infertile Chinese women with polycystic ovary syndrome: a prospective study. Gynecol Endocrinol. 2017;33:462–6.
27. Legro RS, Dodson WC, Kris-Etherton PM, et al. Randomized controlled trial of preconception interventions in infertile women with polycystic ovary syndrome. J Clin Endocrinol Metab. 2015;100:4048–58.
28. Wu H, Ruan X, Jin J, et al. Metabolic profile of Diane-35 versus Diane-35 plus metformin in Chinese PCOS women under standardized life-style changes. Gynecol Endocrinol. 2015;31:548–51.
29. Dokras A, Sarwer DB, Allison KC, et al. Weight loss and lowering androgens predict improvements in health-related quality of life in women with PCOS. J Clin Endocrinol Metab. 2016;101:2966–74.
30. Riley JK, Jungheim ES. Is there a role for diet in ameliorating the reproductive sequelae associated with chronic low-grade inflammation in polycystic ovary syndrome and obesity? Fertil Steril. 2016;106:520–7.
31. McKinnon CJ, Hatch EE, Rothman KJ, et al. Body mass index, physical activity and fecundability in a north American preconception cohort study. Fertil Steril. 2016;106:451–9.
32. Song J, Ruan X, Gu M, et al. Effect of orlistat or metformin in overweight and obese polycystic ovary syndrome patients with insulin resistance. Gynecol Endocrinol. 2018;34:413–7.
33. Ruan X, Song J, Gu M, et al. Effect of Diane-35, alone or in combination with orlistat or metformin in Chinese polycystic ovary syndrome patients. Arch Gynecol Obstet. 2018;297:1557–63.

34. Escobar-Morreale HF, Santacruz E, Luque-Ramirez M, et al. Prevalence of 'obesity-associated gonadal dysfunction' in severely obese men and women and its resolution after bariatric surgery: a systematic review and meta-analysis. Hum Reprod Update. 2017;23:390–408.
35. Lo JC, Feigenbaum SL, Yang J, et al. Epidemiology and adverse cardiovascular risk profile of diagnosed polycystic ovary syndrome. J Clin Endocrinol Metab. 2006;91:1357–63.
36. Cassar S, Misso ML, Hopkins WG, et al. Insulin resistance in polycystic ovary syndrome: a systematic review and meta-analysis of euglycaemic-hyperinsulinaemic clamp studies. Hum Reprod. 2016;31:2619–31.
37. Benham JL, Yamamoto JM, Friedenreich CM, et al. Role of exercise training in polycystic ovary syndrome: a systematic review and meta-analysis. Clin Obes. 2018;8:275–84.
38. American Diabetes Association. Management of diabetes in pregnancy. Diabetes Care. 2017;40(Suppl 1):S114–9.
39. Anagnostis P, Tarlatzis BC, Kauffman RP. Polycystic ovarian syndrome (PCOS): long-term metabolic consequences. Metabolism. 2018;86:33–43.
40. Katulski K, Czyzyk A, Podfigurna-Stopa A, et al. Pregnancy complications in polycystic ovary syndrome patients. Gynecol Endocrinol. 2015;31:87–91.
41. Qin JZ, Pang LH, Li MJ, et al. Obstetric complications in women with polycystic ovary syndrome: a systematic review and meta-analysis. Reprod Biol Endocrinol. 2013;11:56.
42. Naver KV, Grinsted J, Larsen SO, et al. Increased risk of preterm delivery and pre-eclampsia in women with polycystic ovary syndrome and hyperandrogenaemia. BJOG. 2014;121:575–81.
43. Li Y, Ruan X, Wang H, et al. Comparing the risk of adverse pregnancy outcomes of Chinese patients with polycystic ovary syndrome with and without antiandrogenic pretreatment. Fertil Steril. 2018;109:720–7.

Impact of Polycystic Ovarian Syndrome, Metabolic Syndrome, and Obesity on Women's Health

12

Giulia Palla, Maria Magdalena Montt Guevara,
Andrea Giannini, Marta Caretto, Paolo Mannella,
and Tommaso Simoncini

12.1 Introduction

The definition of health given by the World Health Organization is that "Health is a state of complete physical, mental, and social well-being and not merely the absence of disease or infirmity." Being a man or a woman has a significant impact on health, as a result of both biological and gender-related differences.

Cardiovascular disease (CVD) represents the leading cause of death among women in the United States, and it is also the main cause of death in European women in all but two countries (European Cardiovascular Disease Statistics 2017, https://www.cdc.gov/heartdisease/women.htm).

Data have shown that the traditional atherosclerotic CVD risk factors, including diabetes mellitus type 2 (DMT2), smoking, obesity, hypertension, and physical inactivity, present in both women and men, may show a differential impact in women compared to men, as well as the emerging of nontraditional risk factors unique to, or more common in women, may help to recognize the mechanisms leading to gender-specific issues in development and diffusion of CVD between men and women.

For instance, DMT2 and hyperglycemia show a significantly greater risk of coronary death in women compared to men, even after adjusting for age and other CVD risk factors. The etiology of this discrepancy on the basis of gender is unclear; however, one option could be the high prevalence of the metabolic syndrome (MetS) in female diabetic populations. MetS is a well-known risk factor for CVD, and studies have shown that the risk is greater among women than among men, especially after menopause, underlining the strict relationship between steroid hormones, aging, and CVD risk factors.

G. Palla (✉) · M. M. M. Guevara · A. Giannini · M. Caretto · P. Mannella · T. Simoncini
Department of Clinical and Experimental Medicine, University of Pisa, Pisa, Italy

© International Society of Gynecological Endocrinology 2021
A. R. Genazzani et al. (eds.), *Impact of Polycystic Ovary, Metabolic Syndrome and Obesity on Women Health*, ISGE Series,
https://doi.org/10.1007/978-3-030-63650-0_12

In addition, newly identified CVD risk factors, such as gestational diabetes, hypertensive disorders of pregnancy, and polycystic ovarian syndrome (PCOS), may open new and fascinating horizons in understanding emerging, nontraditional CVD risk factors in women.

Furthermore, PCOS, MetS, and obesity determine other health's implications besides CVD risk, including fertility issues, oncology risk, depression, and an overall reduction of quality of life in females.

In this chapter, we aim to evaluate the impact of PCOS, metabolic syndrome, and obesity on women's health.

12.2 Polycystic Ovarian Syndrome (PCOS) and Women's Health

PCOS is one of the most common endocrine disorders in women of reproductive age, affecting up to 10% of adult women.

In women of reproductive age, there are three slightly different definitions of the syndrome. The US National Institutes of Health (NIH) proposed the presence of chronic anovulation and clinical or biochemical hyperandrogenism as diagnostic criteria for PCOS, after having excluded other metabolic or endocrine causes. In 2003, The Rotterdam criteria suggested the presence of polycystic ovarian morphology on ultrasound (12 or more follicles measuring 2–9 mm in diameter in each ovary and/or increased ovarian volume) as additional criteria, with two of three criteria required for the diagnosis. Furthermore, the Androgen Excess and Polycystic Ovary Syndrome Society (AEPCOS) stressed the presence of hyperandrogenism (biochemical or clinical) as main criterion, associated with either chronic oligomenorrhea or polycystic ovarian morphology [1, 2].

PCOS is the main cause of female infertility due to anovulation. This syndrome affects women's health from gestational life until senescence, leading to potential risks that negatively influence quality of life and possibly increase morbidity and mortality rates.

The pathophysiological mechanisms underlying the syndrome are still partially unknown, but probably due to the complex interaction between the functionality of the hypothalamic-pituitary-ovarian axis and metabolic disorders, such as obesity, insulin resistance, and compensatory hyperinsulinemia.

12.2.1 PCOS and Fertility

Infertility, hirsutism, and menstrual disorders are the main clinical problems reported by PCOS women. Regarding infertility, although it is difficult to define the exact pathogenesis of anovulation, many possible mechanisms have been postulated [3]. Ovarian function in infertile PCOS women is mainly characterized by disordered folliculogenesis and anomalous steroidogenesis. Abnormalities in one cause disorder of the other, perpetuating a vicious cycle of anovulation. Ovaries of PCOS women are characterized by multiple small follicles, which are arrested but capable of steroidogenesis. Abnormalities in gonadotrophin and insulin secretion and disordered paracrine function have been identified, including hypersecretion of LH (luteinizing hormone), hyperandrogenemia, and hyperinsulinemia [4]. All these factors seem to be interlinked and together might result in impaired ovarian function. Besides ovarian and central hormonal dysfunctions, with an overactivation of the hypothalamic-pituitary-gonadal axis, other possible anomalies contribute to reproductive failure, namely, obesity. The impact of obesity on reproductive function in PCOS women depends on multiple endocrine mechanisms [5]. Abdominal obesity reflects visceral adiposity, and it is linked to increased circulating insulin levels. Hyperinsulinemia determines reduced sex hormone–binding globulin (SHBG) synthesis with consequent increase of free functional androgen levels. In addition, peripheral adipose tissue is the source of chronic elevation of circulating estrogen caused by the production of estrogens from androgens trough the enzyme aromatase. Hyperleptinemia, which is significantly present in excessive weight, has a detrimental effect on ovarian follicular development and steroidogenesis and thus may contribute to reproduction difficulties in obese women.

Based on these concepts, in the last years, the idea of a PCOS "secondary" to obesity has been postulated [5], as will be further discussed in the following paragraphs.

12.2.2 PCOS and CVD Risk

The presence of insulin resistance and hyperinsulinemia is a common feature in PCOS adult women, with a prevalence of impaired glucose tolerance (IGT) and DMT2, respectively, of 20–37% and 7.5–15%, but the glucose metabolism disorders are probably more frequent when considering only a subset of obese PCOS women [6].

Women with PCOS are more likely to be obese and have an android fat distribution, with higher visceral fat amount, compared with weight-matched controls. Obesity can be found in approximately 50–70% of PCOS adult women. In addition, greater visceral and abdominal adiposity is associated with greater insulin resistance, which is a major predictor of DMT2 and MetS [7].

The cardiometabolic impairment in PCOS starts precociously. Several studies have suggested that adolescent PCOS girls were at substantially higher risk for MetS compared to controls. Besides obesity and insulin resistance, the presence of hyperandrogenemia is an important risk for MetS in young PCOS patients. The odds of having MetS increased approximately fourfold for every quartile increase in free testosterone, independently from BMI and IR [8]. Other data from Hughan et al. showed the presence of increased pulse wave velocity and vascular cell adhesion molecule-1 (VCAM-1) in obese girls with PCOS, which could be the earliest subclinical biomarkers of atherosclerosis [9]. Similarly, young women with PCOS also exhibit a greater risk of hypertension. Several studies indicated an association between hypertension and this endocrinopathy, revealing a twofold prevalence of hypertension in the group with PCOS. The pathogenesis of high blood pressure in PCOS can be determined by the presence of insulin resistance and hyperinsulinemia. They are known to alter vascular smooth muscular cells determining hypertrophy of vascular smooth muscle and reduced compliance, and interfering with the endothelium-related vasodilatation, through the activation of the renin-angiotensin-aldosterone system.

Some studies report that women with PCOS have higher hsCRP (high sensitivity C-reactive protein) levels compared to control, suggesting the hypothesis that cardiometabolic impairment in PCOS patients may be linked to the presence of chronic inflammation [10]. However, it has also been suggested that serum hsCRP concentrations are related to obesity rather than to the presence of PCOS per se, stressing the idea that, at least in a subgroup of PCOS women, obesity is the main determinant of the increased CVD risk.

12.2.3 PCOS and Depression

International research has shown that PCOS has an adverse effect on the patient's quality of life. PCOS women also experience higher rates of depression and anxiety than women in the general population, and this appears to be independent of BMI. Although clinical features of high androgen levels deeply impact health-related quality of life, the association between hirsutism, acne, body image and perception, and depression remain unclear. Similarly, there is limited data on the association between variables such as biochemical hyperandrogenism or infertility and depression [11].

12.2.4 PCOS and Cancer Risk

PCOS is a well-known risk factor for endometrial cancer. The pathogenesis of the increased risk of endometrial cancer in PCOS include multiple determinants, such as obesity, DMT2, hypertension, nulliparity, and familiarity. A meta-analysis including more than 4000 women has evaluated the risk of endometrial cancer in PCOS women compared to the general population [12]. This study underlined that the odds of developing endometrial cancer is almost three times higher in women with PCOS compared to controls. These data translate into a 9% lifetime risk of developing endometrial cancer in PCOS compared to 3% in the general population. Accordingly, a case-control study of endometrial cancer and PCOS has further shown that young women with PCOS (age < 50 years) present a fourfold increased risk of endometrial cancer compared to peers without PCOS. Notably, this increased endometrial cancer risk is halved when adjusted for BMI, emphasizing obesity as a main confounding risk factor for developing endometrial cancer.

There are contradictory evidences regarding the risk of ovarian cancer in PCOS women. A long-term follow-up of UK women with PCOS showed the absence of correlation between PCOS and mortality due to ovarian cancer [13]. However, a case control study reported an increased risk of epithelial ovarian tumor in women with self-reported PCOS compared to controls, even if the pathogenetic mechanism is still unclear.

No associations have been found between PCOS and breast cancer, though obesity and DMT2, which are high prevalent in PCOS, are also major risk factors for breast cancer. Therefore, clinicians should focus their attention on this subset of women to offer correct counselling and possibly apply preventive strategies.

12.3   Metabolic Syndrome (MetS) and Women's Health

MetS is defined in adult population as the presence of three of five of the following criteria: hyperglycemia (glycemia >100 mg/dl), hypertriglyceridemia (triglycerides >150), elevated blood pressure (> 130/85 mmHg), central adiposity (waist circumference >94 cm for white men, >80 cm for white women) [14]. MetS is one of the main health problems, and its worldwide incidence is continually increasing, even if with a large variability among countries.

Even if the prevalence is similar among women and men, the differences within ethnic groups are widely greater in females. There are fewer white women with MetS than white men, but MetS is significantly more frequent in both African American and Mexican American women compared to men. In addition, from the late 1980s to early 2000s, the age-adjusted prevalence of the MetS has increased by 23.5% among women and 2.2% among men, suggesting that the prevalence of MetS in women will quickly outnumber those in men in the near future [15]. Interestingly, increase in blood pressure, waist circumference, and triglyceride levels is the main responsible for the increased MetS prevalence among women.

12.3.1 MetS and Fertility

The effect of MetS on fertility is mainly linked to an altered pituitary-hypothalamic-ovarian function and the presence of overweight and obesity.

Evidences come from studies on diabetic women with secondary amenorrhea due to hypogonadotropic hypogonadism. In diabetic amenorrheic women decreased levels of gonadotropin seem to be related to disorders in gonadotropin-releasing hormone (GnRH) pulse generator, with a decrease in the number of LH pulses, wider pulses, and a decrease in pulse amplitude, compared to eumenorrheic controls [16]. Hyperglycemia is toxic on the neurons of the hypothalamus, and the toxic effect is proportional to the duration of diabetes and GnRH secretion abnormalities. In an immortalized GnRH cell line exposed to hyperglycemia apoptosis results to be increased [17]. In addition to the direct effect of hyperglycemia, other mediators of the central nervous system, including increased opioidergic activity and catecholamine levels, have been implicated in hypogonadism pathophysiology in diabetic patients.

Even in the absence of diabetes, hyperinsulinemia and hyperglycemia play a detrimental role on reproductive female system. Insulin acts on granulosa cells trough insulin receptors, promoting steroidogenesis and follicular development and increasing FSH-stimulated steroid secretion. Moreover, insulin plays a gonadotropic effect on folliculogenesis, driving follicle recruitment and follicular growth.

In addition to the central pituitary effect, hyperglycemia may also determine a negative impact on female fertility due to peripheral effect. Elevated blood glucose is a known determinant of peripheral insulin resistance, which is strongly linked to the pathogenesis of PCOS, as discussed.

Hyperglycemia is also thought to directly affect ovarian function via the presence of advanced glycation products. These molecules link the receptors present in theca and granulosa cells and are probable determinants of impaired ovulatory function in diabetic women.

12.3.2 MetS and CVD Risk

MetS is a complex syndrome in which each component is an independent risk factor for CVD and the combination of these risk factors determines cardiac dysfunction, myocardial infarction, coronary atherosclerosis, endothelial dysfunction, and heart failure, thus increasing the rates and severity of cardiovascular morbidity and mortality. The CVD determinants in MetS include abdominal obesity, high triglycerides, reduced HDL cholesterol, impaired glucose tolerance, and/or hypertension. Besides these factors, other mechanisms have been postulated, including increased circulating levels of pro-inflammatory adipocytokines and the overactivation of the sympathetic nervous system and the renin-angiotensin system. Above all, adipokines have been suggested as key integrative elements linking the traditional CVD risk factors and the molecular mechanisms of increased CVD rates in MetS.

This seems particularly true in peri- and menopausal MetS women. Women in the menopausal transition with excessive body weight and MetS show increased resistin, adipsin, GIP, leptin, IL-6, and FGF21 and PAI-1 levels compared to normal weight ones [18]. Accordingly, several studies found that postmenopausal women with the MetS displayed significantly higher levels of leptin, resistin, adipsin, insulin, and HOMA-IR values in addition to lower adiponectin levels as compared to controls without the MetS [19]. In addition, postmenopausal women with the MetS also displayed higher IL-6 and lower uPA levels, markers of inflammation and endothelial dysfunction, respectively [20]. These detrimental changes may lead to the development and progression of clinically silent atherosclerosis (Fig.12.1).

12.3.3 MetS and Depression

The relationship between depression and MetS has been extensively studied. Several data suggested that a history of major depression is associated with an approximately twofold increased risk of the MetS in both women and men. A 7-year

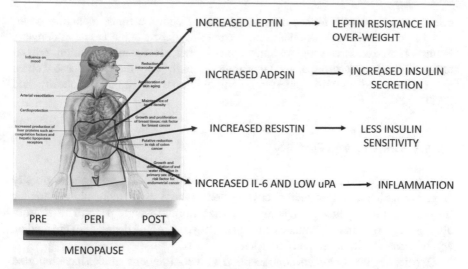

Fig. 12.1 Adipokines and cytokines' effect in insulin metabolism and adiposity during menopausal transition

follow-up study has indicated that women with depressive symptoms at baseline presented a 2.5-fold risk to have MetS at the end of the follow-up, significantly higher compared to men [21].

However, the pathogenesis of the increased risk of MetS in population diagnosed with depression is still unclear. In a recent large population of middle-aged adults, a history of depression was associated with an augmented risk of arterial stiffness assessed peripherally, and this association was partly mediated through MetS. Specifically, approximately one third of the association of depression with arterial stiffness index seemed to be mediated through MetS. In addition, when evaluated the individual components of MetS, abnormal waist circumference was the main contributor of the association between depression and arterial stiffness among women, but not in men [22].

12.4   Obesity: The Key Common Denominator in Women's Health

The rising prevalence of obesity is one of the main concerns in modern society. The World Health Organization estimates that more than 1 billion people are overweight and 300 million are obese. Up to 30% of nonpregnant women ages 20–39 are obese, and 8% of women in reproductive age are extremely obese, putting them at greater risk not only for severe cardiovascular and metabolic disorders but also for pregnancy complications.

Obesity negatively affects women's health in many ways. Being overweight or obese increases the risk of DMT2 and coronary artery disease in women. Furthermore, obesity negatively affects both contraception and fertility. Maternal obesity is linked with higher rates of pregnancy complications, including gestational hypertension and preeclampsia, gestational diabetes, and cesarean delivery. Fetuses from excessive weight women are at higher risk for malformation, prematurity, stillbirth, macrosomia, and labor injury. Finally, children from obese women are at increased risk for long-term complications, as adulthood obesity and DMT2 [23].

12.4.1 Obesity and Fertility

Obesity affects fertility throughout a woman's life. Soon at young age, obesity determines alterations on reproductive system. Obese girls frequently experience the onset of puberty at a younger age than their normal-weight peers. This is probably one of the main determinants, in the last 40 years, of the decrease in the median age of menarche in developed countries.

Obesity negatively affects contraception as well. Previous studies have reported that hormonal contraception methods are less effective in obese women [24]. A retrospective cohort study suggested that women in the highest quartile of body weight had a higher risk of failure than women of lower weight and the risk of failure was greater in women using very low-dose or low-dose oral contraceptives [25]. In contrast, a recent large European cohort study did not demonstrate that BMI alters significantly contraceptive efficacy of oral contraceptive pills [26]. Interesting evidence come from studies evaluating non-oral contraceptive methods in obese women compared to lean controls. A study of more than 1000 women using the levonorgestrel vaginal ring demonstrated increased rates of failure after 1 year of use in the group of heavier patients, weighing 80 kg or more, compared to lean controls. The intrauterine device may be proposed as one of the most reliable contraception options since BMI seems not to influence the efficacy [27].

The association between obesity and menstrual disturbances is strong. Cross-sectional studies report that up to half of overweight and obese women have irregular menses, mostly oligomenorrhea and amenorrhea [28]. In this scenario, the link between obesity and PCOS-related disorders is solid. The potential role of obesity in favoring the development of PCOS has been determined the development of the concept of "PCOS secondary to obesity" [5]. Obesity may impact on the development of PCOS in several ways. The presence of obesity during childhood and adolescence probably plays a key role. It has been extensively suggested that female children and young girls presenting obesity have a significantly higher risk of PCOS compared to lean controls. Moreover, adolescent obese girls with irregular menses present alterations in menses and anovulation which persists for many years, even after weight loss. This can be explained since excess body weight negatively affects hypothalamic-pituitary-gonadal axis during puberty, leading to high LH levels and androgen excess. Adiposity in both girls and boys can determine an early activation of the axis and precocious central activation of puberty. In addition, obesity per se may determine an increased androgen production in both young girls and adults, particularly those with android fat distribution, which is often found in PCOS women. Peripubertal obesity is associated with hyperandrogenemia, evaluated by high total testosterone and/or free androgen index, abnormal LH secretion, and hyperinsulinemia, and BMI is the best indicator for androgen excess [29]. Interestingly, in obese girls, both ovarian and adrenal androgens appear elevated, suggesting that in presence of overweight during puberty, a mixed adrenal and ovarian oversecretion of androgens may favor the development of PCOS.

Another contributing factor for PCOS development in obesity is hyperinsulinemia. Insulin excess is able to directly stimulate adrenal steroidogenesis and increase insulin growth factor-1. In addition, it has been suggested that, in susceptible girls, obesity-related hyperinsulinemia during puberty may cause hyperandrogenemia, by interfering with the normal negative feedback in the hypothalamus and thus enhancing GnRH pulsatility and increasing LH secretion. On the other hand, hyperandrogenemia seems to be able to reduce insulin sensitivity in both fat tissue and muscles. In both subcutaneous tissue and muscles, androgens may interfere with insulin signaling, inhibiting glycogen synthesis and increasing insulin resistance [30].

12.4.2 Obesity and Pregnancy

Obesity has become the major contributor to the global burden of disease worldwide, and its prevalence is growing in pregnant women, even with a large variability among countries and continents. In Australia up to one third of the pregnant women are overweight or obese; accordingly, in the USA it has been recorded a 69% increase in obesity among pregnant women from 1993 to 2003. The obesity rate in pregnant women in Mediterranean countries is far less [31, 32].

Obesity is associated with reduced fecundity mostly but not exclusively related to anovulation. Prolonged time to pregnancy (>12 months) is present also in obese women with regular cycles. Obesity is also linked to poor oocyte and embryos quality in obese women undergoing assisted-reproductive techniques, with a lower live birth rate in obese compared with normal-weight women [33]. Therefore, in overweight and obese women seeking pregnancy, weight-loss interventions, including diet, exercise, and eventually medication treatment, should be addressed as the initial management of infertility women.

Obesity during pregnancy may determine severe complications in both mother, fetus, and newborns, with an overall health-care expenditure, measured by length of hospital stay and use of services to handle long-term complications.

Obese pregnant women have higher risk of fetal anomalies, including neural tube defects and spina bifida, cardiovascular malformations, and cleft lip and palate. Moreover, prepregnancy obesity and excessive gestational weight gain are the main contributor of the development of pregnancy-induced hypertension, late preeclampsia, and gestational diabetes. Obese women are also at higher risk of receiving a cesarean section, and performing obstetrics surgery is more difficult in obese women, besides a higher postoperative thrombotic and infective risk [23].

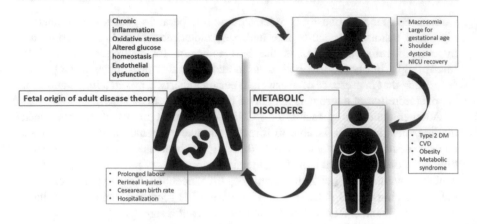

Fig. 12.2 Complex relationship between metabolic disorders in pregnancy and short- and long-term consequences for mother, fetus, and newborn

Bariatric surgery can be the preferred option in obese women seeking pregnancy. Several studies have pointed that after bariatric surgery the possibility of achieving pregnancy is higher and faster. In a large proportion of PCOS women, bariatric surgery determines the normalization of sex hormone levels and the correction of menstrual cycle disorders. Women who had delivered children after surgery showed decreased rates of gestational hypertension, preeclampsia, gestational diabetes, and fetal macrosomia, compared with women who delivered before surgery [34].

In addition, obesity and maternal hyperglycemia during pregnancy may induce intrauterine overnutrition and fetal hyperinsulinemia, resulting in excessive fetal growth. Fetal macrosomia is associated with an increased risk of perinatal morbidity and mortality. Large babies have increased risk of intrapartum complications such as prolonged labor and shoulder dystocia [35]. Moreover, the environmental and metabolic characteristics of intrauterine life deeply influence the individual in the long-term as a child and through adulthood, with possible adverse metabolic consequences, including predisposition to insulin resistance and obesity. Children born to hyperglycemic/hyperinsulinemic intrauterine environment could serve as a unique model of a high-risk population to study fetal programming or early origins of obesity [36] (Fig. 12.2).

12.4.3 Obesity and Cancer Risk

Obesity has been related to a large number of cancers in both women and men. In females, the greater risk is for colon, breast, and endometrium cancer. The physiological mechanisms to explain the effects of adiposity on cancer risk include an increased endogenous production of reactive oxygen species and consequent greater oxidative DNA damage, alterations in carcinogen-metabolizing enzymes, and impairment in endogenous hormone metabolism [37, 38].

In breast and endometrium cancer, abdominal fat may determine alterations in the metabolism of sex steroids, mostly androgens, estrogens, and progesterone. Sex steroids participate in the balance between cellular differentiation, proliferation, and apoptosis, and may also determine the selective growth of preneoplastic and neo-plastic cells.

In addition, obesity, and specifically the accumulation of visceral fat, determines an increased secretion of insulin from pancreas. Consequently, chronically increased insulin levels lead to reduced synthesis of IGF-binding protein-1 and 2 (IGFBP1 and 2), with an increased IGF1 activity. Insulin and IGF1 also strongly stimulate cell proliferation, inhibit apoptosis, and can enhance angiogenesis [39]. Finally, insulin and IGF1 both inhibit the synthesis of SHBG, the major carrier glycoprotein for circulating sex hormones, thus increasing the amount of unbound sex-steroid available for bioactivity, which again can participate in tumorigenesis.

References

1. Broekmans FJ, et al. PCOS according to the Rotterdam consensus criteria: change in prevalence among WHO-II anovulation and association with metabolic factors. BJOG. 2006;113(10):1210–7.
2. Azziz R, et al. The androgen excess and PCOS society criteria for the polycystic ovary syndrome: the complete task force report. Fertil Steril. 2009;91(2):456–88.
3. van der Spuy ZM, Dyer SJ. The pathogenesis of infertility and early pregnancy loss in polycystic ovary syndrome. Best Pract Res Clin Obstet Gynaecol. 2004;18(5):755–71.
4. Bellver J, et al. Polycystic ovary syndrome throughout a woman's life. J Assist Reprod Genet. 2018;35(1):25–39.
5. Pasquali R, Gambineri A. New perspectives on the definition and management of polycystic ovary syndrome. J Endocrinol Investig. 2018;41(10):1123–35.
6. Ehrmann DA, et al. Prevalence of impaired glucose tolerance and diabetes in women with polycystic ovary syndrome. Diabetes Care. 1999;22(1):141–6.
7. Legro RS. Obesity and PCOS: implications for diagnosis and treatment. Semin Reprod Med. 2012;30(6):496–506.
8. Coviello AD, Legro RS, Dunaif A. Adolescent girls with polycystic ovary syndrome have an increased risk of the metabolic syndrome associated with increasing androgen levels independent of obesity and insulin resistance. J Clin Endocrinol Metab. 2006;91(2):492–7.
9. Hughan KS, et al. Early biomarkers of subclinical atherosclerosis in obese adolescent girls with polycystic ovary syndrome. J Pediatr. 2016;168:104–11. e1
10. Oh JY, et al. Serum C-reactive protein levels in normal-weight polycystic ovary syndrome. Korean J Intern Med. 2009;24(4):350–5.
11. Dokras A. Mood and anxiety disorders in women with PCOS. Steroids. 2012;77(4):338–41.
12. Chittenden BG, et al. Polycystic ovary syndrome and the risk of gynaecological cancer: a systematic review. Reprod Biomed Online. 2009;19(3):398–405.
13. Pierpoint T, et al. Mortality of women with polycystic ovary syndrome at long-term follow-up. J Clin Epidemiol. 1998;51(7):581–6.
14. Expert Panel on Detection, E. and A. Treatment of high blood cholesterol in, executive summary of the third report of the National Cholesterol Education Program (NCEP) expert panel on detection, evaluation, and treatment of high blood cholesterol in adults (adult treatment panel III). JAMA, 2001. 285(19): p. 2486–2497.
15. Ford ES, Giles WH, Dietz WH. Prevalence of the metabolic syndrome among US adults: findings from the third National Health and nutrition examination survey. JAMA. 2002;287(3):356–9.

16. Codner E, Merino PM, Tena-Sempere M. Female reproduction and type 1 diabetes: from mechanisms to clinical findings. Hum Reprod Update. 2012;18(5):568–85.
17. Pal L, et al. In vitro evidence of glucose-induced toxicity in GnRH secreting neurons: high glucose concentrations influence GnRH secretion, impair cell viability, and induce apoptosis in the GT1-1 neuronal cell line. Fertil Steril. 2007;88(4 Suppl):1143–9.
18. Palla G, et al. Perimenopause, body fat, metabolism and menopausal symptoms in relation to serum markers of adiposity, inflammation and digestive metabolism. J Endocrinol Investig. 2020;
19. Chedraui P, et al. Circulating leptin, resistin, adiponectin, visfatin, adipsin and ghrelin levels and insulin resistance in postmenopausal women with and without the metabolic syndrome. Maturitas. 2014;79(1):86–90.
20. Chedraui P, et al. Angiogenesis, inflammation and endothelial function in postmenopausal women screened for the metabolic syndrome. Maturitas. 2014;77(4):370–4.
21. Vanhala M, et al. Depressive symptoms predispose females to metabolic syndrome: a 7-year follow-up study. Acta Psychiatr Scand. 2009;119(2):137–42.
22. Dregan, A., et al., Associations between depression, arterial stiffness, and metabolic syndrome among adults in the UK biobank population study: a mediation analysis. JAMA Psychiatry, 2020.
23. ACOG. Practice bulletin no 156: obesity in pregnancy. Obstet Gynecol. 2015;126(6):e112–26.
24. Group, E.C.W. Nutrition and reproduction in women. Hum Reprod Update. 2006;12(3):193–207.
25. Holt VL, Cushing-Haugen KL, Daling JR. Body weight and risk of oral contraceptive failure. Obstet Gynecol. 2002;99(5 Pt 1):820–7.
26. Dinger JC, et al. Oral contraceptive effectiveness according to body mass index, weight, age, and other factors. Am J Obstet Gynecol. 2009;201(3):263.
27. Lash MM, Armstrong A. Impact of obesity on women's health. Fertil Steril. 2009;91(5):1712–6.
28. Practice Committee of American Society for Reproductive, M., Obesity and reproduction: an educational bulletin. Fertil Steril, 2008. 90(5 Suppl): p. S21–9.
29. McCartney CR, et al. Obesity and sex steroid changes across puberty: evidence for marked hyperandrogenemia in pre- and early pubertal obese girls. J Clin Endocrinol Metab. 2007;92(2):430–6.
30. Diamanti-Kandarakis E, Dunaif A. Insulin resistance and the polycystic ovary syndrome revisited: an update on mechanisms and implications. Endocr Rev. 2012;33(6):981–1030.
31. Callaway LK, et al. The prevalence and impact of overweight and obesity in an Australian obstetric population. Med J Aust. 2006;184(2):56–9.
32. Kim SY, et al. Trends in pre-pregnancy obesity in nine states, 1993-2003. Obesity (Silver Spring), 2007 15(4): 986–93.
33. Fedorcsak P, et al. Impact of overweight and underweight on assisted reproduction treatment. Hum Reprod. 2004;19(11):2523–8.
34. American College of, O. and Gynecologists, ACOG practice bulletin no. 105: bariatric surgery and pregnancy. Obstet Gynecol, 2009. 113(6): p. 1405–1413.
35. Committee on Practice, B.-O., Macrosomia: ACOG Practice Bulletin, Number 216. Obstet Gynccol, 2020. 135(1): p. e18-e35.
36. Parlee SD, MacDougald OA. Maternal nutrition and risk of obesity in offspring: the Trojan horse of developmental plasticity. Biochim Biophys Acta. 2014;1842(3):495–506.
37. Manjgaladze M, et al. Effects of caloric restriction on rodent drug and carcinogen metabolizing enzymes: implications for mutagenesis and cancer. Mutat Res. 1993;295(4–6):201–22.
38. Muskhelishvili L, et al. Age-related changes in the intrinsic rate of apoptosis in livers of diet-restricted and ad libitum-fed B6C3F1 mice. Am J Pathol. 1995;147(1):20–4.
39. Khandwala HM, et al. The effects of insulin-like growth factors on tumorigenesis and neoplastic growth. Endocr Rev. 2000;21(3):215–44.

Pregnancy Outcome and Metabolic Syndrome

13

Serena Ottanelli, Serena Simeone, Caterina Serena,
Marianna Pina Rambaldi, Sara Zullino,
and Federico Mecacci

13.1 Introduction

Obesity and metabolic disorders in women of reproductive age is a growing health problem; in the USA, pre-pregnancy obesity in women increased from 13.0% in 1993–1994 to 22.0% in 2002–2003, while the rate of obese European women ranges between 6 and 37% [1, 2].

Recent evidence indicates that approximately 10–30% of obese individuals have no metabolic abnormalities that describe MS (metabolic syndrome) such as impaired glucose tolerance, insulin resistance, dyslipidemia, and hypertension, so despite their excessive body fat, they are "metabolically healthy" [3].

Clinically, overweight risk may differ depending on body adipose tissue distribution, as central or "unhealthy" obesity leads to increased lipolysis, insulin resistance, and reduction of triglycerides storage, in contrast with lower limb adipose distribution with normal level of essential fatty acids (NEFA) or "healthy obesity" [4].

The ectopic fat accumulation is associated with lipotoxicity from lipid oxidation: the consequent oxidative stress causes maternal endothelial/vascular stress, increased inflammation, reduction of trophoblast invasion, and altered placental development [5]. Therefore maternal central obesity is associated with an increased risk of maternal and perinatal complications and also impacts the long-term health of the offspring leading to increased risk of childhood obesity and metabolic disorders given the critical role of intrauterine development [6, 7].

S. Ottanelli (✉) · S. Simeone · C. Serena · M. P. Rambaldi · S. Zullino · F. Mecacci
Division of Obstetrics and Gynecology, Department of Biomedical, Experimental, and Clinical Sciences, Careggi University Hospital, University of Florence, Florence, Italy

© International Society of Gynecological Endocrinology 2021
A. R. Genazzani et al. (eds.), *Impact of Polycystic Ovary, Metabolic Syndrome and Obesity on Women Health*, ISGE Series,
https://doi.org/10.1007/978-3-030-63650-0_13

13.2   Metabolic Syndrome, Obesity, and Pregnancy Complications

MS detection in pregnancy is a controversial issue, because the criteria for identifying MS overlap with the physiologic metabolic changes of pregnancy that disappear after delivery (insulin resistance, increased fat mass, hyperlipidemia, prothrombotic, and proinflammatory state) and some MS markers (obesity, high triglycerides, total cholesterol, and LDL cholesterol levels) show an increasing trend during gestation and there are no defined cut-offs in pregnancy [8].

Therefore there are very few studies about maternal metabolic syndrome in pregnancy examined as a whole phenotype and about its association with birth outcomes.

It is well known that obesity, as the main component of MS, is a relevant risk factor for pregnancy complications from conception to postpartum, and the risks are amplified with a higher maternal BMI. It has been estimated that one quarter of pregnancy complications are attributable to maternal overweight/obesity [9].

Overweight and obese women have an increased risk of spontaneous miscarriage [10] and congenital anomalies [11, 12], and the risks increase with the severity of obesity.

Obesity is strongly associated with the presence of gestational diabetes (GDM), preterm birth (both spontaneous and medically indicated), and intrauterine fetal death [13].

Compared with women with normal pre-pregnancy BMI, obese pregnant women are at increased risk of preeclampsia (PE) and gestational hypertension; the risk of preeclampsia rises as the pre-pregnancy BMI increases, and is closely associated with impaired insulin sensitivity [14, 15].

Several studies have confirmed that maternal obesity increases the risk of fetal macrosomia [16], independent of a diabetic metabolic state [17]. It has been demonstrated that offspring of obese mothers have a significantly higher percent of body fat mass and are more metabolically unhealthy (higher cord blood insulin, leptin, insulin resistance indexes, and IL6).

Furthermore, obesity is associated with increased risk of intrapartum complication; cesarean sections are more commonly performed in obese mothers due to preeclampsia, fetal distress, cephalopelvic disproportion, and failure to progress in labor [18, 19].

These women also have a higher incidence of wound infection and wound healing abnormalities with increased surgery-associated morbidity [20].

Only few studies to date have evaluated metabolic syndrome in pregnancy in relation to reproductive outcomes, and most of the authors have used accepted definition of MS for the adult population.

There is evidence that an unfavorable, atherogenic lipid profile during or prior to pregnancy is associated with increased risk for GDM, PE, large for gestational age (LGA) babies, and spontaneous preterm birth [21–23], and in a small prospective study, multiparous women with MS in early pregnancy had a threefold increased risk for preterm birth [24].

A recent study assessed the association between MS, measured at 15 weeks' gestation, and a range of pregnancy complications in low-risk, nulliparous women recruited to the multicenter, international prospective Screening for Pregnancy Endpoints (SCOPE) study. The research found that 12.3% of women had metabolic syndrome in early pregnancy defined according to the International Diabetes Federation criteria for adults. More than half of the women who had MS in early pregnancy developed a pregnancy complication, compared to one third of those who did not have MS [25].

In particular women with MS were at an increased risk for PE by a factor of 1.63 and for GDM by 3.71, after adjusting for a range of demographic and lifestyle variables; increase in BMI combined with MS increased the risk for GDM and decreased the probability of an uncomplicated pregnancy [26].

13.3   Inflammation, Insulin Resistance, and Oxidative Stress

Metabolic syndrome is characterized with a triad of closely linked metabolic aspects that are implicated in pregnancy complications: inflammation, insulin resistance, and dyslipidemia.

As an organ of exchange and dependent on maternal health, the placenta has a critical role in this metabolic milieu.

Placental dysfunction is implicated in most of the poor pregnancy outcomes associated with maternal obesity, such as preeclampsia or fetal growth anomalies, and is also known to be involved in the programming of later-life diseases.

Inflammation Obesity is a well-known low-grade inflammatory state and can interfere with placental development and function altering inflammatory pathways; it is associated with an increased production of pro-inflammatory mediators by macrophages in the adipose tissue, an increase in circulating levels of inflammatory markers such as tumor necrosis factor alpha (TNFα), interleukin 6 (IL-6) [27, 28], and increased macrophage accumulation in both the adipose tissue and the placenta of obese pregnant women.

An increasing body of both experimental and clinical evidence suggests that pro-inflammatory cytokines stimulate signaling pathways in placental cells (trophoblasts, endothelial cells, and stromal cells), leading to cellular stress and dysfunction and influence placental nutrient transport functions [29, 30]. In particular IL-6 and TNFα stimulate amino acid transport [29, 31] and fatty acid uptake into primary trophoblasts [30].

This proinflammatory milieu in the placenta leads to the impairment of overall placental development and function and produces increased free fatty acid (FFA) delivery to the fetal circulation, which is expected to alter fetal growth and development [32], and has been linked to long-term changes in offspring metabolism [33].

Interesting studies have demonstrated that inflammation is active also in the vasculature of obese women and that it is associated with neutrophil infiltration. Specifically, the percentage of vessels stained for markers of inflammation was highly positively correlated with BMI. In summary, the vessel phenotype of obese women appears to be very similar to the vessel phenotype of preeclamptic women, suggesting that vascular inflammation could act as the underlying connection between obesity and preeclampsia [34].

Insulin resistance Increased insulin resistance is part of the altered physiology of pregnancy. It is necessary to promote fetal growth and development. The physiologic rise in insulin resistance throughout the pregnancy slowly increases during the second half of pregnancy and rapidly decreases after delivery. The progressive insulin resistance during gestation involves a combination of increased maternal adiposity and the effects of the hormonal placental products. Obesity and metabolic syndrome before pregnancy are characterized by higher insulin resistance; therefore these women start pregnancy in a less insulin sensitive state.

It is well known that insulin resistance, together with a reduced beta cell capacity, is the most important feature in GDM pathogenesis and is therefore significantly associated with fetal overnutrition and macrosomia as a consequence of high fetal nutrient availability and placental transport of nutrients [35, 36]. Maternal hyperinsulinemia in the third trimester determines the activation of the main insulin signaling pathways in the placenta (p-ERK and p-Akt) and increases some placental lipid carriers, which might enhance fetal lipid transport and storage, resulting in increased fetal adiposity and probably contributing to the fetal programming of obesity [37].

Maternal insulin resistance has been hypothesized to contribute to altering placental development in pregnancies complicated by obesity and diabetes; in fact recent studies support an association between preeclampsia and increased insulin resistance [38–40], and reduced insulin sensitivity has also been hypothesized to contribute to the pathophysiology of the disease.

There is evidence from recent studies that increased insulin resistance has negative effects on placental growth and efficiency. It is well known that insulin may enhance villous proliferation and increase placental size determining a placental hypertrophy, which is a typical feature of diabetic pregnancies. However villous immaturity, defined as placentas with inadequate or absent terminal villi, was one of the most frequently reported placental abnormalities in pregnancies with increased insulin resistance [41, 42]. A high proportion of immature villi may decrease the efficiency of placental transport resulting in placental insufficiency [43] and consequently higher incidence of preeclampsia, fetal growth restriction, and fetal death.

Moreover insulin resistance can affect maternal endothelial function, and some data show that angiogenic and insulin-dependent pathways may influence each other [44, 45], and it is well known that dysfunction of the vascular endothelium and dysregulation of angiogenesis are thought to play a central role in the pathophysiology of preeclampsia.

Oxidative stress. Oxidative stress has recently been recognized as a key mechanism in insulin resistance; many studies demonstrated that increased oxidative stress is associated with insulin resistance pathogenesis by insulin signals inhibition and adipokine dysregulation [46, 47]. Several studies showed that reactive oxygen species (ROS) levels are increased in obesity, especially in abdominal obesity which is the major component of metabolic syndrome [48, 49].

Pregnancy itself is characterized by increased oxidative stress; in fact ROS regulate many cellular functions including autophagy, differentiation, and inflammation. Excessive ROS production can be harmful, causing oxidative damage to DNA, proteins, and cell membranes. There is evidence that increased placental oxidative stress is a mark of several obstetric pathologies including preeclampsia and intrauterine growth restriction (IUGR) in pregnancies complicated by maternal diabetes or obesity [50].

In recent years an association between chronic oxidative stress and placental senescence has been found; these aspects seem to have an important role in pathogenesis of placental insufficiency and preeclampsia [51, 52]. Moreover excessive ROS production in endothelium can affect vasodilation by inhibiting the expression and function of endothelial nitric oxide synthase [53] and may even be involved with this process in the pathogenesis of preeclampsia [54]. Obesity is associated with excess circulating fatty acids, which can affect placental mitochondrial function. In fact placental villous tissues from overweight and obese women have a 6- and 14-fold increase, respectively, in mitochondrial ROS production [55].

Though data may be limited, oxidative stress and mitochondrial dysfunction can be proposed as mechanisms that mediate placental dysfunction in maternal obesity and insulin resistance.

13.4 Prevention of Adverse Obstetric Complications

Both lifestyle (diet and physical exercise) and pharmacological interventions (metformin, inositol) have been suggested to prevent the development of metabolic complications.

The majority of studies on dietary and lifestyle interventions during pregnancy failed to show significant benefits in maternal and fetal outcomes; potential reasons for these results include the substantial heterogeneity between the characteristics of the participants, the interventions, the settings, the inability to estimate patient adherence, and a tardy intervention start during gestation.

Pre-conceptional and interpregnancy periods should focus on promoting maternal weight loss in overweight and obese women, which may potentially reduce the risk of gestational diabetes and LGA, even with moderate changes [56, 57]. If weight loss is not achieved, it is also important to avoid at least weight gain between pregnancies, as gestational diabetes risk directly increases with a rise in BMI in retrospective cohorts [58].

Concerning polycystic ovary syndrome (PCOS), a recent metanalysis of 12 RCTs comparing 608 women has demonstrated the efficacy of lifestyle interventions plus metformin vs lifestyle interventions plus placebo. Both approaches were significantly associated to lower BMI, lower subcutaneous adipose tissue, and increased number of menstrual cycles after 6 months [59]. Myo-inositol acts on a side pathway influencing insulin sensitivity, and randomized controlled trials have reported its efficacy in reducing basal insulin levels, testosterone concentration, and HOMA index in PCOS [60]. The importance of a pre-conceptional period is underlined by the observation that diet and physical activity in obese women during pregnancy are poorly associated with prevention of adverse outcomes, such as gestational diabetes, as reported by the Limit Study [61, 62]. Multicenter and individualized interventional studies have extended observation to FPG, maternal-neonatal outcomes, risk of CS, and HOMA-IR, demonstrating that in-pregnancy intervention results in no significant preventive effects [63, 64]. According to the Cochrane review on 23 RCTs, the prevention of gestational diabetes mellitus in pregnancy is only potentially associated with reduction in CS, but not with the rate of PE, LGA, and perinatal mortality [65]. In-pregnancy interventions for obese women may be directed toward preventing excessive weight gain rather than reducing BMI, as a gestational weight gain of over 5 kg has been reported as a risk factor for macrosomia (87.8% sensitivity, 54.7% specificity) and hypertensive disorders of pregnancy (70% sensitivity, 48.4% specificity) [66].

The favorable effects of metformin on pregnancy outcome have been extensively studied both in obese and PCOS women. Even if meta-analyses have reported a consistent reduction of GDM risk, recurrent pregnancy loss, and preterm birth [67], other experiences provide conflicting data [68, 69]. One of the most interesting effects of metformin on obese and hyperinsulinemic patients is the prevention of preeclampsia: the reduction of the inflammation state and improvement of endothelial cell function reduce the expression of vascular cell adhesion molecules, and the support of the whole-blood vessel angiogenesis is able to reduce production of sFlt-1 and soluble endoglin, which are strictly involved in the pathogenesis of preeclampsia [35, 70]. Metformin has been suggested to potentially improve the offspring body composition at 2 years of age after gestational diabetes when compared with insulin, lowering the mid-upper arm circumferences, the subscapular, and biceps skinfolds, thus regulating fat distribution by reducing the visceral fat deposition [71]. Nevertheless, long-term effects have not yet been studied.

Myo-inositol is a post-receptorial mediator of insulin. It translocates GLUT4 receptor on the cell membrane and participates in the cholinergic way of insulin secretion [72]. RCTs have reported that its prenatal supplementation is associated with reducing the GDM rate, but has no effect on gestational hypertension, LGA, perinatal mortality, or composite severe neonatal outcome [73–76].

Aspirin seems promising for preventing preeclampsia also in obese women: a body mass index >30 kg/m^2 is classified as a moderate risk factor by ACOG and may be considered a clinical indication for prophylactic administration [77].

References

1. Kim SY, Dietz PM, England L, Morrow B, Callaghan WM. Trends in pre-pregnancy obesity in nine states, 1993–2003. Obesity (Silver Spring) 2007;15:986–993.
2. Berghofer A, Pischon T, Reinhold T, Apovian CM, Sharma AM, Willich SN. Obesity prevalence from a European perspective: a systematic review. BMC Public Health. 2008;8:200.
3. Velho S, Paccaud F, Waeber G, Vollenweider P, Marques-Vidal P. Metabolically healthy obesity: different prevalences using different criteria. Eur J Clin Nutr. 2010;64:1043–51.

4. Denis GV, Obin MS. 'Metabolically healthy obesity': origins and implications. Mol Asp Med. 2013;34:59–70.
5. Jarvie E, Hauguel-de-Mouzon S, Nelson SM, Sattar N, Catalano PM, Freeman DJ. Lipotoxicity in obese pregnancy and its potential role in adverse pregnancy outcome and obesity in the offspring. Clin Sci (Lond). 2010;119(3):123–9.
6. Moussa HN, Alrais MA, Leon MG, Abbas EL, Sibai BM. Obesity epidemic: impact from preconception to postpartum. Future Sci OA. 2016;2(3):FSO137.
7. Catalano PM, Shankar K. Obesity and pregnancy: mechanisms of short term and long term adverse consequences for mother and child. BMJ. 2017 Feb 8;356:j1.
8. Bartha JL, Bugatto FG, Macías RF, González NL, Delgado RC, Vivancos BH. Metabolic syndrome in Normal and complicated pregnancies. Eur J Obstet Gynecol Reprod Biol. 2008;137:178–84.
9. Santos S, Voerman E, Amiano P, Barros H, Beilin LJ, Bergström A. Impact of maternal body mass index and gestational weight gain on pregnancy complications: an individual participant data meta-analysis of European. N Am Aust Cohorts BJOG. 2019;126(8):984.
10. Boots CE, Bernardi LA, Stephenson MD. Frequency of euploid miscarriage is increased in obese women with recurrent early pregnancy loss. Fertil Steril. 2014;102:455–9.
11. Gilboa SM, Correa A, Botto LD, et al; National Birth Defects Prevention Study. Association between prepregnancy body mass index and congenital heart defects. Am J Obstet Gynecol 2010; 202(1):51, e1–e51, e10.
12. Werler MM, Louik C, Shapiro S, Mitchell AA. Prepregnant weight in relation to risk of neural tube defects. JAMA. 1996;275(14):1089–92.
13. Aune D, Saugstad OD, Henriksen T, Tonstad S. Maternal body mass index and the risk of fetal death, stillbirth, and infant death: a systematic review and meta-analysis. JAMA. 2014; 311(15):1536–46.)
14. O'Brien TE, Ray JG, Chan WS. Maternal body mass index and the risk of preeclampsia: a systematic overview. Epidemiology. 2003;14(3):368–74.
15. Bodnar LM, Catov JM, Klebanoff MA, Ness RB, Roberts JM. Prepregnancy body mass index and the occurrence of severe hypertensive disorders of pregnancy. Epidemiology. 2007;18(2):234–9.
16. Yu Z, Han S, Zhu J, Sun X, Ji C, Guo X. Pre-pregnancy body mass index in relation to infant birth weight and offspring overweight/obesity: a systematic review and meta-analysis. PLoS One. 2013;8(4):e61627.
17. Catalano PM, McIntyre HD, Cruickshank JK, McCance DR, Dyer AR, Metzger BE, Lowe LP, Trimble ER, Coustan DR, Hadden DR, Persson B, Hod M, Oats JJ, HAPO Study Cooperative Research Group. The hyperglycemia and adverse pregnancy outcome study: Associations of GDM and obesity with pregnancy outcomes. Diabetes Care. 2012 Apr; 35(4):780–786.
18. Lisonkova S, Muraca GM, Potts J, et al. Association between prepregnancy body mass index and severe maternal morbidity. JAMA. 2017;318:1777–86.
19. Kawakita T, Reddy UM, Landy HJ, Iqbal SN, Huang CC, Grantz KL. Indications for primary cesarean delivery relative to body mass index. Am J Obstet Gynecol. 2016;215:515e1–9.
20. Kim SS, Zhu Y, Grantz KL, et al. Obstetric and neonatal risks among obese women without chronic disease. Obstet Gynecol. 2016;128:104–12.
21. Moayeri M, Heida KY, Franx A, Spiering W, de Laat MW, Oudijk MA. Maternal lipid profile and the relation with spontaneous preterm delivery: a systematic review. Arch Gynecol Obstet. 2017;295:313–23.
22. Ryckman KK, Spracklen CN, Smith CJ, Robinson JG, Saftlas AF. Maternal lipid levels during pregnancy and gestational diabetes: a systematic review and meta-analysis. BJOG. 2015;122:643–51.
23. Barrett HL, Dekker Nitert M, McIntyre HD, Callaway LK. Normalizing metabolism in diabetic pregnancy: is it time to target lipids? Diabetes Care. 2014;37:1484–93.
24. Chatzi L, Plana E, Daraki V, Karakosta P, Alegkakis D, Tsatsanis C, et al. Metabolic syndrome in early pregnancy and risk of preterm birth. Am J Epidemiol. 2009;170:829–36.
25. Grieger JA, Bianco-Miotto T, Grzeskowiak LE, Leemaqz SQ, Poston L, McCowan MLID.

26. Kenny LC, Myers JE, Walker JJ, Dekker GA, Roberts CT. Metabolic syndrome in pregnancy and risk for adverse pregnancy outcomes: A prospective cohort of nulliparous women PLoS Med. 2018:15(12).
27. Cancello R, Clément K. Is obesity an inflammatory illness? Role of low-grade inflammation and macrophage infiltration in human white adipose tissue. BJOG. 2006;113(10):1141–7.
28. Gregor MF, Hotamisligil GS. Inflammatory mechanisms in obesity. Annu Rev Immunol. 2011;29:415–45.
29. Jones HN, Jansson T, Powell TL. IL-6 stimulates system a amino acid transporter activity in trophoblast cells through STAT3 and increased expression of SNAT2. Am J Physiol Cell Physiol. 2009;297:C1228–35.
30. Lager S, Jansson N, Olsson AL, Wennergren M, Jansson T, Powell TL. Effect of IL-6 and TNF-alpha on fatty acid uptake in cultured human primary trophoblast cells. Placenta. 2011;32(2):121–7.
31. Aye IL, Ramirez VI, Gaccioli F, Lager S, Jansson T, Powell T. Activation of placental inflammasomes in pregnant women with high BMI. Reprod Sci. 2013;20(S3):73A–73.
32. Shekhawat P, Bennett MJ, Sadovsky Y, Nelson DM, Rakheja D, Strauss AW. Human placenta metabolizes fatty acids: implications for fetal fatty acid oxidation disorders and maternal liver diseases. Am J Physiol Endocrinol Metab. 2003;284(6):E1098–105.
33. Masuyama H, Hiramatsu Y. Effects of a high-fat diet exposure in utero on the metabolic syndrome-like phenomenon in mouse offspring through epigenetic changes in adipocytokine gene expression. Endocrinology. 2012;153:2823–30.
34. Shah TJ, Courtney EL, Walsh SW. Neutrophil infiltration and systemic vascular inflammation in obese women. Reprod Sci. 2010;17(2):116–24.
35. Romero R, Erez O, Hüttemann M, Maymon E, Panaitescu B, Conde-Agudelo A, Pacora P, Yoon BH, Grossman LI. Metformin, the aspirin of the 21st century: its role in gestational diabetes mellitus, prevention of preeclampsia and cancer, and the promotion of longevity. Am J Obstet Gynecol. 2017 Sep;217(3):282–302.
36. Brett KE, Ferraro ZM, Yockell-Lelievre J, Gruslin A, Adamo KB. Maternal-fetal nutrient transport in pregnancy pathologies: the role of the placenta. Int J Mol Sci. 2014 Sep 12;15(9):16153–85.
37. Ruiz-Palacios M, Ruiz-Alcaraz AJ, Sanchez-Campillo M, Larqué E. Role of insulin in placental transport of nutrients in gestational diabetes mellitus. Ann Nutr Metab. 2017;70:16–25.
38. Valdés E, Sepúlveda-Martínez A, Manukián B. Parra-Cordero M assessment of pregestational insulin resistance as a risk factor of preeclampsia. Gynecol Obstet Investig. 2014;77(2):111–6.
39. Hauth JC, Clifton RG, Roberts JM, Myatt L, Spong CY, Leveno KJ, Varner MW, Wapner RJ, Thorp JM Jr, Mercer BM, Peaceman AM, Ramin SM, Carpenter MW, Samuels P, Sciscione A, Tolosa JE, Saade G, Sorokin Y, Anderson GD. Maternal insulin resistance and preeclampsia. Am J Obstet Gynecol. 2011; 204(4):327
40. Alsnes IV, Janszky I, Forman MR, Vatten LJ, Økland I A population-based study of associations between preeclampsia and later cardiovascular risk factors. Am J Obstet Gynecol. 2014; 211(6):657
41. Huang L, Liu J, Feng L, Chen Y, Zhang J, Wang W. Maternal pre-pregnancy obesity is associated with higher risk of placental pathological lesions. Placenta. 2014;35:563–9.
42. Huynh J, Dawson D, Roberts D, Bentley-Lewis R. A systematic review of placental pathology in maternal diabetes mellitus. Placenta. 2015;36:101–14.
43. Tanaka K, Yamada K, Matsushima M, Izawa T, Furukawa S, Kobayashi Y, Iwashita M. Increased maternal insulin resistance promotes placental growth and decreases placental efficiency in pregnancies with obesity and gestational diabetes mellitus. J Obstet Gynaecol Res. 2018 Jan;44(1):74–80.
44. Autiero M, Waltenberger J, Communi D, Kranz A, Moons L, Lambrechts D, et al. Role of PlGF in the intra-and intermolecular cross talk between the VEGF receptors Flt1 and Flk1. Nat Med. 2003;9:936–43.
45. Thadhani R, Ecker JL, Mutter WP, Wolf M, K. Smirnakis KV, Sukhatme VP. Insulin resistance and alterations in angiogenesis: additive insults that may lead to preeclampsia. Hypertension. 2004;43:988–92.

46. Furukawa S, Fujita T, Shimabukuro M, Iwaki M, Yamada Y, Nakajima Y, Nakayama O, Makishima M, Matsuda M, Shimomura I. J Clin Invest. 2004 Dec;114(12):1752–61.
47. Houstis N, Rosen ED, Lander ES. Reactive oxygen species have a causal role in multiple forms of insulin resistance. Nature. 2006 Apr 13;440(7086):944–8.
48. Vincent HK, Taylor AG. Biomarkers and potential mechanisms of obesity-induced oxidant stress in humans. Int J Obes. 2006;30:400–18.
49. Boden G. Obesity, insulin resistance, and free fatty acids. Curr Opin Endocrinol Diabetes Obes. 2011;18:139–43.
50. Gupta S, Agarwal A, Sharma RK. The role of placental oxidative stress and lipid peroxidation in preeclampsia. Obstet Gynecol Surv. 2005;60(12):807–16.
51. Sultana Z, Maiti K, Dedman L, Smith R. Is there a role for placental senescence in the genesis of obstetric complications and fetal growth restriction? Am J Obstet Gynecol. 2018 Feb;218(2S):S762–73.
52. Sultana Z, Maiti K, Aitken J, Morris J, Dedman L, Smith R Oxidative stress, placental ageing-related pathologies and adverse pregnancy outcomes. Am J Reprod Immunol. 2017;77(5).
53. Farrow KN, Lakshminrusimha S, Reda WJ, Wedgwood S, Czech L, Gugino SF, Davis JM, Russell JA, Steinhorn RH. Superoxide dismutase restores eNOS expression and function in resistance pulmonary arteries from neonatal lambs with persistent pulmonary hypertension. Am J Physiol Lung Cell Mol Physiol. 2008;295(6):L979–87.
54. Matsubara K, Higaki T, Matsubara Y, Nawa A. Nitric oxide and reactive oxygen species in the pathogenesis of preeclampsia. Int J Mol Sci. 2015;16(3):4600–14.
55. Mele J, Muralimanoharan S, Maloyan A, Myatt L. Impaired mitochondrial function in human placenta with increased maternal adiposity. Am J Physiol Endocrinol Metab. 2014;307(5):E419–25.
56. Weight change and the risk of gestational diabetes in obese women. Glazer NL, Hendrickson AF, Schellenbaum GD, Mueller BA. Epidemiology. 2004;15(6):733–7.
57. Villamor E, Cnattingius S. Interpregnancy weight change and risk of adverse pregnancy outcomes: a population-based study. Lancet. 2006;368(9542):1164–70. https://doi.org/10.1016/S0140-6736(06)69473-7.
58. Ehrlich SF, Hedderson MM, Feng J, Davenport ER, Gunderson EP, Ferrara A. Change in body mass index between pregnancies and the risk of gestational diabetes in a second pregnancy. Obstet Gynecol. 2011;117(6):1323–30.
59. Naderpoor N, Shorakae S, de Courten B, Misso ML, Moran LJ, Teede HJ. Metformin and lifestyle modification in polycystic ovary syndrome: systematic review and meta-analysis. Hum Reprod Update. 2015;21(5):560–74.
60. Unfer V, Facchinetti F, Orrù B, Giordani B, Nestler J. Myo-inositol effects in women with PCOS: a meta-analysis of randomized controlled trials. Endocr Connect. 2017 Nov;6(8):647–58.
61. Poston L, Caleyachetty R, Cnattingius S, Corvalán C, Uauy R, Herring S, Gillman MW. Preconceptional and maternal obesity: epidemiology and health consequences. Lancet Diabetes Endocrinol. 2016 Dec;4(12):1025–36.
62. Dodd JM, Cramp C, Sui Z, Yelland LN, Deussen AR, Grivell RM, Moran LJ, Crowther CA, Turnbull D, McPhee AJ, Wittert G, Owens JA, Robinson JS; LIMIT Randomised Trial Group. The effects of antenatal dietary and lifestyle advice for women who are overweight or obese on maternal diet and physical activity: the LIMIT randomised trial. BMC Med 2014;12:161.
63. Simmons D, Devlieger R, van Assche A, Jans G, Galjaard S, Corcoy R, Adelantado JM, Dunne F, Desoye G, Harreiter J, Kautzky-Willer A, Damm P, Mathiesen ER, Jensen DM, Andersen L, Lapolla A, Dalfrà MG, Bertolotto A, Wender-Ozegowska E, Zawiejska A, Hill D, Snoek FJ. Jelsma JG, van Poppel MN effect of physical activity and/or healthy eating on GDM risk: the DALI lifestyle study. J Clin Endocrinol Metab. 2017 Mar 1;102(3):903–13.
64. Koivusalo SB, Rönö K, Klemetti MM, Roine RP, Lindström J, Erkkola M, Kaaja RJ, Pöyhönen-Alho M, Tiitinen A, Huvinen E, Andersson S, Laivuori H, Valkama A, Meinilä J, Kautiainen H, Eriksson JG, Stach-Lempinen B. Gestational diabetes mellitus can be prevented by lifestyle intervention: the Finnish gestational diabetes prevention study (RADIEL): a randomized controlled trial. Diabetes Care. 2016 Jan;39(1):24–30.

65. Shepherd E, Gomersall JC, Tieu J, Han S, Crowther CA, Middleton P. Combined diet and exercise interventions for preventing gestational diabetes mellitus. Cochrane Database Syst Rev. 2017 Nov 13;11(11):CD010443.
66. Barquiel B, Herranz L, Meneses D, Moreno Ó, Hillman N, Burgos MÁ, Bartha JL. Optimal gestational weight gain for women with gestational diabetes and morbid obesity. Matern Child Health J. 2018 Sep;22(9):1297–305.
67. Zeng XL, Zhang YF, Tian Q, Xue Y, An RF. Effects of metformin on pregnancy outcomes in women with polycystic ovary syndrome: a meta-analysis. Medicine (Baltimore). 2016 Sep;95(36):e4526.
68. Chiswick C, Reynolds RM, Denison F, Drake AJ, Forbes S, Newby DE, Walker BR, Quenby S, Wray S, Weeks A, Lashen H, Rodriguez A, Murray G, Whyte S, Norman JE. Effect of metformin on maternal and fetal outcomes in obese pregnant women (EMPOWaR): a randomised, double-blind, placebo-controlled trial. Lancet Diabetes Endocrinol. 2015 Oct;3(10):778–86.
69. Syngelaki A, Nicolaides KH, Balani J, Hyer S, Akolekar R, Kotecha R, Pastides A, Shehata H. Metformin versus placebo in obese pregnant women without diabetes mellitus. N Engl J Med. 2016;374(5):434–43. doi.
70. Brownfoot FC, Hastie R, Hannan NJ, Cannon P, Tuohey L, Parry LJ, Senadheera S, Illanes SE, Kaitu'u-Lino TJ, Tong S. Metformin as a prevention and treatment for preeclampsia: effects on soluble fms-like tyrosine kinase 1 and soluble endoglin secretion and endothelial dysfunction. Am J Obstet Gynecol. 2016;214(3):356.
71. Rowan JA, Rush EC, Plank LD, Lu J, Obolonkin V, Coat S, Hague WM. Metformin in gestational diabetes: the offspring follow-up (MiG TOFU): body composition and metabolic outcomes at 7-9 years of age. BMJ Open Diabetes Res Care. 2018;6(1):e000456.
72. Bizzarri M, Fuso A, Dinicola S, Cucina A, Bevilacqua A. Pharmacodynamics and pharmacokinetics of inositol(s) in health and disease. Expert Opin Drug Metab Toxicol. 2016;12(10):1181–96.
73. Martis R, Crowther CA, Shepherd E, Alsweiler J, Downie MR, Brown J. Treatments for women with gestational diabetes mellitus: an overview of Cochrane systematic reviews. Cochrane Database Syst Rev. 2018;8(8):CD012327.
74. D'Anna R, Scilipoti A, Giordano D, Caruso C, Cannata ML, Interdonato ML, et al. Myoinositol supplementation and onset of gestational diabetes mellitus in pregnant women with a family history of type 2 diabetes: a prospective, randomized, placebo-controlled study. Diabetes Care. 2013;36(4):854–8.
75. D'Anna R, Benedetto A, Scilipoti A, Santamaria A, Interdonato ML, Petrella E, et al. Myoinositol supplementation for prevention of gestational diabetes in obese pregnant women. A randomized controlled trial. Obstetrics. 2015;126(2):310–5.
76. Facchinetti F, Pignatti L, Interdonato ML, Neri I, Bellei G, D'Anna R. Myoinositol supplementation in pregnancies at risk for gestational diabetes. Interim analysis of a randomized controlled trial. Am J Obstet Gynecol 2013;208(Suppl 1):S36.
77. ACOG Practice Bulletin No. 202: Gestational Hypertension and Preeclampsia Obstetrics & Gynecology 2019;133(1):e1-e25.

The Role of Insulin Resistance in Benign Breast Disease

14

Svetlana Vujovic, Miomira Ivovic, Milina Tancic Gajic, Ljiljana Marina, Zorana Arizanovic, Milena Brkic, and Srdjan Popovic

14.1 Principles of Breast Endocrinology

Main regulators of breast metabolism are estradiol, progesterone, prolactin, growth hormone, and insulin-like growth factor 1 (IGF-1) [1]. They control cell function, proliferation, and differentiation activating intracellular signaling cascade (Erk, Akt, JNK, and Ark/Stat) of breast tissue [2]. Estrogen receptor (ER) expression in the breast is stable and differs relatively little in correlation with reproductive status, menstrual cycle phase, or exogenous hormones [3]. Estrogens have apocrine, paracrine, and intercrine effects. Receptors for estradiol are present in fibroblast, epithelial cells, adipocytes, and stromal tissue. Intramammary concentration of estradiol is 20 times higher compared to the level in the blood. Estradiol increases number of progesterone receptors, epithelial proliferation in the luteal phase, galactophore differentiation, connective tissue development, and growth hormone.

Progesterone exerts effects through receptor system, antireceptor system on ER, enzyme effects, and antimitotic activity. Progesterone receptor, part of the steroid thyroid retinoic acid receptor superfamily of transcriptional factors, located on chromosome 11q22–23, uses separate promoters and translation start sites to produce two protein isoforms, PR-A and PR-B. Mammary gland responses to progesterone depend on the ratio of PR-A/PR-B. The single nucleotide polymorphism may alter PR-A to PR-B ratio. The most prominent effects of estradiol and progesterone on breast are shown in Table 14.1. Breast epithelial cells are influenced by many hormones. Receptors for estradiol, progesterone, prolactin, insulin, glucocorticoids, and pituitary hormones were found in the breast tissue [4].

S. Vujovic (✉) · M. Ivovic · M. Tancic Gajic · L. Marina · Z. Arizanovic · M. Brkic · S. Popovic
Faculty of Medicine, University of Belgrade, Belgrade, Serbia

Clinic of Endocrinology, Diabetes and Diseases of Metabolism, Clinical Center of Serbia, Belgrade, Serbia

© International Society of Gynecological Endocrinology 2021
A. R. Genazzani et al. (eds.), *Impact of Polycystic Ovary, Metabolic Syndrome and Obesity on Women Health*, ISGE Series,
https://doi.org/10.1007/978-3-030-63650-0_14

Table 14.1 Some principal effects of estradiol and progesterone in breast tissue

Estradiol Effects	Progesterone Effects
Induction of duct sprout	Induction of ductal development and growth via amphiregulin [5]
Induction of bulbous structures penetration into the fat pad and branches	Lobular development
Stromal tissue growth	Complete maturation of ductal alveolar system
Adipose tissue growth	Increase of estrone sulfur transferase
Increase of nipple-areola complex	Decrease of mineralocorticoid activity
Elongation of terminal duct buds	Decreases number of mitosis
Prolactin increase	Decreases ER and PR

On the breast adipocytes the following receptors were found: estrogen, androgen, insulin, growth hormone, leptin, angiotensin II, glucagon-like peptide-1, gastrin, tumor necrosis factor α, interleukin 6, vitamin D, glucocorticoids, thyroid hormones, thyreostimulating hormone, and glucagon.

The liver is the source of about 80% of IGF-1. Although IGF-1 is responsible for the majority of growth hormone role in mediating breast development, GH itself has been found to play a direct augmentation role, as well as increasing ER expression, in the breast stromal (connective) tissue in contrast to IGF-1. Insulin, cortisol, and thyroxin have permissive role. Estradiol regulates many of the key enzymes involved in mitochondrial bioenergetics, including glucose transporters, hexokinase, pyruvate dehydrogenase, etc. Insulin signaling defects in polycystic ovary syndrome increases cytochrome P450c17 serum kinase. Consequently, progesterone, via 17 alpha hydroxylase, is converted to 17 alpha hydroxyprogesterone, and then to androstenedione (by 17,20 lyase) and testosterone (by 17 β reductase). Insulin response basaly and after 40 g/m^2 oral glucose load in ovulatory hyperandrogenic women leads to hyperinsulinism, higher area under the curve for insulin [6]. Due to such an endocrine milieu, progesterone is lower, and ratio estradiol/progesterone is changed, in favor to estrogens inducing changes in breast tissue response.

Adiponectin acts as insulin sensitizer and has anti-inflammatory effects. It can inhibit proliferation of endothelial cells and has been shown to exert antiproliferative effects on breast tissue [7]. In obese women adiponectin is low and inflammation high. Obesity is considered as chronic pro-inflammatory status. Adipose tissue contributes up to 30% of circulating interleukin 6, as an inflammatory cytokine, which induces hepatic synthesis of C reactive protein.

In normal breast tissue androgen and androgen receptor signaling exerts antiestrogenic growth-inhibitory influences, and the relative levels of circulating sex hormones influence the proliferative capacity of breast epithelial cells. Androgens suppress the action of estradiol by decreasing the expression of ER [8].

Leptin induces epithelial cell proliferation. Calcitriol, via vitamin D receptor, may be a negative regulator of ductal development but a positive regulator of lobuloalveolar development [9]. Vitamin D supplementation decreases cyclooxigenase-2 expression and reduces and increases, respectively, the level of prostaglandin E2 and transforming growth factor beta 2 (TGF β 2), known as inhibitory factors [10]. Overexpression of COX2 induces hyperplasia of breast volume.

Table 14.2 Some of the most important growth factors influencing breast metabolism

Insulin-like growth factor 1 (IGF-1)
Insulin-like growth factor 2 (IGF-2)
Amphiregulin
Epidermal growth factor (EGF)
Fibroblast growth factor (FGF)
Tissue necrosis factor α (TNFα)
Tissue necrosis factor β (TNF β)
Hepatocyte growth factor
Transforming growth factor α (TGF α)
Transforming growth factor β (TGF β)
Heregulin
Wnt
RANKL
Leukemia inhibiting factor (LIF)

Many growth factors are involved in breast metabolism. Some of them are shown in Table 14.2. Epidermal growth factor receptor (EGFR) is a molecular target of EGF, TGF-alpha, amphiregulin, and heregulin. Estradiol and progesterone mediate ductal development through induction of amphiregulin expression and this downstreams EGFR activation.

14.2 Insulin

Insulin resistance is defined as the inability of insulin to exert its physiological effects. It is manifested peripherally (at the tissue levels) or centrally (at the liver levels) through the reduction in the ability of insulin to lower plasma glucose. This can be demonstrated as impaired insulin-stimulated glucose uptake or suppression of lipolysis at the muscles or adipose tissue, hepatic glucose overproduction, and suppression of glycogen synthesis. The mechanisms implicated in the etiology of insulin resistance (IR) include elevated levels of plasma free fatty acids, cytokine (TNFα and IL 6), leptin, resistin, and peroxisome proliferator-activated receptor gamma (PPAR gamma) [11]. A deficiency of D-chiro-inositol (DCI) containing IPG might be at the basis of insulin resistance. DCI is synthesized by an epimerase that converts myo-inositol into DCI, and depending on the specific needs of the two molecules, each tissue has a typical conversion rate [12].

Hyperinsulinism, and IR later, increases androstenedione, bioavailable estrogens, and IGF-1 and decreases sex hormone binding globulin (SHBG), progesterone, and insulin-like growth hormone binding protein 1 (IGFBP-1).

Stressors increase insulin, cortisol, oxidative stress, and cytokines attacking adaptive mechanisms and, frequently, leading to maladaptive response, inducing diseases [13] and shortening telomerase and life expectancy. In such a condition conversion of cortisone to cortisol is increased by 11 β hydroxysteroid dehydrogenase.

Metformin offers many beneficial effects in such a situation like decreasing inflammation by suppressing natural killer cells, decreasing effects on ceramides, DNA damage, cell aging, adiposity, and C reactive protein.

The primary site of metformin action is the mitochondria. The inhibition of mitochondrial complex I of the electron transport chain induces drop in energy charge, resulting in adenosine triphosphate (ATP) decrease. Adenosine monophosphate (AMP) increases bounding of P-site adenylate cyclase enzyme and inhibition of activity leading to defective cAMP protein kinase A (CAMPK) signaling on glucagon receptor. AMPK is an energy sensor and a master coordinator of an integrated signaling network that comprises metabolic growth pathways acting in synchrony to restore cellular energy balance. They switch on catabolic pathways that generate ATP and switch off anabolic pathways. Stimulation of 5'-AMP activated protein kinase confers insulin sensitivity, mainly by modulating lipid metabolism. Metformin increases glucose uptake in skeletal muscles. It blocks insulin receptor/ R/3K/Akt/mTOR signaling in the hyperplastic endometrial tissue inducing GLUT4 expression and inhibits AR expression [14].

Metformin suppresses food intake by increasing levels of glucagon-like peptide 1 and interaction with ghrelin and leptin on the T cell memory by altering fatty acid metabolism [15]. Insulin resistance with increasing LH in the menopause plays a role in adrenal tumorigenesis showing us that early detection and treatment of insulin resistance can be protective for many diseases [16].

Hyperinsulinism induces IR in tumor as a ligand to lower IGF-1 expression and aromatase activity resulting in poor prognosis. Obesity induces inflammatory microenvironment by adipocyte released cytokines to promote cancer cell progression. Leptin, an adipokine, can destable HIF1 α and stimulates hypoxia condition in breast tumor [17].

Insulin resistance induces two major diseases: diabetes mellitus type 2 and cancers (endometrium, breast) by the following mechanisms:

1. When insulin resistance is the primary initiator of pathological processes, reactive hyperinsulinism and hyperandrogenism are fundamental characteristics. Later, the progression of IR results in increased IGF-1, breakthrough of defective insulin receptors, and exhaustion of beta cells, and diabetes mellitus type 2 occurs.
2. Aromatase inhibition leads to estrogen deficiency and insufficient estrogen receptor cxpression and can induce breast carcinoma. As well, aromatase inhibition accumulates androgen precursors, leading to hyperandrogenism, EGF and IGF excess, reactively decreased estrogen receptor expression, estrogen receptor defects, hypoprogesteronemia, and breast carcinoma.

14.3 Benign Breast Disease

Benign breast disease (BBD) represents all benign breast changes in women. About 69% of women experience cyclical breast pain during luteal phase relating to stromal, ductal, and glandular tissue changes. In early reproductive period glandular component may respond to cyclical hormonal stimuli and induce fibroadenoma and cysts formation. In the late reproductive period, glandular tissue becomes hyperplastic with sclerosing adenosis or lobular hyperplasia. During the menopause atrophic changes of glandular, stromal, and fatty tissue occur in hypoestrogenic milieu. During menopause hormone therapy lobular tissue changes persist.

Fibroadenoma represents a benign tumor with epithelial cells arranged in a fibrous stroma and hyperplasia or proliferation of connective tissue. The peak incidence is between 20 and 24 years of age. About 10% of fibroadenoma shrinkage each year. Fibroadenoma completes and finishes growth after reaching 3–4 cm. According to type they can be pericanalicular, intracanalicular, and giant. They are present as painless firm, discrete, round, rubbery tumors with well-shaped borders, freely mobile.

Breast cysts are fluid-filled structures bigger than 3 mm, lined by secretory epithelial cells. They are developed from dilated terminal ducts. In 7–8% of women macrocysts are present resulting from changed ratio estradiol/progesterone in the luteal phase, higher insulin levels, and relatively insufficient luteal phase. They can be divided into three groups [18]:

1. Type 1 cyst: high potassium content, low natrium and chloride (Na:K<3) with increased melatonin (5–23 times higher compared to daytime melatonin in serum) [19], estradiol, dehydroepiandrosterone sulfate, epidermal derived growth factor, and decreased levels of TGF β 2 in cyst fluid.
2. Type 2: low potassium, high natrium and chloride (Na:K>3).
3. Type 3: intermediate electrolyte types.

Pathophysiology of benign breast disease is characterized by increased blood perfusion, capillary permeability, histamine, and prostaglandin E1 and mucocutaneous substances accumulation. Hyalinization, swelling, and organization due to albumin accumulation are key factors developing diffuse synchronous hyperplasia of epithelial tissue and interlobular connective tissue [20]. Vascular, neural, and epithelial factors are involved.

Changes of the ratio of estradiol and progesterone exist even in the ovulatory cycles inducing BBD. In the late reproductive period ovulatory cycles declined resulting in lower progesterone. At the same time hyperinsulinism, due to lifestyle, genetics, and stressors, further decreases progesterone levels. Prior to the menopause, three phases of climacterium are recognized. The first one is manifested by lower progesterone with preserved estradiol levels and regulatory cycles increasing BBD.

Progesterone inhibits estrogen-induced mitosis and prolactin production. Estradiol increases number of mitosis and secretory activity in the pituitary, particularly the proliferation of prolactin secreted cells. High prolactin further suppresses ovulation. Some of the beneficial progesterone roles are protection against benign breast disease, carcinomas, anxiety, etc. It contributes to bone formation and improves sexual drive during menopause. It is well known that progesterone deficiency is the most important etiological factor for premenstrual syndrome, insomnia, early miscarriages, painful or lumpy breasts, infertility, unexplained weight gain, etc. Progesterone has natriuretic effect due to the suppression of renal tubular reabsorption and increment of cell filtration preventing retention of liquid within the breast gland. It decreases capillary permeability and breast tissue edema.

Our study confirmed that progesterone gel, administered twice daily on the breasts (16–26.day), with dietary and lifestyle changes, decreased mastalgia, cysts volume, and number of cysts due to changed ratio of estradiol/progesterone. Estradiol/progesterone ratio before vs. during therapy was on day 21st 12.2 ± 10.7 vs. 10.4 ± 5.5 and on day 24 18.9 ± 23.8 vs. 7.7 ± 6.1. Our latest observations [21] confirmed that hyperinsulinism represents the crucial etiological factor decreasing progesterone levels. Estradiol increases breast cell proliferation by 230%, but progesterone decreases it by 400%. Progesterone inhibited estrogen-induced breast cell proliferation [22].

Nappi C et al. [23] confirmed that micronized progesterone vaginal gel reduced mastalgia by 64.0% compared to 22% reduction of mastalgia in control group. Chang's study confirmed that higher progesterone concentration significantly decrease number of cycling epithelial cells [24].

14.4   Benign Breast Disease and Breast Carcinoma

Estradiol is neither carcinogenic "per se" nor factor inducing DNA mutation. It can be a tumor growth promoter after malignant transformation, increasing mitosis, number and expression of ER and PR, and vascularization. The highest aromatase activity was found in quadrant with breast carcinoma. Progesterone levels are highest during pregnancy when incidence of breast carcinomas is sporadic. Some breast carcinomas were successfully treated by medroxyprogesterone acetate. During reproductive period mitosis and apoptosis are maximal in midluteal phase. In culture tissue in estradiol presence progesterone decreases breast carcinoma cells. Initially progesterone increases number of cells entering S phase after 12 h, and after 24 h a sharp decline of cells entering S phase was detected and effects remained 96 h. In vivo progesterone inhibits proliferation induced by estradiol by aromatase inhibition.

Progesterone induces RANKL. Breast carcinomas with RANKL expression have lower Ki67. Therapy of breast carcinoma with progesterone has the same effects as Tamoxifen therapy. Risk for estrogen-positive breast carcinoma is decreased. Meta-analysis showed correlation between MTHFR gen, C677T in axon 4 on C677T, and breast carcinoma [25]. Hypoestrogenism, high FSH, and insulin resistance in the menopause can induce breast carcinoma in women with inherited genetic mutations [26].

14.5   Conclusion

Dynamic hormonal changes have to be detected in the luteal phase (not only day 21) to confirm diagnosis. Benign breast disease does not represent a "normal finding" and has to be treated depending on etiological factors by progesterone, insulin sensitizers, oral contraceptives, dopaminergic agents, anxiolytics, and eating habit changes. The importance of detecting insulin resistance, especially in the luteal phase, would be obligatory. This completely different approach is more humane, avoiding unnecessary breast surgery and psychological disturbances and offering better quality of life.

References

1. Hynes NE, Watson CJ. Mammary gland growth factors: roles in normal development and in cancer. Cold Spring Herb Perspect Bio. 2010;2:8–11.
2. Rawlings JS, Rosler KM, Harrison DA. The JAK/STST signaling pathway. J Cell Sci. 2004;117:1281–3.
3. Haslam S, Osuch J. Hormones and breast cancer in postmenopausal women. Breast Dis. 2006;42:69.
4. Houdebine LM. Djiane J, Dusanter-Fourt et al.Hormonal action controlling mammary activity. J Daily Sci. 1985;68:489–560.
5. Aupperlee MD, Leipprandt JR, Bennet JM, et al. Amphiregulin mediates progesterone induced mammary ductal development during puberty. Breast Cancer Res. 2013;15:44–7.
6. Diamanti Kandarakis E, Dunaif A. The effects of old, new and emergency medicines on metabolic abberation in PCOS. Endocr Rev 2012; l33:981–1030.
7. Catsburg C, Gunter M, Chen C, et al. Insulin, estrogen, inflammatory markers and risk of benign proliferative breast disease. Cancer Res. 2014;74:3248–58.
8. Zhou J, Ng S, Adesanya-Famuiya O, et al. Testosterone inhibits estrogen-induced mammary epithelial proliferation and suppress estrogen receptor expression. FASEB J. 2000;14:1725–30.
9. Welsh J. Vitamin D metabolism in mammary gland and breast cancer. Mol Cell Enbdocrinol. 2011;347:55–60.
10. Qin W, Smith C, Jensen M, et al. Vitamin D favourably alters the cancer promoting prostaglandin cascade. Anticancer Res. 2013;33:4496–9.
11. Kahn DB, Flier JS. Obeslty and insulin resistance. Clin Invest. 2000;106:473–81.
12. Genazzani AD, Ricchieri F, Prati A, et al. Differential insulin response to myoinositol administration in obese PCOS patients. Gynecol Endocrinol. 2012;28:969–73.
13. Slijepcevic D. Stres. Ur. Sekanic D, Kremen, Beograd, 1993.
14. Pernicova I, Korbonis M. Metforin – mode of action and clinical implications for diabetes and cancer. Nat Rev Endocrinol. 2014;10:577–86.
15. Pearce EL. Enhance CD-8 T-cell memory by modulating fatty acid metabolism. Nature. 2009;460:103–7.
16. Marina LJ, Ivovic M, Vujovic S, et al. Luteinizing hormone and insulin resistance in menopausal patients with adrenal incidentalomas. The cause-effect relationship? Clin Endocrinol. 2018;4:541–8.
17. Chu DT, Phuong TN. The effect of adipocytes on the regulation of breast in the tumor microinvorenment: an update. Cell. 2019;8:857–60.
18. Ness J, Sedghinasab M, Moe RE, et al. Identification of multiple proliferative growth factors in breast cyst fluid. Am J Surg. 2014;166:237–43.
19. Burch JB, Walling M, Rush A, et al. Melatonin and estrogen in breast cyst fluid. Breast Cancer Res Treat. 2007;103:331–41.
20. Vujovic S. Benign Breast disease during women;s life. In ISGE series: Pre-menopause, menopause and Beyond. Vol 5, Frontiers in Gynecological endocrinology. Editors: Birkhauser M, Genazzani AR, Springer, 2018: 215–221.
21. Brkic M, Vujovic S, Franic-Ivanisevic M, et al. The influence of progesterone gel therapy in the treatment of fibrocystic breats disease. Open J Obstet Gynecol. 2016;6:334–41.
22. Foidart JM, Cohn C, Denoo X. Estrogen and progesterone result the proliferation of human breast epithelial cells. Fertil Steril. 1998;69:963–9.

23. Nappi C, Affinitio PO, Carlo D, et al. Double blind control trial of progesterone vaginal cream treatment of cyclical mastalgia in women with benign breast disease. J Endocrinol Investig. 1992;15:801–6.
24. Chang KJ, Lee TT, Linares-Cruz G, et al. Et al. influences of percutaneous administration of estradiol and progesterone on human breast epithelial cell cycle in vivo. Fertil Steril. 1995;63:735–91.
25. Yan W, Zhang Y, Zhao E, et al. Association between the MTHFR C667T polymorphism and breast carcinoma risk: a meta analysis of 23 case control studies. The Breast J. 2016;22:593–4.
26. Carrol JS, Hickey TE, Tarulli GA, et al. Deciphering the divergent roles of progesterone in breast cancer. Nat Rev Cancer. 2017;17:54–64.

Polycystic Ovary Syndrome and Inflammation

15

Peter Chedraui and Faustino R. Pérez-López

15.1 Introduction

The polycystic ovary syndrome (PCOS) is the most prevalent endocrine disorder in adolescents and young women, and it is expressed by four clinical and metabolic phenotypes. The dominant clinical manifestation of women with PCOS is hyperandrogenism that affects the functioning of granulosa cells and follicular development (e.g., abnormal folliculogenesis without a dominant follicle). Androgen excess contributes to weight gain, insulin resistance, hirsutism, acne, and androgenic alopecia. The prevalence of the metabolic syndrome (MetS) is higher in women with Rotterdam criteria PCOS [1] as compared to controls (15.8% vs. 10.1%), although the differences are not significant after controlling for body mass index (BMI) [2]. Hence, an interaction between PCOS and BMI is suggested. To date, the four recognized PCOS phenotypes are i) hyperandrogenism + oligoanovulation + polycystic ovarian morphology; ii) hyperandrogenism + oligoanovulation; iii) hyperandrogenism + polycystic ovarian morphology; and iv) oligoanovulation + polycystic ovarian morphology, each of these with different long-term health and metabolic implications [3].

P. Chedraui (✉)
Instituto de Investigación e Innovación en Salud Integral, Facultad de Ciencias Médicas, Universidad Católica de Santiago de Guayaquil, Guayaquil, Ecuador

Facultad de Ciencias de la Salud, Universidad Católica "Nuestra Señora de la Asunción", Asunción, Paraguay
e-mail: peter.chedraui@cu.ucsg.edu.ec

F. R. Pérez-López
Department of Obstetrics and Gynecology, Faculty of Medicine, Instituto de Investigación Sanitaria de Aragón, University of Zaragoza, Zaragoza, Spain

© International Society of Gynecological Endocrinology 2021
A. R. Genazzani et al. (eds.), *Impact of Polycystic Ovary, Metabolic Syndrome and Obesity on Women Health*, ISGE Series,
https://doi.org/10.1007/978-3-030-63650-0_15

15.2 Obesity and the PCOS

Central fat accumulation and androgen metabolic alterations are fundamental for the clinical evolution of the PCOS and its metabolic and inflammatory complications. Puder et al. [4] reported that PCOS women, as compared to non-PCOS controls matched for BMI, have increased trunk fat mass, insulin resistance (in the homeostasis model assessment of insulin resistance [HOMA-IR]), and higher inflammatory alterations (higher C-reactive protein [CRP], tumor necrosis factor α [TNF-α], procalcitonin, and white blood cell count). This was found even after adjusting for total body fat.

The presence of both visceral fat hypertrophy and androgen excess correlates with the degree of insulin resistance, the worse PCOS phenotype, and cardiovascular risk factors. The abnormal secretion of many adipocyte-derived products (adipokines) will produce a state of chronic low-intensity inflammation that progressively creates a lifetime vicious circle that will affect every organ and system [5]. Thus, PCOS women display increased circulating CRP, TNF-α and interleukin 6 (IL-6), and HOMA-IR values [6]. Despite this, inflammation and insulin resistance seems to be increased in PCOS women regardless of their BMI. Therefore, early intervention, aimed at improving lifestyle, is essential to prevent cardiovascular and other organ and system complications.

15.3 Inflammation and PCOS

PCOS is associated with hyperandrogenism that will cause insulin to exacerbate many endocrine and metabolic alterations [7]. These steroids seem to contribute to inflammation through the promotion of adipocyte hypertrophy and the stimulation of mononuclear cells to release TNF-α and IL-6 [8]. In addition, hyperandrogenism will then promote abdominal fat accumulation and further exacerbate insulin resistance. The progressive accumulation of fat mass and the MetS is accompanied by chronic low-grade inflammation activated by adipose expansion, which permanently alters the immune system through a pro-inflammatory status in different organs (e.g., pancreas, liver, gut, bone, muscle, brain) and systems (e.g., cardiovascular, reproductive) [9, 10]. Chronic inflammation is closely related to the MetS, insulin resistance, type 2 diabetes mellitus (T2DM), dynapenia, and sarcopenia. The early identification, prevention, and management/treatment of this increased inflammatory status in PCOS women is a major task (Fig. 15.1). This should be done before the MetS is fully developed.

15.3.1 Inflammation during Reproductive Life

Premenopausal women who are close to the menopause display impaired glucose metabolism, increased androgen secretion, and inflammation, situation that will persist after the onset of the menopause [11]. In young women, obesity is an important determinant of circulating serum inflammatory markers related to

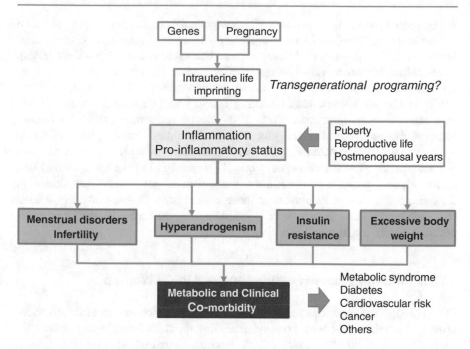

Fig. 15.1 The PCOS is probably determined by genes and pregnancy factors that imprint a pro-inflammatory condition or inflammation. This alteration will be expressed starting in puberty and persisting during reproductive and postmenopausal years. The main clinical alteration will be expressed by menstrual disorders, amenorrhea and infertility, hyperandrogenism, insulin resistance, and excessive body weight. The syndrome is associated to metabolic and clinical co-morbidity, including an increased risk of developing the metabolic syndrome, insulin resistance, and diabetes mellitus, as well as cardiovascular and cancer risks, and other clinical conditions

cardiovascular risk [12]. These markers are currently not included as diagnostic criteria of PCOS. Obese PCOS women have increased CRP and IL-6 levels when compared to lean counterparts; and there are inverse correlations between insulin sensitivity and several inflammatory markers (CRP, IL-6, TNF-α, and soluble intercellular cell adhesion molecule-1). After controlling for BMI, a weak correlation persists between insulin sensitivity and CRP [12]. It is important to take into account that obese and non-obese PCOS women have more visceral adipose tissue than women without PCOS, and this fat tissue correlates positively with total free androgens levels [13]. Therefore, androgens are closely associated with obesity in PCOS women.

Young PCOS women display higher total testosterone, dehydroepiandrosterone sulfate (DHEA-S), and androstenedione levels, both in the obese and lean ones, when compared to those without PCOS. Also, sexual hormone binding globulin (SHBG) levels are significantly lower while CRP, TNF-α, and α-1 acid glycoprotein are increased in all PCOS patients [14]. This profile is compatible with a pro-inflammatory status.

The majority of evidence linking PCOS with chronic inflammation has been described during the fasting state. Martínez-Garcia et al. [15] recruited PCOS women (obese and non-obese), non-PCOS women (obese and non-obese), and men (obese and non-obese) in order to analyze postprandial inflammatory status after providing different nutrient challenges (e.g., isocaloric oral macronutrient loads). Authors found that serum IL-6 decreased after glucose and protein load, while there was a slight increase after oral lipid intake. However, leukocyte IL6 expression was not altered by macronutrients. Circulating TNF-α levels decreased in a similar pattern after macronutrient load while TNF-α expression increased. The highest increase was observed after oral glucose. Obesity did not have a global effect on postprandial secretion patterns of IL-6 or TNF-α. Circulating IL-18 concentrations decreased after all oral challenges, while IL-10 (anti-inflammatory cytokine) was increased; as a possible compensatory mechanism of postprandial inflammation. This situation seems to be blunted in those with obesity. In this study, the authors conclude that glucose, as opposed to protein load, was the main trigger of the postprandial expression of inflammatory genes [15].

15.3.2 Inflammation in Postmenopausal PCOS Women

PCOS clinical manifestations are usually reduced after menopause, although endocrine and metabolic alterations remain, including the risk of developing atherosclerosis [16]. In postmenopausal PCOS women, impaired glucose metabolism enhances ovarian androgen secretion and chronic inflammation found in premenopausal women [11]. Basal circulating androgens tend to decrease slightly before the menopause in normal women, and then remain stable during the menopausal transition [17]. Contrary to this, postmenopausal women with PCOS maintain higher androgenic secretory capacity in comparison to normal women. This persistent production of androgens is mainly of adrenal origin. On the other hand, SHBG decreases after the menopause in normal women, levels which are lower than those observed in PCOS women [11]. Dexamethasone suppression test in postmenopausal PCOS women suggests that DHEAS and total testosterone are partially of adrenal origin [18].

15.4   Effect of Diet and Exercise on Inflammation

Diet, weight management, and physical activity are pivotal in PCOS women [19]. Patients may benefit from a ketogenic diet that may reduce inflammation and insulin resistance [20, 21]. This may obviate the need of pharmaceutical options. The reduction of carbohydrate intake may improve insulin sensitivity, and secondarily reduce circulating insulin and inflammation that stimulate androgen production [22]. Ketones also have anti-oxidant properties and may downregulate the activity of major-inflammation-controlling genes [23].

The ketogenic Mediterranean diet based on phytoextracts used for several weeks has been associated with changes in body weight and endocrine and metabolic improvements. Paoli et al. [24] reported that after a 12-week ketogenic diet, overweight PCOS women displayed a reduction in body weight (−9.43 kg), BMI (−3.35 kg/m^2), visceral adipose tissue, blood glucose and insulin levels, and HOMA-IR values. They also observed a significant reduction of triglyceride, total cholesterol, and low-density-lipoprotein-cholesterol (LDL-C) levels, along with a rise in high-density-lipoprotein-cholesterol (HDL-C). The LH/FSH ratio, LH, testosterone (total and free), and DHEAS blood levels were also significantly reduced, whereas estradiol and SHBG increased. Therefore, appropriate nutrition is a relevant intervention to maintain endocrine and metabolic well-being.

Physical activity and programmed exercise may improve metabolic and endothelial dysfunction and also clinical outcomes in healthy pre- and postmenopausal women as well as those with PCOS and inflammation. These interventions have been endorsed by PCOS Societies for the prevention of cardiovascular disease [25]. The meta-analysis of Benham et al. [26] reported that exercise improves waist perimeter, systolic blood pressure, fasting insulin, and lipid profiles.

The effect of aerobic exercise in young PCOS women with excessive body weight (overweight and obese) has been reported by Dantas et al. [27]. They excluded those with T2DM, smokers, or oral contraceptive users. Included participants were restrained from alcohol consumption and vigorous physical activity for at least 48 h before the study. A large panel of serum and muscle cytokines were measured before and after the exercise sessions. They also measured skeletal muscle protein inflammatory signals (c-Jun N-terminal kinase [JNK] α/β and IκB kinase B [IKKβ]) that impair the effect of insulin over muscle. Interestingly, PCOS women had significantly higher muscle TNF-α (+62%) and plasma IL-1β (+76%) as compared to controls. Exercise decreased plasma and muscle TNF-α (−14% and −46%, respectively) and increased plasma and muscle IL-4 (+147%, and + 62%, respectively) and plasma IL-10 (+38%, $p = 0.0029$) in PCOS women. Exercise reduces skeletal muscle IKKβ and JNKα/β levels approaching to that of controls. This study suggests that PCOS women can decrease their inflammatory status and this effect (anti-inflammatory) may be considered an interesting intervention to reduce cardiometabolic risk in PCOS women.

15.5 Effect of Probiotic and Synbiotic on Inflammation

Studies have reported that probiotic bacteria may improve glucose homeostasis in PCOS women. Ahmadi et al. [28] carried out a randomized control trial (RCT) to analyze the effect of probiotic supplementation or placebo on weight, glycemia, and lipid profiles in PCOS women. Consumption of probiotic supplements resulted in a significant reduction of weight and BMI as compared to placebo. Moreover, probiotic administration was associated with a significant decrease in fasting blood glucose, insulin, triglycerides, and HOMA-IR values, in addition to a significant increase of insulin sensitivity.

In another RCT, Karimi et al. [29] assessed the effect of supplementing synbiotic or placebo for 12 weeks over glucose and insulin-related outcomes in PCOS women (aged 19–37). Synbiotic supplementation significantly decreased serum apelin 36 and CRP levels, with no effect on plasma glucose, glycated hemoglobin, HOMA-IR values, and the quantitative insulin sensitivity check index (QUICKI).

A meta-analysis of six RCTs [30] regarding the effects of probiotic supplementation on glucose control, lipid profiles, weight loss, and CRP levels in PCOS women found a beneficial decrease in fasting blood insulin, triglyceride, and very low-density lipoprotein-cholesterol (VLDL-C) levels, with an increase of QUICKI scores. In another more recent meta-analysis, Hadi et al. [31] reported that probiotics and synbiotics significantly reduced blood glucose, insulin, CRP and total testosterone levels, and HOMA-IR values in PCOS women. The improvement of glucose hemostasis, insulin sensitivity, and inflammation was not associated with changes in body weight in PCOS women.

15.6   Effect of Soy on Inflammation

There are a few studies addressing the effect of soy in PCOS women. Jamilian et al. [32] performed a RCT in PCOS women (aged 18–40) allocated to 50 mg/day soy isoflavones or placebo for 12 weeks. After the study period, women receiving isoflavones showed a significant reduction of circulating insulin and HOMA-IR values, with an increase in the insulin sensitivity index. In addition, when compared to placebo, isoflavone intervention was associated to a reduction of the free androgen index and serum triglycerides. There was no significant effect of soy isoflavones on other lipids.

Karamali et al. [33] studied the effect of soy intake on weight loss, glucose control, lipid profile, and inflammation and oxidative stress biomarker levels in PCOS women. They carried out a RCT in 60 PCOS women to receive for 8 weeks either a test (n = 30) or a control diet (n = 30). Test group participants consumed a diet containing 0.8 g protein/kg body weight (35% animal proteins, 35% soy protein, and 30% vegetable proteins), and the control group consumed a similar diet containing 70% animal proteins and 30% vegetable proteins. Adherence to the test diet, as compared to the control diet, significantly decreased BMI, glucose control, total testosterone, triglycerides, and malondialdehyde, while increasing nitric oxide and glutathione levels.

15.7   Vitamin D Supplementation

Few studies have addressed the effect of vitamin D supplementation in PCOS women. A RCT carried out by Maktabi et al. [34] studied the effect of vitamin D supplementation (50,000 IU/twice a week for 12 weeks) or a placebo in women with PCOS aged 18–40 with vitamin D deficiency (serum levels <20 ng/mL). Compared to placebo, vitamin D intervention was associated with a reduction of fasting blood glucose, insulin, and CRP levels. HOMA-IR values and plasma malondialdehyde levels (-0.1 ± 0.5 vs. $+0.9 \pm 2.1\,\mu$mol/l, $p = 0.01$) were also reduced.

The Akbari et al. [35] meta-analysis based on seven RCTs found that vitamin D supplementation in PCOS women was associated with a reduction of high-sensitivity

CRP and malondialdehyde levels which was related to a significant increase of total antioxidant capacity. Vitamin D supplementation had no significant effect on nitric oxide and total glutathione levels.

Despite the abovementioned, there are conflicting results regarding the effect of vitamin D supplementation in PCOS women. A more recent RCT [36] reported results from 180 European PCOS women with 25(OH)D < 75 nmol/L, who were randomized to receive 20,000 IU of cholecalciferol weekly or placebo for 24 weeks. The primary outcome was the between group difference area under the curve (AUC) of glucose at the end of the intervention and adjusting for baseline levels in the 123 participants that completed the study [age 25.9 ± 4.7 years; BMI 27.5 ± 7.3 kg/m^2; baseline 25(OH)D 48.8 ± 16.9 nmol/L, baseline fasting glucose 84 ± 8 mg/dL]. Although vitamin D supplementation significantly increased 25(OH)D levels (mean treatment effect 33.4 nmol/L, increased to 42.2 nmol/L; $p < 0.001$), the treatment had no significant effect on AUC glucose (mean treatment effect -9.19; 95% CI -21.40 to 3.02; $p = 0.139$). The treatment was associated with a significant decrease in plasma glucose during the oral tolerance test. It seems that there are controversial results or confounding factors among studies from different populations and latitudes that should be delineated.

15.8   Effect of Mineral Supplementation on Inflammation

Various minerals, alone or associated to vitamins, have been proposed to decrease inflammation in PCOS women. Jamilian et al. [37] compared in a double-blind RCT the effect of selenium supplementation (200 µg per day) versus placebo for 8 weeks on glucose and lipid metabolism in PCOS women (aged 18–40). At the end of the intervention, as compared to placebo-treated women, those receiving selenium displayed significantly higher QUICKI scores together with lower serum insulin, HOMA-IR, and homeostatic model assessment-beta-cell function (HOMA-B) values. In addition, supplementation with selenium resulted in a significant reduction in serum triglycerides and VLDL-C concentrations.

One RCT assessed the effect of zinc supplementation (50 mg/day for 8 weeks) or placebo over insulin resistance and lipids in PCOS women (aged 18–40) [38]. Compared to placebo-treated women, those who received the zinc supplement significantly increased their blood zinc levels and QUICKI scores, while reducing blood glucose, insulin, triglyceride, VLDL-C, and HOMA-IR values.

Jamilian et al. [39] compared the effects of co-supplementing magnesium and vitamin E (250 and 400 mg/day, respectively) or placebo for 12 weeks in PCOS women. The combined supplementation was related to a significant reduction in serum insulin and HOMA-IR values and a significant increase in the QUICKI scores. Furthermore, the consumed co-supplement significantly decreased serum triglyceride and VLDL-C levels when compared to placebo. A borderline trend ($p = 0.05$) for a decrease in total cholesterol levels was observed in the co-supplemented group as compared to the placebo one.

15.9 Coenzyme Q10 Supplementation

One RCT studied the effect of coenzyme Q10 supplementation (100 mg/day) or placebo for 12 weeks in PCOS women over insulin and metabolic outcomes [40]. Coenzyme Q10 treatment was associated with a significant increase in QUICKI scores and a reduction of blood glucose, insulin, cholesterol (total and low density), HOMA-IR, and HOMA-B values. When values were adjusted for biochemical parameters and baseline BMI, serum LDL-C became non-significant while other outcomes were not altered. Coenzyme Q10 supplementation upregulates gene expression of peroxisome proliferator-activated receptor gamma and downregulates gene expression of oxidized low-density lipoprotein receptor 1, IL-1, IL-8, and TNF-α in peripheral blood mononuclear cells of PCOS women [41].

15.10 Final Remarks

As occurs with many syndromes, the PCOS is a complex process with imprecise limits and heterogeneous clinical and evolutionary characteristics. Inflammation is one of the initial and sustained alterations. Anti-inflammatory treatment may be one approach to detain the syndrome's progression and prevent irreversible clinical complications. Different supplements may aid in the management of some of the metabolic alterations of the PCOS. Despite this, there is an urgent need of treatment options focused on anti-inflammation that should be free of side effects.

Conflicts of Interest The authors report no conflicts of interest.

Improve to This document was partially supported by the *Sistema de Investigación y Desarrollo and the Vice-Rectorado de Investigación & Postgrado of the Universidad Católica de Santiago de Guayaquil, Guayaquil, Ecuador*, through grants No. SIU-318–853-2014 (The Omega II, Women's Health Project 2014) and SIU-554-56-2020 (The Omega III project) provided to Peter Chedraui.

Funding This document was partially supported by the *Sistema de Investigación y Desarrollo and the Vice-Rectorado de Investigación & Postgrado of the Universidad Católica de Santiago de Guayaquil, Guayaquil, Ecuador,* through grant No. SIU-318–853-2014 (The Omega II, Women's Health Project 2014) provided to Peter Chedraui.

References

1. Rotterdam ESHRE/ASRM-Sponsored PCOS Consensus Workshop Group. Revised 2003 consensus on diagnostic criteria and long-term health risks related to polycystic ovary syndrome. Fertil Steril. 2004;81(1):19–25.
2. Panidis D, Macut D, Tziomalos K, Papadakis E, Mikhailidis K, Kandaraki EA, Tsourdi EA, Tantanasis T, Mavromatidis G, Katsikis I. Prevalence of metabolic syndrome in women with polycystic ovary syndrome. Clin Endocrinol. 2013;78(4):586–92.

3. Aziz M, Sidelmann JJ, Faber J, Wissing ML, Naver KV, Mikkelsen AL, Nilas L, Skouby SO. Polycystic ovary syndrome: cardiovascular risk factors according to specific phenotypes. Acta Obstet Gynecol Scand. 2015;94(10):1082–9.
4. Puder JJ, Varga S, Kraenzlin M, De Geyter C, Keller U, Muller B. Central fat excess in polycystic ovary syndrome: relation to low-grade inflammation and insulin resistance. J Clin Endocrinol Metab. 2005;90(11):6014–21.
5. Delitala AP, Capobianco G, Delitala G, Cherchi PL, Dessole S. Polycystic ovary syndrome, adipose tissue and metabolic syndrome. Arch Gynecol Obstet. 2017;296:405–19.
6. Souza Dos Santos AC, Soares NP, Costa EC, de Sá JC, Azevedo GD, Lemos TM. The impact of body mass on inflammatory markers and insulin resistance in polycystic ovary syndrome. Gynecol Endocrinol. 2015;31(3):225–8.
7. Legro R. Obesity and PCOS: implications for diagnosis and treatment. Semin Reprod Med. 2012;30(6):496–506.
8. Ebejer K, Calleja-Agius J. The role of cytokines in polycystic ovarian syndrome. Gynecol Endocrinol. 2013;29(6):536–40.
9. O'Neill S, O'Driscoll L. Metabolic syndrome: a closer look at the growing epidemic and its associated pathologies. Obes Rev. 2015;16(1):1–12.
10. Saltiel AR, Olefsky JM. Inflammatory mechanisms linking obesity and metabolic disease. J Clin Invest. 2017;127(1):1–4.
11. Puurunen J, Piltonen T, Morin-Papunen L, Perheentupa A, Järvelä I, Ruokonen A, Tapanainen JS. Unfavorable hormonal, metabolic, and inflammatory alterations persist after menopause in women with PCOS. J Clin Endocrinol Metab. 2011;96(6):1827–34.
12. Escobar-Morreale HF, Villuendas G, Botella-Carretero JI, Sancho J, San Millán JL. Obesity, and not insulin resistance, is the major determinant of serum inflammatory cardiovascular risk markers in pre-menopausal women. Diabetologia. 2003;46(5):625–33.
13. Jena D, Choudhury AK, Mangaraj S, Singh M, Mohanty BK, Baliarsinha AK. Study of visceral and subcutaneous abdominal fat thickness and its correlation with Cardiometabolic risk factors and hormonal parameters in polycystic ovary syndrome. Indian J Endocrinol Metab. 2018;22(3):321–7.
14. Nehir Aytan A, Bastu E, Demiral I, Bulut H, Dogan M, Buyru F. Relationship between hyperandrogenism, obesity, inflammation and polycystic ovary syndrome. Gynecol Endocrinol. 2016;32(9):709–13.
15. Martínez-García MÁ, Moncayo S, Insenser M, Montes-Nieto R, Fernández-Durán E, Álvarez-Blasco F, Luque-Ramírez M, Escobar-Morreale HF. Postprandial inflammatory responses after oral glucose, lipid and protein challenges: influence of obesity, sex and polycystic ovary syndrome. Clin Nutr. 2020;39(3):876–85.
16. Anagnostis P, Paschou SA, Lambrinoudaki I, Goulis DG. Polycystic ovary syndrome-related risks in postmenopausal women. In: Pérez-López FR, editor. Postmenopausal diseases and disorders. Cham: Springer; 2019. p. 249–59.
17. Spencer JB, Klein M, Kumar A, Azziz R. The age-associated decline of androgens in reproductive age and menopausal black and white women. J Clin Endocrinol Metab. 2007;92(12):4730–3.
18. Markopoulos MC, Rizos D, Valsamakis G, Deligeoroglou E, Grigoriou O, Chrousos GP, Creatsas G, Mastorakos G. Hyperandrogenism in women with polycystic ovary syndrome persists after menopause. J Clin Endocrinol Metab. 2011;96(3):623–31.
19. Moran LJ, Brown WJ, McNaughton SA, Joham AE, Teede HJ. Weight management practices associated with PCOS and their relationships with diet and physical activity. Hum Reprod. 2017;32(3):669–78.
20. Boden G, Sargrad K, Homko C, Mozzoli M, Stein TP. Effect of a low-carbohydrate diet on appetite, blood glucose levels, and insulin resistance in obese patients with type 2 diabetes. Ann Intern Med. 2005;142(6):403–11.
21. Forsythe CE, Phinney SD, Fernandez ML, Quann EE, Wood RJ, Bibus DM, Kraemer WJ, Feinman RD, Volek JS. Comparison of low fat and low carbohydrate diets on circulating fatty acid composition and markers of inflammation. Lipids. 2008;43(1):65–77.

22. McGrice M, Porter J. The effect of low carbohydrate diets on fertility hormones and outcomes in overweight and obese women: a systematic review. Nutrients. 2017;9(3):204.
23. Youm YH, Nguyen KY, Grant RW, Goldberg EL, Bodogai M, Kim D, D'Agostino D, Planavsky N, Lupfer C, Kanneganti TD, Kang S, Horvath TL, Fahmy TM, Crawford PA, Biragyn A, Alnemri E, Dixit VD. The ketone metabolite β-hydroxybutyrate blocks NLRP3 inflammasome-mediated inflammatory disease. Nat Med. 2015;21(3):263–9.
24. Paoli A, Mancin L, Giacona MC, Bianco A, Caprio M. Effects of a ketogenic diet in overweight women with polycystic ovary syndrome. J Transl Med. 2020;18(1):104.
25. Wild RA, Carmina E, Diamanti-Kandarakis E, Dokras A, Escobar-Morreale HF, Futterweit W, et al. Assessment of cardiovascular risk and prevention of cardiovascular disease in women with the polycystic ovary syndrome: a consensus statement by the androgen excess and polycystic ovary syndrome (AE-PCOS) society. J Clin Endocrinol Metab. 2010;95(5):2038–49.
26. Benham JL, Yamamoto JM, Friedenreich CM, Rabi DM, Sigal RJ. Role of exercise training in polycystic ovary syndrome: a systematic review and meta-analysis. Clin Obes. 2018;8(4):275–84.
27. Dantas WS, Neves WD, Gil S, Barcellos CRG, Rocha MP, de Sá-Pinto AL, Roschel H, Gualano B. Exercise-induced anti-inflammatory effects in overweight/obese women with polycystic ovary syndrome. Cytokine. 2019;120:66–70.
28. Ahmadi S, Jamilian M, Karamali M, Tajabadi-Ebrahimi M, Jafari P, Taghizadeh M, Memarzadeh MR, Asemi Z. Probiotic supplementation and the effects on weight loss, glycaemia and lipid profiles in women with polycystic ovary syndrome: a randomized, double-blind, placebo-controlled trial. Hum Fertil (Camb). 2017;20(4):254–61.
29. Karimi E, Moini A, Yaseri M, Shirzad N, Sepidarkish M, Hossein-Boroujerdi M, Hosseinzadeh-Attar MJ. Effects of synbiotic supplementation on metabolic parameters and apelin in women with polycystic ovary syndrome: a randomised double-blind placebo-controlled trial. Br J Nutr. 2018;119(4):398–406.
30. Hadi A, Moradi S, Ghavami A, Khalesi S, Kafeshani M. Effect of probiotics and synbiotics on selected anthropometric and biochemical measures in women with polycystic ovary syndrome: a systematic review and meta-analysis. Eur J Clin Nutr. 2020;74(4):543-547.
31. Liao D, Zhong C, Li C, Mo L, Liu Y. Meta-analysis of the effects of probiotic supplementation on glycemia, lipidic profiles, weight loss and C-reactive protein in women with polycystic ovarian syndrome. Minerva Med. 2018;109(6):479–487.
32. Jamilian M, Asemi Z. The effects of soy isoflavones on metabolic status of patients with polycystic ovary syndrome. J Clin Endocrinol Metab. 2016;101(9):3386–94.
33. Karamali M, Kashanian M, Alaeinasab S, Asemi Z. The effect of dietary soy intake on weight loss, glycaemic control, lipid profiles and biomarkers of inflammation and oxidative stress in women with polycystic ovary syndrome: a randomised clinical trial. Hum Nutr Diet. 2018;31(4):533–43.
34. Maktabi M, Chamani M, Asemi Z. The effects of vitamin D supplementation on metabolic status of patients with polycystic ovary syndrome: a randomized, double-blind, placebocontrolled trial. Horm Metab Res. 2017;49(7):493–8.
35. Akbari M, Ostadmohammadi V, Lankarani KB, Tabrizi R, Kolahdooz F, Heydari ST, Kavari SH, Mirhosseini N, Mafi A, Dastorani M, Asemi Z. The effects of vitamin D supplementation on biomarkers of inflammation and oxidative stress among women with polycystic ovary syndrome: a systematic review and meta-analysis of randomized controlled trials. Horm Metab Res. 2018;50(4):271–9.
36. Trummer C, Schwetz V, Kollmann M, Wölfler M, Münzker J, Pieber TR, Pilz S, Heijboer AC, Obermayer-Pietsch B, Lerchbaum E. Effects of vitamin D supplementation on metabolic and endocrine parameters in PCOS: a randomized-controlled trial. Eur J Nutr. 2019;58(5):2019–28.
37. Jamilian M, Razavi M, Fakhrie Kashan Z, Ghandi Y, Bagherian T, Asemi Z. Metabolic response to selenium supplementation in women with polycystic ovary syndrome: a randomized, double-blind, placebo-controlled trial. Clin Endocrinol. 2015;82(6):885–91.

38. Foroozanfard F, Jamilian M, Jafari Z, Khassaf A, Hosseini A, Khorammian H, Asemi Z. Effects of zinc supplementation on markers of insulin resistance and lipid profiles in women with polycystic ovary syndrome: a randomized, double-blind, placebo-controlled trial. Exp Clin Endocrinol Diabetes. 2015;123(4):215–20.
39. Jamilian M, Sabzevar NK, Asemi Z. The effect of magnesium and vitamin E co-supplementation on glycemic control and markers of cardio-metabolic risk in women with polycystic ovary syndrome: a randomized, double-blind. Placebo-Controlled Trial Horm Metab Res. 2019;51(2):100–5.
40. Samimi M, Zarezade Mehrizi M, Foroozanfard F, Akbari H, Jamilian M, Ahmadi S, Asemi Z. The effects of coenzyme Q10 supplementation on glucose metabolism and lipid profiles in women with polycystic ovary syndrome: a randomized, double-blind, placebo-controlled trial. Clin Endocrinol. 2017;86(4):560–6.
41. Rahmani E, Jamilian M, Samimi M, Zarezade Mehrizi M, Aghadavod E, Akbari E, Tamtaji OR, Asemi Z. The effects of coenzyme Q10 supplementation on gene expression related to insulin, lipid and inflammation in patients with polycystic ovary syndrome. Gynecol Endocrinol. 2018;34(3):217–22.

Metabolic Changes at the Menopausal Transition

16

Marta Caretto, Andrea Giannini, Giulia Palla,
and Tommaso Simoncini

16.1 Introduction

The age of the natural menopause among women in developed countries is between
50 and 52 years [1, 2], whereas, in the less developed countries, it is 3–4 years less
[3]. Deprivation of sex steroid hormones is an important consequence of normal
aging and gonadal failure that potentially increases vulnerability to disease in
hormone-responsive tissues, including the brain, bone, and the cardiovascular system. Energy metabolism also changes during menopausal transition, which is
important and yet does not receive enough attention. Clinical surveys observed a
trend of weight gain, increased food intake, intra-abdominal fat accumulation,
increased low-density lipoprotein cholesterol and triglycerides, insulin resistance,
and reduced energy expedition. Obesity is a growing worldwide problem, which
exacerbates several chronic diseases: After menopause, several chronic pathologies
may occur, and these include metabolic disease, CVD, osteoporosis, and cancer [4].
In menopausal women, the incidence of insulin resistance and diabetes has risen
exponentially: this translates into an increased risk of CVD and death. If estrogen
deprivation leads to altered fat distribution, menopausal hormone therapy (MHT)
appears to decrease the incidence of diabetes and also improves diabetes control as
indicated by assessment of glycosylated hemoglobin concentrations [5]. CVD is the
most common cause of death in women over the age of 50 years: prior studies have
investigated the relationship between menopause and CVD [6]. Major primary prevention measures are smoking cessation, weight loss, blood pressure reduction,
regular aerobic exercise, and diabetes and lipid control. How do hormonal changes
in menopause lead to alterations in lipid and glucose metabolism, fat distribution,

M. Caretto · A. Giannini · G. Palla · T. Simoncini (✉)
Division of Obstetrics and Gynecology, Department of Clinical and Experimental Medicine,
University of Pisa, Pisa, Italy
e-mail: tommaso.simoncini@med.unipi.it

© International Society of Gynecological Endocrinology 2021
A. R. Genazzani et al. (eds.), *Impact of Polycystic Ovary, Metabolic Syndrome
and Obesity on Women Health*, ISGE Series,
https://doi.org/10.1007/978-3-030-63650-0_16

and food intake? It is also interesting to review the latest progress of the MHT and how it influences fat redistribution, and metabolism of MHT has the potential for improving the cardiovascular risk profile through its beneficial effects on vascular function, lipid levels, and glucose metabolism.

16.2   Fat Distribution, Obesity, and Metabolic Syndrome (MS)

The WHO (World Health Organization) defines obesity as a chronic condition, characterized by an excessive weight gain due to an extreme fat mass deposition with great negative effects on health and quality of life (QoL). More or less 25–30% of women are overweight or obese [7]. There are two different kinds of obesity: visceral or central obesity (android) and peripheral obesity (gynoid). The central obesity, typical of men and of postmenopausal women, is characterized by an increase of waist circumference, as measured with the waist/hip ratio (WHR) being normal below 0.80. In the gynoid obesity, typical of the fertile women, fat is mainly fixed on the thighs and buttocks, and these different fat distributions reflect the different body structures between male and female, due to the ancestral different roles of the two genders: abdominal obesity permits manhunting, running, and escaping, while the gynoid fat distribution in women provides protection during pregnancy from the mechanical and metabolic point of view [8]. Moreover, around menopausal transition, many women experience weight gain and increase in central adiposity. The central/visceral obesity is associated with important changes of lipids and glucose profiles, insulin-resistance, and/or diabetes mellitus, with an increase of metabolic and cardiovascular risk. The central and the peripheral fat mass show also structural differences in the fat cell: the adipocyte of the gynoid obesity has a small size, a higher insulin sensibility, and a more estrogenic receptor density, thus promoting a higher fat mass deposition than in the android fat cells. On the contrary, the latter result more responsive to androgenic stimulation and produce and release a greater amount of pro-inflammatory adipocitokines in the portal circulation. The different estrogenic or androgenic responsiveness of the fat cells, depending on the site of fat deposition, may explain the reason of the different obesity site in the two genders and during the women life [9]. A positive relationship exists between the waist girth increase and the worsening of cardiovascular profile, also in normal-weight people, especially in women [10]. In fact, more than BMI (body mass index), the main positive predictive factor of the negative obesity impact on health is the abdominal fat. According to the International Diabetes Federation (IDF) criteria, the waist circumference is the main diagnostic element of the metabolic syndrome (MS), which links the visceral adiposity with the worsening of metabolic profile (Fig. 16.1).

The MS represents a whole heterogeneous disorder, which correlates to high mortality and morbidity rates and high economics and social costs. The syndrome affects 20–25% of the general population with an increased prevalence with aging,

WHO Clinical Criteria for Metabolic Syndrome

Insulin resistance, identified by one of the following:

- Type 2 diabetes

- Impaired fasting glucose

- Impaired glucose tolerance

- or for those with normal fasting glucose levels (<6.1 mmol/L), glucose uptake below the lowest quartile for the background population under investigation under hyperinsulinemic, euglycemic conditions

Plus any two of the following:

- Antihypertensive medication and/or high blood pressure (≥140 mm Hg systolic or ≥90 mm Hg diastolic)

- Plasma triglycerides ≥1.7 mmol/L

- HDL cholesterol <0.9 mmol/L in men or <1.0 mmol/L in women

- BMI >30 kg/m² and/or waist:hip ratio >0.9 in men, >0.85 in women

- Urinary albumin excretion rate ≥20 μg/min or albumin:creatinine ratio ≥3.4 mg/mmol

Fig. 16.1 International Diabetes Federation (IDF) criteria for MS

in particular among the 50–60-year-old people. The characteristics of MS are visceral obesity, abnormal lipid and glucose pro les, and high blood pressure: the specific physiopathological feature is represented by the insulin resistance which can explain each of the metabolic impairments; the insulin resistance promotes the storage of fat tissue at visceral level which becomes less sensitive to insulin action, and as a consequence, a higher lipolytic activity takes place, and this increases the NEFA (non-esterified fatty acids) release into liver circulation. NEFA cause an abnormal glucose and triglycerides synthesis that in turn compromises the hepatic insulin clearance. Furthermore, the fat mass is not considered as a simple energetic store but an active endocrine tissue that releases a large number of adipocitokines, some of which have pro-inflammatory and pro-atherogenic functions (such as TNF-α, IL-6, leptin, adiponectin, omentin) [11] with an active role on the modulation of the insulin sensitivity: in fact the reduced secretion of adiponectin has a crucial role in inducing insulin resistance and in determining the increase of triglycerides and of small, dense LDL particles.

The insulin resistance can be triggered also by other problems: an intrinsic/structural cell disorder, due to receptorial or post-receptorial function defects, or an acquired disorder, such as an excessive weight (overweight or obesity), that increases the amount of fat and induces a change of the receptor-binding ability of hormones. It can depend also on familial predisposition, especially when there are diabetic relatives and often on the combination of many elements above described. Moreover insulin resistance promotes sodium retention at the kidney level, with a consequent negative impact on blood pressure homeostasis [12].

16.3 Relationship between Obesity, MS, and Menopausal Transition

The menopausal transition is characterized by an early (more or less 10 years before the menopause) and progressive increase of FSH levels, linked to a decrease of inhibin production by the ovaries; at the same time, the higher frequency of anovulatory cycles induces a progesterone fall during the luteal phase, thus resulting in a relative hyperestrogenism, followed by a stable hypoestrogenism when menopause finally takes place. In general weight changes depend on an increase of energetic input and/or a decrease of energy consumption, mostly due to physical activity and to the resting energy expenditure. It's well known that women after 45–50 years old, in the presence of no changes of their lifestyle (feeding and physical activity), show a progressive body weight increase. Whereas weight gain per se cannot be attributed to the menopause transition, the change in the hormonal milieu at menopause is associated with an increase in total body fat, and in particular there is an increase in abdominal fat [13]. Lovejoy et al. [14] showed that all along the perimenopausal interval, there is an increase of abdominal fat mass, concomitant with climacteric hypoestrogenism, with a slow increase of body weight despite the slightly reduced amount of total calories intake. The gonadal steroid hormones have specific metabolic effects during perimenopausal transition. As mentioned before, menopausal transition is characterized by low level of estrogens and/or hyperestrogenism associated to low luteal progesterone levels. This event is greatly related to the higher amount of anovulatory menstrual cycles. Indeed, during the luteal phase of the menstrual cycle, the typical increase of progesterone/estrogens ratio induces the increase of body temperature of about 0.4 °C [15]: this temperature rise causes an elevation of basal metabolism of about 200 Jk (50 kcal) a day [16]. On the contrary, the absence of progesterone increase, during the menopausal transition, determines the lack of such energy consumption in resting conditions typical of the luteal phase (about 50 kcal a day, for 12–14 days: approximately 600–700 kcal every month). This event is at the basis of the increased fat mass deposition during perimenopause [17] that can be interpreted as a reduction of the physiological burning of fat during the luteal phase. This decline of the energetic consumption seems to be not exclusively dependent from the progesterone deficiency but also from other factors, such as the amount of lean mass, the sympathetic nervous system (SNS) activity, the endocrine status, and the aging-mediated physiological changes. In fact the decline of basal metabolism observed in postmenopausal women may depend also form aging [18]. Probably estrogen depletion contributes to accelerate the basal metabolism decrease during menopausal transition [19].

As the perimenopause becomes menopause, the progressive reduction of estrogen levels induces a progressively worsening of the insulin resistance that is also increased by the concomitant cortisol rise (typical of aging and menopause). This latter event physiologically induces gluconeogenesis, a typical compensatory mechanism that starts to occur to people above 55–60 years of age, and later promotes the increase of insulin resistance. In addition hypoestrogenism partly induces also the fall of GH levels that facilitates the storage of abdominal fat mass with a decrease of lipid metabolism [20, 21]. In addition the lack of estrogens during the menopausal transition promotes the different fat storage: instead of mainly in the gluteal and femoral subcutaneous region, fat is mainly stored at the abdominal level [22], and thus estrogen deficiency is expected to result in decreased peripheral fat mass [23]. The decrease of basal metabolism induces the gain in fat mass which, in turn, may contribute to improve the incidence of obesity-related diseases, such as worsening of cardiovascular profile and a higher risk to develop type II diabetes. The increase of visceral adiposity further worsens the insulin sensibility, in particular at the liver level so that higher amounts of insulin are needed to control glucose intake at tissue levels. All these changes determine the increase of the rate of incidence of the MS in overweight/obese women during the menopausal transition.

Recently, it has been suggested that another possible link between menopausal hypoestrogenism, appetite control, and weight gain is the increase of orexin-A plasma levels [23]. This hypothalamic neuropeptide is involved in the regulation of feeding behavior, of sleep-wake rhythm, and of neuroendocrine homeostasis [24, 25]. In postmenopausal women, while estrogens show low levels, plasma orexin-A levels are significantly higher, and this seems to participate in the increase of the cardiovascular risk factors, such as high glycemia, abnormal lipid profile, increased blood pressure, and high BMI [26].

16.3.1 Lipid Metabolism and Menopausal Transition

It is well known that estrogen has a significant effect on modulate lipid metabolism. A variety of research show that total cholesterol (TC), triglycerides (TG), low-density lipoprotein cholesterol (LDL-C), and apolipoprotein B (Apo B) increased in perimenopausal women, while menopause-related alternation in high-density lipoprotein cholesterol (HDL-C) is inconsistent [27–29]. Some studies reported a significant reduction, others found an increase in menopausal transition, and rest showed no changes in HDL-C [30].

The underlying mechanisms that estrogen and lipid interact at a molecular level to contribute to the risk of CVD are not clear. It has been reported that estrogen-related receptor γ (ERRγ) regulates hepatic TG metabolism through the action phospholipase A2G12B [31], and polymorphic hepatic lipase is associated with estrogen modulate lipolysis of TG [32]. Della Torre et al. showed that liver ERα activity was essential for balanced lipid and TC metabolism and lack of ERα might lead to hepatic fat accumulation and nonalcoholic fatty liver disease. Several research studies have suggested that estrogen can reduce circulating LDL-C but not cholesterol synthesis by downregulation of hepatic and plasma PCSK9, which is a suppressor of LDL receptors, in both animals and humans [33, 34].

Recent evidence emphasizes the gender differences and age independent on the lipid changes around the final menstrual period and suggest that ovarian hormone may influence the hepatic lipid synthesis, reduce the lipid circulation, upregulate the lipolysis, and lead to protective cardiometabolic effects. Growing body of literatures indicated several related functional proteins might play a crucial role in sex hormone's regulation of lipid metabolism. Therefore, the complex association of menopause, ovarian hormone, especially estrogen, and lipid metabolism needs further extensive experimentation.

Prevention of weight gain and lipid metabolic disorder is important components in the healthcare of postmenopausal women. Although the latest guideline from International Menopause Society (IMS) indicated that MHT may ameliorate perimenopausal intra-abdominal fat accumulation, whether the MHT might maintain the lipid level during menopause transition has not been mentioned [35]. Numerous studies have attempted to understand the metabolic consequences of MHT use and define the effects of different MHT regimens. Major studies have consistently found MHT decrease LDL-C, TC, and lipoprotein (a) levels; however, findings regarding TG and HDL-C levels have been inconsistent [32]. Godsland reviewed the effect of different MHT regimens, estrogen alone, estrogen plus progestogen, raloxifene, or tibolone on plasma lipid and lipoprotein levels and found estrogen alone raise HDL-C and lower LDL-C and TC. Oral and transdermal estrogen had opposite effect on TG. The increases in HDL-C and TG when using estrogen alone were opposed according to the additional progesterone type. Specifically, effects arranged from the least to the greatest are dydrogesterone, medrogestone, progesterone, cyproterone acetate, medroxyprogesterone acetate, transdermal norethindrone acetate, norgestrel, and oral norethindrone acetate [36]. Stevens et al. suggested that MHT-related metabolic pathways are linked to multiple cellular processes, and the different MHT regimens might lead to distinct intracellular signal transduction events which contributed to the disparate risks for some diseases, e.g., CVD and cancer, in menopausal women with MHT [37]. In conclusion, different MHT regimens have different effects on lipid metabolism, exerting favorable and unfavorable changes. The choice for a particular regimen should consider individual demands, indications, complications, and lipid profile.

16.3.2 The Management of Obesity and MS during Perimenopause

The management of overweight/obese premenopausal women has to start from a careful anamnesis investigating the age of the onset of obesity, and the weight changes occurred in the last months, if there are diabetic members of a family suffering from any other endocrinological diseases and/or obesity. The purpose of this check is to exclude any clinical cause that might need specific therapeutical approaches, like some uncommon secondary obesities, due to genetic, neurological, or psychiatric conditions.

It's important to know if the patient suffered in the past for PCOS and/or premenstrual syndrome and premenstrual dysphoric disease (PMS and PMDD). It is well recognized that insulin resistance is a frequent feature of the PCOS and that 50–60% of the patients are overweight/obese [38]. A recent manuscript demonstrated [39] that patients with PCOS and insulin resistance have double chance to suffer from PMS/PMDD and mood disorders up to depression, during their reproductive life and more frequently during the menopausal transition. This condition seems to be due to a reduced production of neurosteroids, in particular of allopregnanolone, which is considered the most powerful endogenous anxiolytic and antidepressant substance derived from progesterone metabolism. PCOS and hyperinsulinemic patients, during menopausal transition, have a higher risk to suffer from more intense climacteric symptoms, in particular those due to neurosteroids deficiency (i.e., allopregnanolone), like mood disorders, depression, and anxiety, if they don't reduce insulin resistance and their weight [40].

In the presence of overweight/obesity, it is necessary to assess the presence of insulin resistance, even in nonobese women; in fact, perimenopausal women may have a normal weight, thanks to their lifestyle, though they have an insulin resistance predisposition, which can be disclosed only by an OGTT (oral glucose tolerance test). This test is usually done over 4 h, but it can be performed also with two blood samples, at time 0 (i.e., before drinking the glucose) and 60 or 90 min after glucose load of 75 g of sugar dissolved in a glass of water: a hyperinsulinism is diagnosed when insulin response is higher than 60 microU/ml [41]. In women with a history of PCOS, an insulin resistance is frequently confirmed both during pre- and postmenopause [42].

The therapeutical approaches for women during menopausal transition have to consider the body weight at the moment of the perimenopausal transition: the normal-weight women and the overweight/obese women should be treated differently. In the first case, the approach is targeted to the weight gain's prevention, while in latter group, it is important to avoid a further weight increase and/or to treat the metabolic abnormalities. In both cases, the first recommendation is the modification of lifestyle, through the combination of a hypocaloric diet and a correct choice of nutrients with physical activity.

An endurance training (aerobic exercise for 45 min a day, three times a week) has been shown to promote body weight and fat mass losses and to reduce both waist girth and blood pressure in overweight/obese women. Moreover, these interventions decrease plasma triglyceride, total cholesterol, and low-density lipoprotein levels and increase high-density lipoprotein plasma concentrations [43]. The best improvement in metabolic risk profile has been observed in women with two or more determinants of the MS but still with no coronary heart disease [44]. In addition, the physical exercise amplifies the triggers on anorectic response limiting food's introduction [45]. Unfortunately, the association of diet and physical activity results effective in the short period and shows an increasing lower compliance and higher difficulty to maintain the weight loss in the long term. Quite often, in these cases, a psychological support is needed.

In normal-weight women with climacteric symptoms, the hormonal replacement therapy (HRT) has been successfully demonstrated to protect against perimenopausal changes of body composition [46, 47]. In these patients, no significant variations in weight, fat mass content, and distribution have been observed probably also, thanks to the route of administration of HRT. In particular transdermal estrogens seem to be more protective against fat mass increase and android fat distribution. Oral estrogens have been associated with a small increase in fat mass and a decrease in lean mass [48]. Similar effects on body composition and on fat tissue have been observed when administering tibolone and raloxifene.

In obese women during menopausal transition, behavioral therapy is essential to achieve the weight control on long term, but there exists some medication like metformin, orlistat, and inositol that might help and facilitate weight control and/or weight loss. Metformin, a well-known antidiabetes drug, reduces insulin levels improving insulin sensitivity, through an increase of glucose cell uptake. It is frequently administered to hyperinsulinemic PCOS women during fertile age. Also myo-inositol, alone or in combination with chiro-inositol or alpha-lipoic acid, administration can enhance insulin sensibility through an improvement of postreceptorial pathways' functions. On the contrary, orlistat represents a specific antiobesity treatment since it reduces the absorption of dietary fats, promoting their fecal elimination.

Overweight, obesity, and metabolic syndrome are tightly linked with the changing of the hormonal pattern during the menopausal transition. In fact, as previously mentioned, the progressive decline of estrogens and progesterone plasma levels promotes some metabolic impairment, such as the worsening of insulin resistance or the increasing of central fat mass storage. At the same time, obesity is an important factor that affects the changes of hormonal profiles during menopausal transition since women with higher BMI were more likely to start the perimenopause earlier though moving slower towards the menopause if compared to those with a lower BMI [49]. If during fertile age, these women had PCOS and overweight/obesity, it is more likely that insulin resistance led them not only to a MS predisposition but also to mood disorders that might be more severe as soon as menopausal transition occurs. Recent findings sustain such hypothesis since it has been reported that menopausal women who suffered from PCOS have higher adiponectin and lower leptin [50] and a higher insulin response to OGTT than menopausal women with no history of PCOS.

16.3.3 How to Prevent Weight Gain

When dealing with prevention of weight gain, the only logical solutions include physical activity, caloric-restricted diet, and, eventually, specific antiobesity drugs or bariatric surgery. As previously mentioned, physical activity is relevant to counteract the body weight increase, independently from age and menopausal condition. It is important to point out that physical activity cannot block or prevent weight gain related to aging, but it can protect against the development of obesity. An activity of 45 min at least three times in a week really improves the control of body weight and maintains elasticity and lean mass despite the decrease of fat mass [13].

It is obvious that calorie restriction induces reduction of body weight and fat similar to physical exercise. If the body weight is reduced to 5% or more, this reduces the risk factors for CVD, that is, hypertension and dyslipidemia, and diabetes [51]. When being obese during menopause, the diet should provide a low amount of calories but not below 800 Kcal/day [52]. Whatever the diet is, the adherence to the diet is the most important factor for the success, independently from the nutrient composition. Ideally the diet should try to avoid the loss of proteins, promoting the use of fat as source of energy. If the diet is low in carbohydrate, mono- and polyunsaturated fat and protein from fish, nuts, and legumes should be suggested.

Regarding antiobesity drugs, these compounds are substances that suppress appetite and give the sense of satiety, increasing the metabolism but mainly interfering on the absorption of the nutrients of the food. Among these substances, there are orlistat, sibutramine, and rimonabant. All of them have been demonstrated to improve body weight, but only one (orlistat) is now available, being sibutramine and rimonabant withdrawn due to severe side effects. Obviously natural remedies can be helpful such as herbal preparations and can be used as supplements to aid weight loss [13]. Last but not least important to mention is metformin. This drug has been approved for the treatment of diabetes, and a great use has been done to control weight gain in young women with obesity and PCOS [38], but only when compensatory hyperinsulinism is present, metformin administration is highly effective on metabolism [53]. Though it cannot be considered as a drug to induce weight loss, metformin is relevant to counteract the risk of diabetes and maintain a lower level of insulinemia [13].

Bariatric surgery should be considered as the last attempt to reduce body weight since it is cost-effective, and it should be proposed only for very obese women. There are various surgical procedures such as the gastric bypass, the vertical banded gastroplasty, the adjustable gastric banding, and the laparoscopic sleeve gastrectomy. When compared, gastric bypass was reported to be more effective than the others [13].

16.4   Cardiovascular Disease and Menopause

Screening for CVD at regular intervals after menopause is extremely important. This includes measurement of blood pressure, lipids, and perhaps inflammatory markers, BMI, and ascertainment of lifestyle factors such as activity level and smoking status. In addition, a family history of heart disease and stroke is important. Risk assessment tools allow to calculate the 10-year risk of a myocardial infarction based on gender and race for individuals aged 40–79 years [54]. The main risk calculators used are the Framingham model [55] and a new one from the American Heart Association [56]. The latter is also used as part of the algorithm to decide about initiating statin therapy. The main components of these risk models are age, sex, race, total cholesterol, HDL cholesterol, systolic blood pressure, treatment for high blood pressure, diabetes, and smoking status. Interventions to reduce the risk of CVD after menopause include smoking cessation, weight control through diet and exercise, aggressive treatment of elevated blood pressure, and therapies directed at elevated cholesterol and thrombosis risks. The American Heart Association has outlined diet and lifestyle recommendations to reduce CVD, resulting in better population health. The prevailing belief is that statins reduce CHD events and all-cause mortality under primary and secondary prevention conditions in women and men. However, careful examination and meta-analyses of randomized controlled trial (RCT) data do not provide clear evidence that statins reduce CHD events or all-cause mortality in women under primary prevention conditions. The sex-specific effects are similar for aspirin. In meta-analyses of primary CHD prevention trials, aspirin significantly reduced myocardial infarction (MI) by approximately 32%, with a null effect on stroke in men, whereas, in women, aspirin had a null effect on MI but significantly reduced ischemic stroke by approximately 17% [57]. The primary CHD prevention trials and sex-specific meta-analyses of primary prevention trials show no evidence that aspirin therapy relative to placebo reduces CHD events or all-cause mortality in women. Evidence has clearly established a link between the menopause and increased cardiovascular risk. Estrogen deficiency, which is responsible for the vasomotor and urogenital symptoms and osteoporosis in menopausal women, is also responsible for changes in metabolism and physiology to a more android pattern. The European Society of Hypertension–European Society of Cardiology guidelines recommended increasing physical activity, stopping smoking, and maintaining moderate alcohol consumption: the first interventions are lifestyle change such as changes in diet can also have a favorable effect on dyslipidemia. Many women will require pharmacological intervention with the use of antihypertensives to reduce blood pressure and statins to improve LDL cholesterol profiles, but statins have only a moderate beneficial effect on HDL cholesterol. According to the most recent guidelines of Menopause International Society, personal and familial risk of CVD, stroke, and VTE should be considered before starting MHT. For healthy symptomatic women aged younger than 60 years or who are within 10 years of menopause onset, the more favorable effects of MHT on CHD and all-cause mortality should be considered against potential rare increases in risks of breast cancer, VTE, and stroke. However, FDA doesn't indicate MHT for primary or secondary cardioprotection. Women who initiate MHT when aged older than 60 years and/or who are more than 10 years, and clearly by 20 years, from menopause onset are at higher absolute risks of CHD, VTE, and stroke than women initiating MHT in early menopause.

16.5   Conclusions

Prevention of weight gain and lipid metabolic disorder is important components in the healthcare of postmenopausal women. Numerous studies have attempted to understand the metabolic consequences of MHT use and define the effects of different MHT regimens. With the aging of world population, the health issue of postmenopausal women has been an unprecedented concern. Obesity is associated with a decline of lifespan. Especially, the increased risk of weight gain, central accumulation of body fat, and energy metabolism disorders during the menopausal transition lead to further CVD and rise of overall mortality in women. An early intervention of MHT perimenopause is recommended, which may control the energy metabolic homeostasis and increase the average life expectancy (Fig. 16.2). More studies are

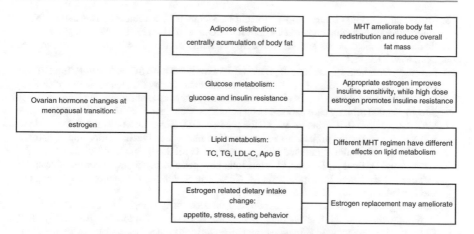

Fig. 16.2 An overview of the metabolic changes at the menopausal transition

necessary to characterize the complex effects of ovarian hormone on the energy metabolism, in which multiple organs and systems are involved.

Conflicts of Interest   No conflicts of interest to disclose.

References

1. Gold EB, Bromberger J, Crawford S, Samuels S, Greendale GA, Harlow SD, Skurnick J. Factors associated with age at natural menopause in a multiethnic sample of midlife women. Am J Epidemiol. 2001;153(9):865–74.
2. Dratva J, Gómez Real F, Schindler C, Ackermann-Liebrich U, Gerbase MW, Probst-Hensch NM, Svanes C, Omenaas ER, Neukirch F, Wjst M, Morabia A, Jarvis D, Leynaert B, Zemp E. Is age at menopause increasing across Europe? Results on age at menopause and determinants from two population-based studies. Menopause. 2009;16(2):385–94.
3. Kriplani A, Banerjee K. An overview of age of onset of menopause in northern India. Maturitas. 2005;52(3–4):199–204.
4. Lobo RA, Davis SR, De Villiers TJ, Gompel A, Henderson VW, Hodis HN, Lumsden MA, Mack WJ, Shapiro S, Baber RJ. Prevention of diseases after menopause. Climacteric. 2014;17(5):540–56.
5. Manson JE, Chlebowski RT, Stefanick ML, Aragaki AK, Rossouw JE, Prentice RL, Anderson G, Howard BV, Thomson CA, LaCroix AZ, Wactawski-Wende J, Jackson RD, Limacher M, Margolis KL, Wassertheil-Smoller S, Beresford SA, Cauley JA, Eaton CB, Gass M, Hsia J, Johnson KC, Kooperberg C, Kuller LH, Lewis CE, Liu S, Martin LW, Ockene JK, O'Sullivan MJ, Powell LH, Simon MS, Van Horn L, Vitolins MZ, Wallace RB. Menopausal hormone therapy and health outcomes during the intervention and extended poststopping phases of the Women's Health Initiative randomized trials. JAMA. 2013;310(13):1353–68.
6. Wellons M, Ouyang P, Schreiner PJ, Herrington DM, Vaidya D. Early menopause predicts future coronary heart disease and stroke: the multi-ethnic study of atherosclerosis. Menopause. 2012;19(10):1081–7.
7. Flegal KM, Carroll MD, Ogden CL, Curtin LR. Prevalence and trends in obesity among US adults, 1999–2008. JAMA. 2010;303(3):235–41.

8. Genazzani AD, Vito G, Lanzoni C, Strucchi C, Mehmeti H, Ricchieri F, Mbusnum MN. La Sindrome Metabolica menopausale. Giorn It Ost Gin. 2005;11(12):487–93.
9. Ibrahim M. Subcutaneous and visceral adipose tissue: structural and functional differences. Obes Rev. 2010;11:11–8.
10. Balkau B, Deanfield JE, Després JP, Bassand JP, Fox KA, Smith SC Jr, Barter P, Tan CE, Van Gaal L, Wittchen HU, Massien C, Haffner SM. International day for the evaluation of abdominal obesity (IDEA): a study of waist circumference, cardiovascular disease, and diabetes mellitus in 168,000 primary care patients in 63 countries. Circulation. 2007;116(17):1942–51.
11. Sites CK, Toth MJ, Cushman M, L'Hommedieu GD, Tchernof A, Tracy RP, Poehlman ET. Menopause-related differences in in ammation markers and their relationship to body fat distribution and insulin-stimulated glucose disposal. Fertil Steril. 2002;77:128–35.
12. Genazzani AD, Prati A, Despini G. Metabolic changes and metabolic syndrome during the menopausal transition. In: Birkhaeuser M, Genazzani A, editors. Pre-menopause, menopause and beyond. Cham: ISGE Series. Springer; 2018.
13. Davis SR, Castelo-Branco C, Chedraui P, Lumsden MA, Nappi RE, Shah D, Villaseca P. Writing Group of the International Menopause Society for World Menopause Day 2012. Understanding weight gain at menopause. Climacteric. 2012;15(5):419–29.
14. Lovejoy JC, Champagne CM, De Longe L, Xie H, Smith SR. Increased visceral fat and decreased energy expenditure during the menopausal transition. Int J Obes. 2008; 32(6):949–58.
15. Cagnacci A, Volpe A, Paoletti AM, Melis GB. Regulation of the 24-hour rhythm of body temperature in menstrual cycles with spontaneous and gonadotropin-induced ovulation. Fertil Steril. 1997;68(3):421.
16. Webb P. 24-hour energy expenditure and the menstrual cycle. Am J Clin Nutr. 1986;44:14.
17. Gambacciani M, Ciaponi M, Cappagli B, Benussi C, DeSimone L, Genazzani AR. Climacteric modifications in body weight and fat tissue distribution. Climateric. 1999;2(1):37–44.
18. Roubenoff R, Hughes VA, Dallal GE, Nelson ME, Morganti C, Kehayias JJ, Singh MA, Roberts S. The effect of gender and body composition method on the apparent decline in lean mass-adjusted resting metabolic rate with age. J Gerontol A Biol Sci Med Sci. 2000;55(12):M757–60.
19. Ravussin E, Lillioja S, Knowler WC, Christin L, Freymond D, Abbott WG, Boyce V, Howard BV, Bogardus C. Reduced rate of energy expenditure as a risk factor for body-weight gain. N Engl J Med. 1988;318(8):467–72.
20. Veldhuis JD, Bowers CY. Sex-steroid modulation of growth hormone (GH) secretory control: three-peptide ensemble regulation under dual feedback restraint by GH and IGF- I. Endocrine. 2003;22(1):25–40.
21. Walenkamp JD, Wit JM. Genetic disorders in the growth hormone-insulin-like growth factor-I axis. Horm Res. 2006;66(5):221–30.
22. Peppa M, Koliacki C, Dimitriadis G. Body composition as an important determinant of metabolic syndrome in postmenopausal women. Endocrinol Metabol Syndr. 2012;2:1.
23. Messina G, Viggiano A, DeLuca V, Messina A, Chief S, Monda M. Hormonal changes in menopause and orexin-a action. Obst Gynecol Int. 2013;2013:1–5.
24. Willie JT, Chemelli RM, Sinton CM, Yanagisawa M. To eat or to sleep? Orexin in the regulation of feeding and wakefulness. Ann Rev Neurosci. 2001;24:429–58.
25. Kukkonen JP, Holmqvist T, Ammoun S, Akerman KEO. Functions of the orexinergic/hypocretinergic system. Am J Phys. 2002;283(6):C1567–91.
26. El-Sedeek M, Korish AA, Deef MM. Plasma orexin-a levels in postmenopausal women: possible interaction with estrogen and correlation with cardiovascular risk status. BJOG. 2010;117(4):488–92.
27. Derby CA, Crawford SL, Pasternak RC, Sowers M, Sternfeld B, Matthews KA. Lipid changes during the menopause transition in relation to age and weight: the study of Women's health across the nation. Am J Epidemiol. 2009;169(11):1352–61.
28. Carr MC, Kim KH, Zambon A, Mitchell ES, Woods NF, Casazza CP, Purnell JQ, Hokanson JE, Brunzell JD, Schwartz RS. Changes in LDL density across the menopausal transition. J Investig Med. 2000;48(4):245–50.

29. Matthews KA, Crawford SL, Chae CU, Everson-Rose SA, Sowers MF, Sternfeld B, Sutton-Tyrrell K. Are changes in cardiovascular disease risk factors in midlife women due to chronological aging or to the menopausal transition? J Am Coll Cardiol. 2009;54(25):2366–73.
30. El Khoudary SR. HDL and the menopause. Curr Opin Lipidol. 2017;28(4):328–36.
31. Chen L, Wu M, Zhang S, Tan W, Guan M, Feng L, Chen C, Tao J, Chen L, Qu L. Estrogen-related receptor γ regulates hepatic triglyceride metabolism through phospholipase A2 G12B. FASEB J. 2019;33(7):7942–52.
32. Pulchinelli A Jr, Costa AM, de Carvalho CV, de Souza NC, Haidar MA, Andriolo A, da Silva ID. Positive association of the hepatic lipase gene polymorphism c.514C > T with estrogen replacement therapy response. Lipids Health Dis. 2011;10:197.
33. Ghosh M, Gälman C, Rudling M, Angelin B. Influence of physiological changes in endogenous estrogen on circulating PCSK9 and LDL cholesterol. J Lipid Res. 2015;56(2):463–9. https://doi.org/10.1194/jlr.M055780. Epub 2014 Dec 22. Erratum in: J Lipid Res. 2018;59(11):2253.
34. Persson L, Henriksson P, Westerlund E, Hovatta O, Angelin B, Rudling M. Endogenous estrogens lower plasma PCSK9 and LDL cholesterol but not Lp(a) or bile acid synthesis in women. Arterioscler Thromb Vasc Biol. 2012;32(3):810–4.
35. Baber RJ, Panay N. Fenton a; IMS writing group. 2016 IMS recommendations on women's midlife health and menopause hormone therapy. Climacteric. 2016;19(2):109–50.
36. Godsland IF. Effects of postmenopausal hormone replacement therapy on lipid, lipoprotein, and apolipoprotein (a) concentrations: analysis of studies published from 1974-2000. Fertil Steril. 2001;75(5):898–915.
37. Stevens VL, Wang Y, Carter BD, Gaudet MM, Gapstur SM. Serum metabolomic profiles associated with postmenopausal hormone use. Metabolomics. 2018;14(7):97.
38. Genazzani AD, Ricchieri F, Lanzoni C. Use of metformin in the treatment of polycystic ovary syndrome. Womens Health. 2010;6(4):577–93.
39. Monteleone P, Luisi S, Tonetti A, Bernardi F, Genazzani AD, Luisi M, Petraglia F, Genazzani AR. Allopregnanolone concentrations and premenstrual syndrome. Eur J Endocrinol. 2000;142(3):269–73.
40. Kerchner A, Lester W, Stuart SP, Dokras A. Risk of depression and other mental health disorders in women with polycystic ovary syndrome: a longitudinal study. Fertil Steril. 2009;91:207–12.
41. Genazzani AD, Lanzoni C, Ricchieri F, Jasonni VM. Myo-inositol administration positively affects hyperinsulinemia and hormonal parameters in overweight patients with polycystic ovary syndrome. Gynecol Endocrinol. 2008;24(3):139–44.
42. Puurunen J, Piltonen T, Morin-Papunen L, Perheentupa A, Järvelä I, Ruokonen A, Tapanainen JS. Unfavorable hormonal, metabolic, and inflammatory alterations persist after menopause in women with PCOS. J Clin Endocrinol Metab. 2011;96(6):1827–34.
43. Roussel M, Garnier S, Lemoine S, Gaubert I, Charbonnier L, Auneau G, Mauriège P. Influence of a walking program on the metabolic risk pro le of obese postmenopausal women. Menopause. 2009;16(3):566–75.
44. Martins C, Kulseng B, King NA, Holst JJ, Blundell JE. The effects of exercise-induced weight loss on appetite-related peptides and motivation to eat. J Clin Endocrinol Metab. 2010;95:1609–16.
45. Genazzani AR, Gambacciani M. Effect of climacteric transition and hormone replacement therapy on body weight and body fat distribution. Gynecol Endocrinol. 2006;22(3):145–50.
46. Tommaselli GA, DiCarlo C, Di Spiezio SA, Bifulco CG, Cirillo D, Guida M, Papasso R, Nappi C. Serum leptin levels and body composition in postmenopausal women treated with tibolone and raloxifene. Menopause. 2006;13:660–8.
47. Di Carlo C, Tommaselli GA, Sammartino A, Bifulco G, Nasti A, Nappi C. Serum leptin levels and body composition in postmenopausal women: effects of hormone therapy. Menopause. 2004;11:466–73.
48. dos Reis CM, de Melo NR, Meirelles ES, Vezozzo DP, Halpern A. Body composition, visceral fat distribution and fat oxidation in postmenopausal women using oral or transdermal oestrogen. Maturitas. 2003;46:59–68.

49. Morris DH, Jones ME, Schoemaker MJ, McFadden E, Ashworth A, Swerdlow AJ. Body mass index, exercise, and other lifestyle factors in relation to age at natural menopause: analyses from the breakthrough generations study. Am J Epidemiol. 2012;175:998–1005.

50. Krents AJ, von Muhlen D, Barret-Connor E. Adipocytokine pro les in a putative novel post-menopausal polycystic ovary syndrome (PCOS) phenotype parallel those in premenopausal PCOS: the rancho Bernardo study. Metabolism. 2012;61:1238–41.

51. Douketis JD, Macie C, Thabane L, Williamson DF. Systematic review of long-term weight loss studies in obese adults: clinical significance and applicability to clinical practice. Int J Obes. 2005;29:1153–67.

52. Freedman MR, King J, Kennedy E. Popular diets: a scientific review. Obes Rev. 2001;9(Suppl 1):1–40S.

53. Genazzani AD, Lanzoni C, Ricchieri F, Baraldi E, Casarosa E, Jasonni VM. Metformin administration is more effective when non-obese patients with polycystic ovary syndrome show both hyperandrogenism and hyperinsulinemia. Gynecol Endocrinol. 2007;23:146–52.

54. Collins P, Rosano G, Casey C, Daly C, Gambacciani M, Hadji P, Kaaja R, Mikkola T, Palacios S, Preston R, Simon T, Stevenson J, Stramba-Badiale M. Management of cardiovascular risk in the perimenopausal women: a consensus statement of European cardiologists and gynecologists. Climacteric. 2007;10(6):508–26.

55. Lerner DJ, Kannel WB. Patterns of coronary heart disease morbidity and mortality in the sexes: a 26-year follow-up of the Framingham population. Am Heart J. 1986;111:383–90.

56. Grundy SM, Brewer HB Jr, Cleeman JI, Smith SC Jr, Lenfant C. Definition of metabolic syndrome: report of the National Heart, lung, and BloodInstitute/ American Heart Association conference on scientific issues related to definition. Circulation. 2004;109:433–8.

57. Hodis HN, Mack WJ. The timing hypothesis: a paradigm shift in the primary prevention of coronary heart disease in women: part 1, comparison of therapeutic efficacy. J Am Geriatr Soc. 2013;61(6):1005–10.

Cardiovascular Impact of Metabolic Abnormalities

17

Sophia Tsiligiannis and John C. Stevenson

17.1   Introduction

There are numerous cardiovascular risk factors in women – these can be genetic including family history or related to ethnic origin. They can also be metabolic including diabetes mellitus, dyslipidemia, and hypertension. Lifestyle factors including diet (consumption of fruits, vegetables, and alcohol), smoking, change in body fat distribution, obesity, and exercise (or lack thereof) also contribute with known links to socio-economic status. These risks account for most of the risk of myocardial infarction (MI) worldwide in all age groups for both women and men [1].

The traditional metabolic syndrome is a cluster of risk factors for CVD and type 2 diabetes mellitus (T2DM) which occur more often than by chance alone [2]. Any three of the following five risk factors constitute a diagnosis of metabolic syndrome – elevated waist circumference (population and country specific), elevated fasting triglycerides ≥1.7 mmol/L (or drug treatment for elevated triglycerides), reduced high-density lipoprotein cholesterol (HDLc) <1.3 mmol/L in women (or drug treatment for reduced HDLc), elevated blood pressure systolic ≥130 mm Hg or diastolic ≥80 mm Hg (or antihypertensive treatment), and elevated fasting glucose or ≥5.6 mmol/L (or drug treatment for elevated glucose) [2]. Clustering of three or more risk factors has been shown to be associated with 48% of CHD events in women [3].

S. Tsiligiannis
Chelsea and Westminster Hospital, London, UK

J. C. Stevenson (✉)
National Heart and Lung Institute, Imperial College London, Royal Brompton Hospital, London, UK
e-mail: j.stevenson@imperial.ac.uk

© International Society of Gynecological Endocrinology 2021
A. R. Genazzani et al. (eds.), *Impact of Polycystic Ovary, Metabolic Syndrome and Obesity on Women Health*, ISGE Series,
https://doi.org/10.1007/978-3-030-63650-0_17

Table 17.1 Review of the literature surrounding the effects of the menopause provides evidence for the following metabolic changes occurring at or after the menopause [4]

Lipids	Insulin	Fat distribution	Vascular function	Clotting changes	Hormonal changes
↑ total cholesterol ↑ triglycerides	↑ insulin resistance	↑ android fat distribution	Impaired vascular function	↑ factor VII and fibrinogen	↓ sex-hormone binding globulin
↓ HDLc ↓ HDL2c	↓ insulin secretion				
↑ LDLc particularly in the small dense subfraction	↓ insulin elimination				
↑ lipoprotein (a)					

There are however specific metabolic effects of menopause as shown in Table 17.1.

Many of these changes themselves affect other adverse metabolic risk factors, and an identification of a menopause-specific metabolic syndrome could help guide clinical practice [4].

Preliminary data from the Women's Health Initiative (WHI) trial showed possible early harm from CHD in women receiving combined estrogen and progestogen [5]. Subsequently follow-up data from the WHI published in 2013 showed no detrimental effect of combined HRT on CHD and a significant reduction in events with estrogen-alone HRT initiated below 60 years of age [6].

There is therefore evidence that estrogen therapy may be cardioprotective if started around the time of the menopause (often referred to as the "window of opportunity") [7]. More specifically to reduce CHD and overall mortality, initiation of HRT would be prior to 60 years of age and/or within 10 years of the menopause [8].

The potential improvements in CVD risk in HRT users are in part due to the beneficial effect on lipids, vascular function, and glucose metabolism [9].

17.2   Lipids and Lipoproteins: What Happens in Menopause

Loss of sex steroids with perimenopause/menopause correlates with changes in lipids and lipoproteins which directly increase the risk of CHD [10, 11].

Low-density lipoprotein cholesterol (LDLc) is a key causal factor of atherosclerosis and therefore CHD [12]. There is a positive correlation between menopause and LDLc [13], and there is an increase in more dense LDLc particles with menopause [13, 14].

HDLc is however inversely associated with CHD [15]. Triglycerides are a further independent risk factor for CHD particularly in women [16] of which there are increases with the loss of ovarian function. There is a positive correlation between atherosclerosis and increased lipoprotein (a) [17]. Lipoprotein (a) especially in association with increased LDL levels is another independent risk factor for CHD [18], and menopause results in an increase in lipoprotein (a) levels [19].

A study by Stevenson et al. measured lipoprotein concentrations and fasting serum lipids in 542 healthy non-obese pre- and post-menopausal women aged 18–70 years. Post-menopausal women had significantly higher concentrations of total cholesterol, triglycerides, LDLc, and high-density lipoprotein subfraction 3 cholesterol (HDL3c), while HDLc and high-density lipoprotein subfraction 2 cholesterol (HDL2c) were significantly lower. Most importantly these potentially adverse changes were independent of age and body mass index (BMI) [10]. Furthermore a cross-sectional database analysis of 515 pre-menopausal women and 518 post-menopausal women again showed a more atherogenic lipid profile with lower HDL2c but no difference in HDL3c [11].

A Swedish 19-year follow-up study of 1372 women with no prior cardiovascular disease showed a 1 mmol increase in cholesterol was associated with a 51% increased risk of MI and/or revascularization [20] and a 1 mmol increase in triglycerides was associated with 49% increased risk of MI [1].

17.3   Lipids and Lipoproteins: Effect of HRT on Lipids

All conjugated equine estrogen (CEE) and CEE/medroxyprogesterone acetate (MPA) regimens demonstrate favorable effects on lipid profiles, including reductions in LDLc and increase in HDLc although triglyceride increases have been observed with oral HRT therapy [21]. Godsland analyzed studies published from 1974 to 2000 looking at the effect of HRT on serum lipids. Analysis of 248 studies showed that all estrogen-only regimes raised HDLc and lowered LDLc [22]. This analysis also showed oral estrogens raised triglycerides but transdermal estradiol lowered triglyceride levels. Furthermore the study showed that addition of progestogens has little effect on estrogen-induced reductions in total cholesterol and LDLc; androgenic progestogens blunt the estrogen-induced increase in HDLc, but this effect was not seen with the non-androgenic dydrogesterone [22].

A further study indicated sequential combinations of 1 mg or 2 mg 17β-estradiol with dydrogesterone are associated with long-term favorable changes in serum lipid profile, and again there was no evidence that dydrogesterone compromised the estradiol-induced improvements [23].

The SMART trials were a series of phase-3 trials of a tissue-selective estrogen complex (TSEC), partnering a selective estrogen receptor modulator with an estrogen. CEE 0.45 mg/bazedoxifene (BZA) 20 mg and CEE 0.625 mg/BZA 20 mg were shown to have generally positive effects on most lipid parameters for up to 2 years of treatment although there was some blunting of the estrogen-induced rise in HDLc [24].

A cross-sectional study of 96 women showed post-menopausal women not taking HRT had significantly higher cholesterol, LDLc, and lipoprotein (a) compared to postmenopausal women taking HRT and to premenopausal women [25].

A study conducted over 4 years confirmed common findings of significantly higher total cholesterol, LDLc, and lipoprotein (a) and significantly lower HDLc in postmenopausal women and also demonstrated the serum lipoprotein (a) concentration decreased significantly in women taking CEE and MPA. Results in the transdermal estradiol and MPA group were unchanged [17].

There are several studies evaluating the effect of HRT with transdermal estradiol on serum lipoprotein (a) concentrations; however consistent results are lacking [17]. There is a suggestion that oral estrogen is more effective in lowering lipoprotein (a) concentrations [17]. The greatest decreases in lipoprotein (a) are seen with cyclical CEE (0.625 mg/day) and MPA (5 mg/day or 10 mg/day) [22] and also with cyclical or continuous treatment with oral estradiol (2 mg/day) and norethisterone (1 mg/day) [22].

17.4 Glucose: What Happens in Menopause

Glucose and insulin metabolism are affected by sex hormone deficiency with postmenopausal women becoming both increasingly insulin resistant and hyperinsulinemic. The loss of hormones reduces both insulin secretion and elimination, but insulin resistance increases resulting in a net increase in circulating insulin concentrations. These increased insulin concentrations are frequently found in women and men with CHD [26, 27]. Hyperinsulinemia may increase the risk of CHD by stimulating atherogenesis [28], and insulin propeptides may have a role in this process [29]. Menopausal age (measured in months since menopause) has been shown to be positively associated with plasma insulin concentrations (fasting insulin and postglucose challenge areas under the curve), and this relationship was not found with chronological age and was not confounded by alcohol consumption, physical exercise, BMI, or smoking [30]. This may be due to alterations in the clearance of circulating insulin from the plasma [30].

Insulin resistance and subsequent hyperinsulinemia can also lead to adverse changes in lipids and lipoproteins including an increase in triglycerides and reduction in HDLc and HDL2c [27].

Insulin resistance is also related to hypertension [27] as hyperinsulinemia is correlated with hypertension [31] with Ferrannini et al. showing a direct correlation with the severity of hypertension [31].

Women are more adversely affected by diabetes as demonstrated by a higher incidence of CHD in diabetic women than in their male counterparts [32], and menopause is known to increase the risk of T2DM. Both premature or early menopause have been shown to increase the risk of T2DM [33, 34], and furthermore lower serum estradiol levels in the perimenopause have shown an association with increased risk of T2DM [35].

17.5 Glucose: Effect of HRT on Glucose

Overall HRT in transdermal preparation, CEE, or oral esterified estrogens – alone or in combination with progestogens – reduces insulin resistance [36]. The androgenic progestogens such as MPA [37] and norethisterone acetate [38] have been shown to have adverse effects on glucose and insulin metabolism; however, dydrogesterone DOES not appear to oppose the potentially beneficial effects of estradiol on insulin [39].

17.5.1 Hypertension: What Happens in Menopause

There is a direct correlation between increased blood pressure and CHD death in all age groups [40] and although blood pressure increases with chronological age in both women and men [41], the loss of ovarian hormones results in an increase in blood pressure independent of one's chronological age and BMI [42]. Early menopause is associated with an increased risk of hypertension [43]. A recent systematic review and meta-analysis involving 273,994 women with 76,853 cases of arterial hypertension confirmed women who had early menopause at age <45 years were at higher risk of arterial hypertension than those women with menopause >45 years of age. This finding was not confounded by smoking status, age, BMI, or the use of HRT or oral contraception [43].

There are multiple theories about the pathogenesis of this relationship. It may be due to oxidative stress caused by endothelial dysfunction influenced by increases in vasoconstrictor endothelin 1 (a potent vasoconstrictor and mitogen for vascular smooth muscle cells) and reductions in nitric oxide (NO) which is a vasodilator [44]. The lowering of both estrogen concentrations and the estrogen to androgen ratio are also thought to lead to increased production of angiotensinogen [36]. These factors may therefore contribute to renal vasoconstriction [36, 44].

17.5.2 Hypertension: Effect of HRT on Hypertension

Most studies have shown little effect of HRT on blood pressure. However, HRT containing estradiol with drospirenone has been shown to decrease blood pressure in women who had elevated blood pressure at baseline [45]. This involved a decrease in both the mean systolic and diastolic blood pressures.

17.5.3 Obesity: What Happens in Menopause

Central or abdominal adipose tissue is known as android fat, whereas lower body segment adipose tissue is known as gynoid fat. There is an observed redistribution of body fat with menopause which results in relatively increased android fat and relatively decreased gynoid fat [46]. There is a known association between android fat and higher risk of CHD but no such relationship with gynoid fat [47]. Therefore, there would be an expected increase in CHD risk from the observed changes in body fat distribution with loss of ovarian hormones. Distribution of fat is associated with CHD risk independent of obesity itself. This is likely due to the fact that android fat distribution represents an increase in visceral fat which is known to be linked to increases in free fatty acid fluxes into the portal vein which result in adverse metabolic outcomes. For example, a negative correlation exists between HDLc and HDL2c and android fat mass but a positive correlation with triglycerides [48].

17.5.4 Obesity: Effect on HRT on Weight

Most studies show that overall there is no significant increase in weight with HRT, but there is a beneficial effect on body fat distribution, with a significant reduction in android fat [49].

17.5.5 Inflammatory Markers: What Happens in Menopause

There is a linear relationship between plasma high sensitivity C-reactive protein (CRP) and the risk of ischemic heart disease in the general population [50]. However, there does not appear to be an independent association with menopause in which case there does not seem to be value in measuring this in a clinical setting [51].

17.5.6 Inflammatory Markers: Effect of HRT on Inflammatory Markers

It has been suggested that HRT is associated with an increased inflammatory response, as oral HRT is associated with an increase in CRP. Silvestri et al. investigated this relationship; the results showed that compared to baseline HRT increased CRP but reduced plasma levels of all other markers of inflammation (soluble intracellular adhesion molecule-1, soluble vascular cell adhesion molecule-1, interleukin-6, plasma E-selectin, s-thrombomodulin). Therefore, it was concluded that HRT is associated with an overall decrease in vascular inflammation [52].

17.5.7 Vascular Function/VTE: What Happens in Menopause

As vessels age there are associated arterial stiffening and endothelial dysfunction which are major risk factors for CHD. During the first few years after the menopause there is an increase in carotid artery waveform pulsatility index which reflects increased stiffness/reduced arterial compliance [53].

One study showed a protective effect of endogenous estrogens on endothelial function by measuring acetylcholine induced forearm blood flow responses [54]. Moreau et al. measured endothelial dependent vasodilation (a marker of endothelial function) by brachial artery flow-mediated dilation using ultrasound. Function was highest in the premenopausal group with significantly progressive decrements in perimenopausal women (17% impairment) and postmenopausal women (35% impairment). Adjustment for existing risk factors and vasomotor symptoms did not alter the association [55].

Estrogen is thought to have cardiovascular protective properties. A significant proportion of the beneficial effects that estrogens demonstrate on vasculature are thought to be mediated via direct effects on the vascular wall. Estrogen acts directly on the vascular endothelium to increase nitric oxide (NO) synthase levels and hence the production of NO [56]. It also reduces the release of endothelin-1 [57]. Therefore, the loss of estrogen would be associated with an increase in endothelin-1 and a decrease in endothelial NO resulting in impaired endothelial function and vasoconstriction.

The vascular, neuroendocrine, and physiological changes with flushing also appear to be linked to CHD risk, most likely due to greater adverse changes in vascular and metabolic parameters in symptomatic women [58].

17.6 Vascular Function/VTE: Effect of HRT on Vascular Function

HRT has been shown to restore NO-dependent endothelial function, increase endothelial NO synthase production, and reduce endothelial endothelin-1 release. HRT inhibits calcium channels and enhances potassium-dependent channels thereby promoting vasodilatation, reducing ACE activity, and reducing smooth muscle cell proliferation [59].

The risk of venous thromboembolism (VTE) is increased by oral HRT relative to baseline population risk [6]. Conversely, epidemiological studies have not identified a risk of VTE above baseline population risk with the use of transdermal HRT preparations [60–62]. This is likely due to the fact that transdermal delivery avoids first pass liver metabolism of estrone in the liver which is known to increase thrombin generation [63]. The ESTHER study however demonstrated no significant association between VTE and oral micronized progesterone [64]. The observational studies have also confirmed the importance of the type of progestogen association with estradiol when defining VTE risk [64]. The use of MPA combined with oral estrogen may be associated with increased risk of VTE, and furthermore continuous combined regimes may pose a greater risk than sequential regimes [7].

A recent case control study confirmed that transdermal HRT preparations are not associated with VTE risk. The highest risk of VTE was demonstrated with CEE combined with MPA. In contrast, the only oral combined HRT regimen that did not show a significant increased risk was estradiol plus dydrogesterone [65].

17.7 Conclusion

CHD increases during and after menopause with RCTs, meta-analyses, and observational studies all supporting primary prevention with HRT as a worthwhile approach. Therefore, risk factor assessment for menopausal women is a crucial part of holistic care to ensure minimization of metabolic factors and a subsequent decrease in CVD [66]. This should be done via a multidisciplinary approach (general practitioners, gynecologists, cardiologists, metabolic physicians).

References

1. Yusuf S, Hawken S, Ounpuu S, Dans T, Avezum A, Lanas F, et al. Effect of potentially modifiable risk factors associated with myocardial infarction in 52 countries (the INTERHEART study): case-control study. Lancet (London, England). 2004;364(9438):937–52.
2. Alberti KGMM, Eckel RH, Grundy SM, Zimmet PZ, Cleeman JI, Donato KA, et al. Harmonizing the metabolic syndrome: a joint interim statement of the International Diabetes Federation Task Force on Epidemiology and Prevention; National Heart, Lung, and Blood Institute; American Heart Association; World Heart Federation. Int Circulation. 2009;120(16):1640–5.
3. Wilson PWF, Kannel WB, Silbershatz H, D'Agostino RB. Clustering of metabolic factors and coronary heart disease. Arch Intern Med. 1999;159(10):1104.
4. Spencer CP, Godsland IF, Stevenson JC. Is there a menopausal metabolic syndrome? Gynecol Endocrinol. 1997;11(5):341–55.
5. Rossouw JE, Anderson GL, Prentice RL, et al. Risks and benefits of estrogen plus progestin in healthy postmenopausal women: principal results from the Women's health initiative randomized controlled trial. JAMA. 2002;288:321–33.
6. Manson JE, Chlebowski RT, Stefanick ML, Aragaki AK, Rossouw JE, Prentice RL, et al. Menopausal hormone therapy and health outcomes during the intervention and extended post-stopping phases of the Women's health initiative randomized trials. JAMA. 2013;310:1353–68.
7. Baber RJ, Panay N, Fenton A. 2016 IMS recommendations on women's midlife health and menopause hormone therapy. Climacteric. 2016;19:109–50.
8. Hodis HN, Collins P, Mack WJ, Schierbeck LL. The timing hypothesis for coronary heart disease prevention with hormone therapy: past, present and future in perspective. Climacteric. 2012;15(3):217–28.
9. Lobo RA, Davis SR, De Villiers TJ, Gompel A, Henderson VW, Hodis HN, et al. Prevention of diseases after menopause. Climacteric. 2014;17(5):540–56.
10. Stevenson JC, Crook D, Godsland IF. Influence of age and menopause on serum lipids and lipoproteins in healthy women. Atherosclerosis. 1993;98(1):83–90.
11. Anagnostis P, Stevenson JC, Crook D, Johnston DG, Godsland IF. Effects of menopause, gender and age on lipids and high-density lipoprotein cholesterol subfractions. Maturitas. 2015;81(1):62–8.
12. Ference BA, Ginsberg HN, Graham I, Ray KK, Packard CJ, Bruckert E, et al. Low-density lipoproteins cause atherosclerotic cardiovascular disease. 1. Evidence from genetic, epidemiologic, and clinical studies. A consensus statement from the European atherosclerosis society consensus panel. Eur Heart J. 2017;38(32):2459–72.
13. Campos H, McNamara JR, Wilson PW, Ordovas JM, Schaefer EJ. Differences in low density lipoprotein subfractions and apolipoproteins in premenopausal and postmenopausal women. J Clin Endocrinol Metab. 1988;67(1):30–5.
14. Carr MC, Kim KH, Zambon A, et al. Changes in LDL density across the menopausal transition. J Investig Med. 2000;48:245–50.
15. Emerging Risk Factors Collaboration DA, Di Angelantonio E, Sarwar N, Perry P, Kaptoge S, Ray KK, et al. Major lipids, apolipoproteins, and risk of vascular disease. JAMA. 2009;302(18):1993–2000.
16. McBride P. Triglycerides and risk for coronary artery disease. Curr Atheroscler Rep. 2008;10(5):386–90.
17. Ushioda M, Makita K, Takamatsu K, Horiguchi F, Aoki D. Serum lipoprotein(a) dynamics before/after menopause and long-term effects of hormone replacement therapy on lipoprotein(a) levels in middle-aged and older Japanese women. Horm Metab Res. 2006;38(09):581–6.
18. Danesh J, Collins R, Peto R. Lipoprotein(a) and coronary heart disease. Meta-analysis of prospective studies. Circulation. 2000;102(10):1082–5.
19. Anagnostis P, Karras S, Lambrinoudaki I, Stevenson JC, Goulis DG. Lipoprotein(a) in postmenopausal women: assessment of cardiovascular risk and therapeutic options. Int J Clin Pract. 2016;70(12):967–77.

20. Johansson S, Wilhelmsen L, Lappas G, Rosengren A. High lipid levels and coronary disease in women in Göteborg--outcome and secular trends: a prospective 19 year follow-up in the BEDA*study. Eur Heart J. 2003;24(8):704–16.
21. Lobo RA, Bush T, Carr BR, Pickar JH. Effects of lower doses of conjugated equine estrogens and medroxyprogesterone acetate on plasma lipids and lipoproteins, coagulation factors, and carbohydrate metabolism. Fertil Steril. 2001;76(1):13–24.
22. Godsland IF. Effects of postmenopausal hormone replacement therapy on lipid, lipoprotein, and apolipoprotein (a) concentrations: analysis of studies published from 1974-2000. Fertil Steril. 2001;75(5):898–915.
23. Stevenson JC, Rioux JE, Komer L, Gelfand M. 1 and 2 mg 17beta-estradiol combined with sequential dydrogesterone have similar effects on the serum lipid profile of postmenopausal women. Climacteric. 2005;8(4):352–9.
24. Stevenson JC, Chines A, Pan K, Ryan KA, Mirkin S. A pooled analysis of the effects of conjugated estrogens/Bazedoxifene on lipid parameters in postmenopausal women from the selective estrogens, menopause, and response to therapy (SMART) trials. J Clin Endocrinol Metab. 2015;100(6):2329–38.
25. Abbey M, Owen A, Suzakawa M, Roach P, Nestel PJ. Effects of menopause and hormone replacement therapy on plasma lipids, lipoproteins and LDL-receptor activity. Maturitas. 1999;33(3):259–69.
26. Rönnemaa T, Laakso M, Pyörälä K, Kallio V, Puukka P. High fasting plasma insulin is an indicator of coronary heart disease in non-insulin-dependent diabetic patients and nondiabetic subjects. Arterioscler Thromb a J Vasc Biol. 1991;11(1):80–90.
27. Ley CJ, Swan J, Godsland IF, Walton C, Crook D, Stevenson JC. Insulin resistance, lipoproteins, body fat and hemostasis in nonobese men with angina and a normal or abnormal coronary angiogram. J Am Coll Cardiol. 1994;23(2):377–83.
28. Stout RW. Insulin and atheroma. 20-yr perspective. Diabetes Care. 1990;13(6):631–54.
29. Båvenholm P, Proudler A, Tornvall P, Godsland I, Landou C, de Faire U, et al. Insulin, intact and split proinsulin, and coronary artery disease in young men. Circulation. 1995;92(6):1422–9.
30. Proudler AJ, Felton C V, Stevenson JC. Ageing and the response of plasma insulin, glucose and C-peptide concentrations to intravenous glucose in postmenopausal women. Vol. 83, Clinical Science. 1992.
31. Ferrannini E, Buzzigoli G, Bonadonna R, Giorico MA, Oleggini M, Graziadei L, et al. Insulin resistance in essential hypertension. N Engl J Med. 1987;317(6):350–7.
32. Abbott WG, Lillioja S, Young AA, Zawadzki JK, Yki-Järvinen H, Christin L, et al. Relationships between plasma lipoprotein concentrations and insulin action in an obese hyperinsulinemic population. Diabetes. 1987;36(8):897–904.
33. Shen L, Song L, Li H, Liu B, Zheng X, Zhang L, et al. Association between earlier age at natural menopause and risk of diabetes in middle-aged and older Chinese women: the Dongfeng-Tongji cohort study. Diabetes Metab. 2017;43(4):345–50.
34. Brand JS, van der Schouw YT, Onland-Moret NC, Sharp SJ, Ong KK, Khaw K-T, et al. Age at menopause, reproductive life span, and type 2 diabetes risk: results from the EPIC-InterAct study. Diabetes Care. 2013;36(4):1012–9.
35. Park SK, Harlow SD, Zheng H, Karvonen-Gutierrez C, Thurston RC, Ruppert K, et al. Association between changes in oestradiol and follicle-stimulating hormone levels during the menopausal transition and risk of diabetes. Diabet Med. 2017;34(4):531–8.
36. Salpeter SR, Walsh JME, Ormiston TM, Greyber E, Buckley NS, Salpeter EE. Meta-analysis: effect of hormone-replacement therapy on components of the metabolic syndrome in postmenopausal women. Diabetes Obes Metab. 2006;8(5):538–54.
37. Lindheim SR, Presser SC, Ditkoff EC, Vijod MA, Stanczyk FZ, Lobo RA. A possible bimodal effect of estrogen on insulin sensitivity in postmenopausal women and the attenuating effect of added progestin. Fertil Steril. 1993;60(4):664–7.
38. Spencer C, Godsland I, Cooper A, Ross D, Whitehead M, Stevenson J. Effects of oral and transdermal 17beta-estradiol with cyclical oral norethindrone acetate on insulin sensitivity, secretion, and elimination in postmenopausal women. Metabolism. 2000;49(6).

39. Crook D, Godsland IF, Hull J, Stevenson JC. Hormone replacement therapy with dydroges-terone and 17 beta-oestradiol: effects on serum lipoproteins and glucose tolerance during 24 month follow up. Br J Obstet Gynaecol. 1997;104(3):298–304.
40. Lewington S, Clarke R, Qizilbash N, Peto R, Collins R. Prospective studies collaboration. Age-specific relevance of usual blood pressure to vascular mortality: a meta-analysis of indi-vidual data for one million adults in 61 prospective studies. Lancet. 2002;360(9349):1903–13.
41. Wiinberg N, Høegholm A, Christensen HR, Bang LE, Mikkelsen KL, Nielsen PE, et al. 24-h ambulatory blood pressure in 352 normal Danish subjects, related to age and gender. Am J Hypertens. 1995;8(10 Pt 1):978–86.
42. Staessen J, Bulpitt CJ, Fagard R, Lijnen PAA. The influence of menopause on blood pressure. J Hum Hypertens. 1989;3:427–33.
43. Anagnostis P, Theocharis P, Lallas K, Konstantis G, Mastrogiannis K, Bosdou J, et al. Early menopause is associated with increased risk of arterial hypertension: a systematic review and meta-analysis. Maturitas. 2020;135
44. Coylewright M, Reckelhoff JF, Ouyang P. Menopause and hypertension: an age-old debate. Hypertension. 2008;51(4):952–9.
45. Archer DF, Thorneycroft IH, Foegh M, Hanes V, Glant MD, Bitterman P, et al. Long-term safety of drospirenone-estradiol for hormone therapy: a randomized, double-blind, multicenter trial. Menopause. 2005;12(6):716–27.
46. Ley CJ, Lees B, Stevenson JC. Sex- and menopause-associated changes in body-fat distribu-tion. Am J Clin Nutr. 1992;55(5):950–4.
47. McCarty MF. A paradox resolved: the postprandial model of insulin resistance explains why gynoid adiposity appears to be protective. Med Hypotheses. 2003;61(2):173–6.
48. Stevenson JC, Lees B, Bruce R, Ley C CD. Influence of body composition on lipid metabolism in postmenopausal women. Christ C, Overgaard K Eds Osteoporos 1990, Osteopress ApS Copenhagen. 1990;pp 1837–8.
49. Gambacciani M, Ciaponi M, Cappagli B, Piaggesi L, De Simone L, Orlandi R, et al. Body weight, body fat distribution, and hormonal replacement therapy in early postmenopausal women. J Clin Endocrinol Metab. 1997;82(2):414–7.
50. Zacho J, Tybjaerg-Hansen A, Jensen JS, Grande P, Sillesen H, Nordestgaard BG. Genetically ele-vated C-reactive protein and ischemic vascular disease. N Engl J Med. 2008;359(18):1897–908.
51. Kim HC, Greenland P, Rossouw JE, Manson JE, Cochrane BB, Lasser NL, et al. Multimarker prediction of coronary heart disease risk: the Women's health initiative. J Am Coll Cardiol. 2010;55(19):2080–91.
52. Silvestri A, Gebara O, Vitale C, Wajngarten M, Leonardo F, Ramires JAF, et al. Increased levels of C-reactive protein after oral hormone replacement therapy may not be related to an increased inflammatory response. Circulation. 2003;107(25):3165–9.
53. Gangar KF, Vyas S, Whitehead M, Crook D, Meire H, Campbell S. Pulsatility index in internal carotid artery in relation to transdermal oestradiol and time since menopause. Lancet (London, England). 1991;338(8771):839–42.
54. Taddei S, Virdis A, Ghiadoni L, Mattei P, Sudano I, Bernini G, et al. Menopause is associated with endothelial dysfunction in women. Hypertens (Dallas, Tex 1979). 1996;28(4):576–82.
55. Moreau KL, Hildreth KL, Meditz AL, Deane KD, Kohrt WM. Endothelial function is impaired across the stages of the menopause transition in healthy women. J Clin Endocrinol Metab. 2012;97(12):4692–700.
56. Wingrove CS, Garr E, Pickar JH, Dey M, Stevenson JC. Effects of equine oestrogens on mark-ers of vasoactive function in human coronary artery endothelial cells. Mol Cell Endocrinol. 1999;150(1–2):33–7.
57. Wingrove CS, Stevenson JC. 17 beta-Oestradiol inhibits stimulated endothelin release in human vascular endothelial cells. Eur J Endocrinol. 1997;137(2):205–8.
58. Sturdee DW, Hunter MS, Maki PM, Gupta P, Sassarini J, Stevenson JC, et al. The menopausal hot flush: a review. Climacteric. 2017;20(4):296–305.

59. Stevenson JC. HRT for the primary prevention of coronary heart disease. In: Brinton R, Genazzani A, Simoncini T, Stevenson J, editors. Sex steroids' effects on brain. Heart and Vessels ISGE Series Cham: Springer; 2019. p. 257–64.
60. Canonico M. Hormone therapy and risk of venous thromboembolism among postmenopausal women. Maturitas. 2015;82:304–7.
61. Canonico M, Fournier A, Carcaillon L, Olié V, Plu-Bureau G, Oger E, et al. Postmenopausal hormone therapy and risk of idiopathic venous thromboembolism. Arterioscler Thromb Vasc Biol. 2010;30(2):340–5.
62. Renoux C, Dell'Aniello S, Suissa S. Hormone replacement therapy and the risk of venous thromboembolism: a population-based study. J Thromb Haemost. 2010;8(5):979–86.
63. Mueck AO. Postmenopausal hormone replacement therapy and cardiovascular disease: the value of transdermal estradiol and micronized progesterone. Climacteric. 2012;15(Suppl 1):11–7.
64. Canonico M, Oger E, Plu-Bureau G, Conard J, Meyer G, Lévesque H, et al. Hormone therapy and venous thromboembolism among postmenopausal women. Circulation. 2007;115(7):840–5.
65. Vinogradova Y, Coupland C, Hippisley-Cox J. Use of hormone replacement therapy and risk of venous thromboembolism: nested case-control studies using the QResearch and CPRD databases. BMJ. 2019;364:k4810.
66. Collins P, Webb C, de Villiers T, Stevenson J, Panay N, Baber R. Cardiovascular risk assessment in women - an update. Climacteric. 2016;19(4).

How to Prevent, Diagnose, and Treat Gynecological Cancer in PCO Patients?

18

Catherine Galopin, Geraldine Brichant, Linda Tebache, and Michelle Nisolle

18.1 Introduction

Polycystic ovaries syndrome (PCOS) was first described in 1935 by Stein and Leventhal. Fourteen years later, an association between PCOS and endometrial cancer (EC) in young women was published by Speert [1]. When analyzing the risks of cancer in patients with micropolycystic ovaries, the most common is endometrial cancer. The meta-analysis of Haoula et al. in [2] includes five studies with a total of 4605 patients. Eighty-eight women had PCOS of whom 47 had EC and 4517 did not have PCOS of whom 773 had endometrial cancer. According to these results, women with PCOS are about three times more likely at risk to develop endometrial cancer (OR: 2.89). If analyzing results depending on the age, patients under the age of 50 would have an even greater risk. This translates into a 9% lifetime risk of EC in Caucasian women with PCOS compared with 3% in women without it. Although most women (91%) with PCOS will not develop endometrial cancer, this study has shown that they are at higher risk. The same year, Fauser et al. [3] confirmed that there were moderate quality data to support that women with PCOS have a 2.7-fold (95% CI 1.0–7.3) increased risk for EC (level B). Most EC are well differentiated and have a good prognosis. Limited data suggest that PCOs women are not at increased risk of ovarian cancer nor breast cancer (level B).

In [4], Barry et al., analyzing five studies comparing women with PCOS and non-PCOS, demonstrated that PCOS patients are at greater risk of presenting EC (OR = 2.79) and even greater if under the age of 54 (OR: 4.05). Compiling results from three comparative studies, no increased risk of ovarian cancer was found in women suffering from PCOS (OR 1,41). Subsequent analysis showed that women under the age of 54 had an increased OR of 2.52. However, this difference was

C. Galopin · G. Brichant · L. Tebache · M. Nisolle (✉)
Department of Gynecology and Obstetrics, University of Liège, Liège, Belgium
e-mail: michelle.nisolle@uliege.be

© International Society of Gynecological Endocrinology 2021
A. R. Genazzani et al. (eds.), *Impact of Polycystic Ovary, Metabolic Syndrome and Obesity on Women Health*, ISGE Series,
https://doi.org/10.1007/978-3-030-63650-0_18

found in a single study, and the authors concluded that no significant evidence showed an increased risk of ovarian cancer in PCOS patients.

Concerning the risk of breast cancer, it was evaluated in three comparative studies, and no significant differences could be shown whether analyzing the entire group population (OR 0.95) or the less than 54 years patients group (OR 0.78).

Concerning the other gynecological cancers, there is insufficient evidence to evaluate any association between PCOS and vaginal cancer, vulvar cancer, cervical cancer, and uterine leiomyosarcoma.

18.2 Endometrial Cancer Overview

Endometrial cancer is the most common gynecological cancer in North American and European women. It's the fourth most common cancer in women, 319,500 cases and 76,000 deaths being reported worldwide annually. The incidence rate has increased by ± 50% in Europe since the early 1990s. The EC is predominant in postmenopausal women as the peak incidence is observed between 50 and 60 years. Concerning the histological classification two types of EC are described, the type 1 endometrioid representing 80–90% of all EC. Type 1 EC is estrogen-induced, has a good prognosis, and is associated to PCOS. A pre-invasive status with an atypical hyperplasia is described. On the contrary, type 2 EC (serous, clear cell, mucinous) is estrogen-independent and of poor prognosis.

Clinical presentation of EC is usually the presence of AUB which allows the diagnosis at an early stage. The prognosis is related to the histology and to the stage. The estimated overall 5-year survival rate is 81.5% and 97.6% in cases of well-localized endometrioid EC [5]. Risk factors for developing EC include PCOS, obesity, nulliparity, type-2 diabetes, insulin resistance, tamoxifen use, and exposure to unopposed estrogen therapy.

18.3 Etiological and Molecular Mechanisms

The understanding of molecular mechanisms is needed to develop clinical strategies to prevent EC in PCOS. The type 1 EC is explained by an imbalance between estrogen and progesterone. The cumulative exposure to estrogen is higher in case of early menarche, late menopause, or nulliparity. The estrogen is increased for the age in postmenopausal obesity. In PCOS, there is an insufficient progesterone secretion due to a chronic anovulation leading to a prolonged endometrial exposure to unopposed estrogen. The latter promotes endometrial growth and proliferation with a higher probability of random mutations in oncogenes and tumor suppressor genes.

The World Health Organization (WHO) and the International Society of Gynecological Pathologists (ISGP) established a pathological classification of atypical endometrial hyperplasia (EH). The simple EH is similar to a normal proliferative endometrium with an abnormal glandular growth despite the presence of a normal gland-to-stroma ratio. The complex EH is characterized by an increased complexity in the glandular architecture, with glandular proliferation and a consequent disproportion in the gland-to-stroma ratio, with the former increasing relative to the latter. The presence of cytological atypia identifies the third and fourth categories: simple atypical EH and complex atypical EH.

Yang et al. [6] developed an interesting animal model to understand the link between endometrial hyperplasia (EH), endometrial cancer, and hormonal stimulation. They induced EH in a mouse model with a subcutaneous estradiol-sustained releasing pellet. The authors were able to demonstrate the assessment of local and systemic hormone effects after 2, 4, 6, 8, and 10 weeks post-E2 stimulation and the evolution towards EC.

Four weeks after the implantation of E2 pellets, disordered proliferative endometrium was observed, non-atypical hyperplasia after 6 weeks, localized atypical endometrial hyperplasia after 8 weeks, and diffuse atypical hyperplasia after 10 weeks. The expression of hormone receptors was found to be altered as EH progressed to atypical hyperplasia. An increase in nuclear PR expression was noted after E2 expression, but a total loss in PR occurred in some endometrial glands when simple EH was observed. The expression of nuclear ER was found to be reduced in disordered proliferation but increased when EH progressed to atypical EH. This animal model, easily reproducible, could be used for testing therapeutic agents to investigate and to improve the management of EH which remains a serious health problem.

Insulin resistance reduces receptor binding and decreases insulin receptor-mediated transduction. This leads to a hyperinsulinemia which causes an inhibition in the liver of sex hormone binding globulin (SHBG) secretion. This decrease of SHBG reduces the production of insulin growth factor binding protein (IGFBP) which causes exaggerated bioactivity of insulin growth factors (IGF). All these mechanisms promote the ovarian steroidogenesis and the androgen production in theca cells.

PCOS women are often obese, and it has been demonstrated that obesity is strongly related to endometrial carcinoma risk [7]. Of all obesity-related cancers occurring among women, higher body mass index (BMI) is most strongly related to EC risk. The obese women have a two- to five-fold elevated risk of EC. This applies to both menopausal and premenopausal patients. The relative risk of EC is 1.59 times higher for each 5 kg/m^2 increase in BMI [8]. Each 5 kg increase in adult weight gain was associated with a 39% increase in postmenopausal EC risk among non-users of menopausal hormones.

Different hypotheses have been suggested. First, postmenopausal obesity is associated with an increased circulating estrogens rate due to aromatization of androgens in adipose tissue and to higher levels of bioavailable estrogen because of decreased SHBG levels. Premenopausal obesity may lead to a higher frequency of anovulatory cycles and relative progesterone deficiency when compared to the high estrogen levels. Second, the obesity contributes to insulin resistance and vice versa. Finally, obesity also induces non-hormonal modifications such as inflammation, immune dysfunction, and cell signaling pathway errors contributing to an increased risk of endometrial cancer [5].

18.4   Prevention of Endometrial Cancer

The perfect prevention for endometrial hyperplasia and endometrial cancer is not known. The recommendations established in 2018 by the international evidence-based guideline for the assessment and management of PCOS claimed that "The health professionals and women with PCOS should be aware of a 2- to 6- fold increase risk of endometrial cancer, which often presents before menopause; however, absolute risk of endometrial cancer remains relatively low. The health professionals require a low threshold for investigation of endometrial cancer in women with PCOS or a history of PCOS, with investigation by transvaginal ultrasound and/or endometrial biopsy recommended with persistent thickened endometrium and/or risk factors including prolonged amenorrhea, abnormal vaginal bleeding or excess weight. However, routine ultrasound screening of endometrial thickness in PCOS is not recommended."

18.5   Place of Hormonal Prevention

A pragmatic approach could include combined oral contraceptive (COC) or progestin therapy in patients with cycles longer that 90 days [9].

Progestins inhibit proliferative pathways by modulation of endometrial glands' secretory differentiation, inhibition of estrogen receptor function, and endometrial cell mitosis. Progestins are pro-apoptotic and also anti-angiogenic thanks to a stimulation of stromal insulin-like growth factor binding protein-1 (IGFBP-1), which inhibits insulin-like growth factor-1 (IGF-1) expression and activity. This is significant as IGF-1 is proliferative and anti-apoptotic, with increased expression in EH [10].

According to the ESHRE recommendations, specific types or dose of progestins, estrogens, or combination of COC cannot be suggested in adults and adolescents with PCOS. The 35-microgram ethinylestradiol plus cyproterone acetate preparation should not be considered as first-line therapy in PCOS, due to adverse effects such as venous thromboembolic risks (especially in overweight women).

Nevertheless, it is well-known that the women with PCOS taking COC daily for 21 days per month reduce by 50% the risk of EC compared with non-users. The risk reduction is observed after at least 1 year of use. The increasing duration of COC use is significantly related to a greater protection, and this risk reduction after discontinuation is persisting for up to 20 years [5]. Furthermore, COC is associated with a reduction risk of ovarian cancer in all women [11]. The risk reduction is about 20% for every 5 years of COC use. A reduction of 50% occurs after 15 years of use. The benefit is already observed after 1 year of use and remains significant after discontinuation. Other contraceptive methods like injectable contraceptive, implant, or transdermal patch need more studies to be evaluated.

A decrease of the combined postmenopausal hormone therapy use was observed in the United States [12] after the initial women's health initiative (WHI) report in 2002 [13]. This decrease was followed by an endometrial cancer increase, which can be attributed to this hormone therapy decrease. In [14], Chlebowski et al.

evaluated the effect of continuous combined estrogen plus progestin on EC in the WHI randomized trial. Women aged 50–79 years old with normal endometrial biopsy at entry were randomly assigned to once – daily 0.625 mg conjugated equine estrogen plus 2.5 mg medroxyprogesterone acetate (n = 8506) as a single pill or matching placebo (n = 8102).

They observed that the use of continuous combined estrogen plus progestin for 5.6 years in postmenopausal women with normal endometrial biopsy at entry of the therapy resulted in a statistically significant reduction in endometrial cancer incidence [15]. Indeed, the continuous estrogen plus progestin use is associated to a 35% lower endometrial cancer risk compared to non-users. The greatest risk reduction occurred among obese women.

The progestin dose, schedule, and duration have to be taken into consideration in the prevention of EC. Indeed, sequential regimens with fewer days of progestin exposure are less effective in reducing endometrial cancer risk. In 2014, Briton and Felix [16] studied the effect of various hormonal regimens on the risk of developing EC. The data revealed that the use of estrogen plus sequential progestin for less than 10 days per month was linked to a higher risk of EC (OR = 1.32, 95% CI = 1.06 to 1.65), while the progestin sequential use for 10–14 days didn't have an impact, positive nor negative (OR = 1.32, 95% CI = 0.84 to 1.3). The addition of micronized progesterone to estrogen is less associated to breast cancer in some studies. However, the latter association provides few to no protection against EC (HR = 2.42 95% CI = 1.53 to 3.83).

Taking into account that progestogenic potency varies as normethyltestosterone derivatives are more potent on the endometrium than pregnane and micronized progesterone, rules for optimal endometrial protection have been published by Gompel in [17] as follows:

1. Adapt the dose of progestogen to dose/duration of estrogen treatment.
2. Inform the woman of the importance of taking the progestogen pill.
3. Check regularly woman's compliance on the progestogen.
4. Adapt the dose to body mass index.
5. Prefer continuous treatment rather than sequential.

18.5.1 Place of Weight Control

It has been clearly demonstrated that obesity has a linear relationship with all cancer types [7]. As obesity and an increased BMI are strongly associated with the incidence and mortality of endometrial cancer, the weight control is very important in the prevention of EC. A moderate physical activity is associated with 20–30% reduction in EC risk. An increase of 1 h a week in physical activity is related to a 5% lower risk of EC. The benefits of physical activity are multiple: weight control, increase in SHBG levels leading to less bioavailable estrogen, decrease of inflammation, reducing adipose storages, improving insulin sensitivity, and also immune function.

18.5.2 Place of Metformin

Metabolic syndrome, a triad including obesity, hyperinsulinemia, and diabetes, is commonly observed in PCOS women and seems to be the key mechanism of EC pathogenesis. Metformin is an insulin sensitizer agent and could have a chemo-protective, anti-proliferative effect and could also increase the expression of proges-terone receptor.

Metformin directly activates adenosine monophosphate (AMP)-activated protein kinase (AMPK) via oxidative phosphorylation inhibition which reduces adenosine triphosphate (ATP). Metformin also promotes AMPK activation by liver kinase B1 (LBKI), and murine models have shown that this AMPK activation inhibits cancer incidence [18].

Metformin is safe, widely available, licensed for type-2 diabetes and may help to lose weight. It has been shown to be of value in reversing endometrial hyperplasia in both animal and human studies and could therefore be used to prevent EC in PCOS. In [19], Shafiee et al. summarized the literature and identified only three human studies including five patients with regression of atypical endometrial hyper-plasia. According to the Cochrane Database of Systematic Reviews of [20], there is no evidence to support or not the use of Metformin alone or in association with progestins for the treatment of EH.

18.6 Diagnosis of Endometrial Hyperplasia and Cancer

The average age at diagnosis is 62 years with a peak of incidence from 50 to 60 years of age. AUB is the cardinal symptom in peri- or postmenopausal women. The diag-nosis can also be made on cervical cytology or can be an incidental finding on imag-ing (transvaginal ultrasound, TVUS).

TVUS is the first-line imaging modality used to examine clinical cases consid-ered suspicious for endometrial hyperplasia. There is a high sensitivity in the mea-surement of endometrial thickness in the longitudinal plane of the scan. The thresholds used are the following: 4 mm in postmenopausal women and 12 mm in childbearing age women. Indeed, in postmenopausal women an endometrial thick-ness of more than 4 mm has an 85% positive predictive value for endometrial anom-alies, with 96% of specificity and 100% of sensitivity [5].

In [21], Park et al. established predictable clinical factors for endometrial disease in women with PCOS. As described earlier, endometrial disease includes several stages of evolution: simple hyperplasia, complex hyperplasia (with or without cyto-logic atypia), and adenocarcinoma. This study performed in a series of 117 women with PCOS demonstrated that in predicting endometrial disease, an endometrial thickness >8.5 mm has a 77.8% sensitivity and 56.7% specificity. Moreover, age >25.5 years has a 70.4% sensitivity and 55.6% specificity. It is important to note that in their series the incidence of endometrial disease was as high as 23.1%, including EH in 21.4% and EC in 1.7% of cases.

Office hysteroscopy is a very good method to evaluate the endometrium with a direct view of the cavity and the possibility of performing biopsies. The no-touch procedure makes examination more comfortable for patients. The principal morphological criteria serving as hysteroscopic predictors of endometrial hyperplasia (78% of sensitivity) are inhomogeneous polypoid or papillary endometrial thickening (focal or diffuse), abnormal vascular patterns, and presence of glandular cysts or glandular outlets demonstrating abnormal architectural features (thickening, irregular gland density, dilatation). It should be noted that these criteria have not been defined based on scientific evidence resulting from controlled randomized clinical trials, but rather stem from retrospective trials published between 1987 and 1996 [22]. Each of the following hysteroscopic criteria can reasonably be linked to an endometrial hyperplasia context. However, taken individually, each of them is entirely unspecific. Some specific hysteroscopic features suggestive of an endometrial malignancy are also described: whitish or green-gray coloration, areas of necrosis, hemorrhage and microcalcifications, atypical vascularization, irregular or ulcerated surface, and soft consistency (Figs. 18.1 and 18.2).

Endometrial biopsy performed during office hysteroscopy or operative hysteroscopy is required if a woman has persistent post-menopausal bleeding or abnormal menstrual bleeding regardless the endometrial thickness.

Specifically, in women at high risk of developing EC, such as Lynch syndrome or Cowden disease, the screening is recommended at 30 years old by evaluating the endometrial thickness by TVUS and also by performing an endometrial biopsy [5].

Very recently, the risk factors for EC or EH in adolescents and women 25 years old or younger have been described, demonstrating that PCOS was frequently associated to endometrial pathologies such as complex EH with or without atypia and also EC. This study pointed out the importance of endometrial evaluation in young patients suffering from abnormal uterine bleeding [23].

Fig. 18.1 Office hysteroscopy: simple endometrial hyperplasia

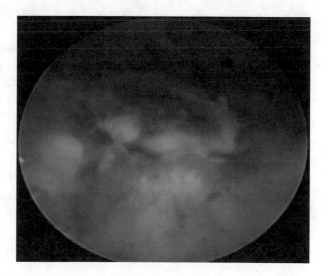

Fig. 18.2 Office
hysteroscopy:
endometrioid tumor
grade III

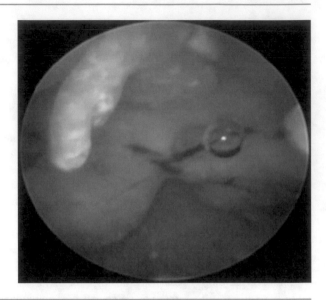

18.7 Risk of Progression of Endometrial Hyperplasia

The risk of progression of simple EH is low as 80% of cases will regress spontaneously. Simple EH is associated with 3% rate of progression to complex EH and 8% to simple atypical EH. The risk of progression of atypical EH to EC is estimated at 52% [24].

18.8 Treatment of Endometrial Hyperplasia and Cancer

18.8.1 Endometrial Hyperplasia

The treatment options for EH depend on patient's age, the presence of cytological atypia, and the desire of pregnancy. EH without atypia responds well to several progestins such as medroxyprogesterone acetate, megestrol acetate, levonorgestrel, and norethisterone acetate. A systematic review and meta-analysis of RCT comparing the administration of oral progestins versus the levonorgestrel-releasing intra-uterine system for non- atypical EH demonstrated better therapeutic effects of LNG-IUS at 3, 6, 12, and 24 months [25].

Surgical procedures are favored in cases of EH with atypia especially if there is no desire of fertility. Conservative treatment by using endometrial ablation is possible only in simple and complex non-atypical EH. If atypical EH is diagnosed in postmenopausal women, hysterectomy with concomitant bilateral salpingo-oophorectomy is recommended.

18.8.2 Endometrial Cancer

The current standard management of endometrial cancer is surgery with total hysterectomy with or without oophorectomy. Depending on the stage of the disease, radical hysterectomy will be performed (total hysterectomy with a pelvic and para-aortic lymphadenectomy). If there is an advanced pathologic stage, an adjuvant therapy is needed with radiation, vaginal brachytherapy, and/or chemotherapy.

The steady increase in EC cases among young women of reproductive age means that a nonsurgical management is needed. A fertility-sparing therapy is possible with oral progestins or levonorgestrel-releasing intrauterine system. The fertility-sparing therapy was studied [26] with 34 observational studies involving 408 patients with early clinical stage and well-differentiated EC (group 1) and 141 patients with atypical complex EH (group 2). The pooled regression rate was 76.2% in the group 1 and 85.6% in the group 2. The relapse rate was 40.6% in the group 1 and 26% in the group 2. The live birth rate was 28% in the group 1 and 26.3% in the group 2. During the follow-up, 3 to 4% of ovarian malignancies (concurrent or metastatic) have been diagnosed. A progression of disease to higher than stage 1 has been observed in 2% and 2 deaths have been reported. For the group 2, the regression has been better with the LNG-IUS than with the oral progestagens. This systematic review and meta-analysis established essential conditions for the successful completion of this treatment. The duration of the treatment must be at least 3 months and up to 12 months [27, 28]. A repeat biopsy is needed to confirm the regression before a pregnancy. To obtain pregnancy, it is recommended to undertake assisted reproduction treatment in order to maximize the chances and to avoid the prolonged unopposed estrogen period and to minimize the delay for performing hysterectomy. The recommendations are to undergo staging hysterectomy with bilateral salpingo-oophorectomy once the family is complete. The follow-up must last at least 5 years and the risk of relapse should not be underestimated.

18.9   Conclusion

Women with PCOS will about three times more likely develop endometrial cancer, and patients under the age of 50 are at even greater risk. It is difficult to separate the effects of PCOS from its component factors such as obesity and insulin resistance. The prevention consists of COC, progestin or IUD, and hormonal therapy after menopause. There is also a very important role of weight loss and maybe of Metformin. Facing a patient suffering from PCOS, even if it is a young patient, the health professionals should not hesitate to do an endometrial evaluation by transvaginal ultrasound and a biopsy especially if there is a complaint of abnormal uterine bleeding.

References

1. Speert H. Carcinoma of the endometrial in young women. Surg Gynec Obst. 1949;88:332.
2. Haoula Z, Salman M, Atiomo W. Evaluating the association between endometrial cancer and polycystic ovary syndrome. Hum Reprod. 2012;27(5):327–1331.
3. Fauser B, Tarlatzis BC, Rebar RW, et al. Consensus on women's health aspects of polycystic ovary syndrome (PCOS): the Amsterdam ESHRE/ASRM-sponsored 3rd PCOS consensus workshop group. Hum Reprod. 2012;27(1):14–24.
4. Barry JA, Azizia MM, Hardiman PJ. Risk of endometrial, ovarian and breast cancer in women with polycystic ovary syndrome: a systematic review and meta-analysis. Hum Reprod. 2014;20(5):748–58.
5. Ellenson LH, editor. Molecular genetics of endometrial carcinoma, Advances in experimental medicine and biology, vol. 943. Heidelberg: Springer; 2017.
6. Yang CH, Almomen A, Wee YS, et al. An estrogen-induced endometrial hyperplasia mouse model recapitulating human disease progression and genetic aberrations. Cancer Med. 2015;4(7):1039–50.
7. Reeves GK, Pirie K, Beral V, et al. Cancer incidence and mortality in relation to body mass index in the Million Women Study: cohort study. BMJ. 2007;335:1134.
8. Renehan AG, Tyson M, Egger M, et al. Body-mass index and incidence of cancer: a systematic review and meta-analysis of prospective observational studies. Lancet. 2008;371(9612):569–78. https://doi.org/10.1016/S0140-6736(08)60269-X.
9. Teede HJ, Misso ML, Costello MF, et al. Recommendations from the international evidence-based guideline for the assessment and management of polycystic ovary syndrome. Hum Reprod. 2018;33(9):1602–18.
10. Kim ML, Seong SJ. Clinical applications of levonorgestrel-releasing intrauterine system to gynecologic diseases. Obstet Gynecol Sci. 2013;56:67–75.
11. Beral V, Doll R, Hermon C, et al. Ovarian cancer and oral contraceptives: collaborative reanalysis of data from 45 epidemiological studies including 23,257 women with ovarian cancer and 87,303 controls. Lancet. 2008;371:303–14.
12. Hersh AL, Stefanick ML, Stafford RS. National use of menopausal hormone therapy: annual trends and response to recent evidence. JAMA. 2004;291(1):47–53.
13. Rossouw JE, Anderson GL, Prentice RL, et al. Risks and benefits of estrogen plus progestin in healthy postmenopausal women. JAMA. 2002;288(3):321–33.
14. Chlebowski RT, Anderson GL, Sarto GE, et al. Continuous combined estrogen plus progestin and endometrial cancer: the women's health initiative randomized trial. J Natl Cancer Inst. 2016;108(3):djv350.
15. Nwanodi O. Progestin intrauterine devices and metformin: endometrial hyperplasia and early stage endometrial Cancer medical management healthcare. 2017;5(30). https://doi.org/10.3390/healthcare5030030.
16. Briton BA, Felix AS. Menopausal hormone therapy and risk of endometrial cancer. J Steroid Biochem Mol Biol. 2014;142:83–9.
17. Gompel A. Progesterone, progestins and the endometrium inperimenopause and in menopausal hormone therapy. Climacteric. 2018;21(4):321–5. https://doi.org/10.1080/13697137.2018.1446932.
18. Tabrizi AD, Melli MS, Foroughi M, et al. Antiproliferative effect of metformin on the endometrium–a clinical trial. Asian Pac J Cancer Prev. 2014;15:10067–70.
19. Shafiee MN, Khan G, Ariffin R, et al. Preventing endometrial cancer risk in polycystic ovarian syndrome (PCOS) women: could metformin help? Gynecol Oncol. 2014;132:248–53.
20. Clement NS, Oliver TRW, Shiwani H, et al. Metformin for endometrial hyperplasia. Cochrane Database Syst Rev. 2017;10:CD012214. https://doi.org/10.1002/14651858.CD012214.pub2.
21. Park JC, Lim SY, Jang TK, et al. Endometrial histology and predictable clinical factors for endometrial disease in women with polycystic ovary syndrome. Clin Exp Reprod Med. 2011;38(1):42–6.

22. Nappi C, Di Spiezio SA. State-of-the-art Hysteroscopic approaches to pathologies of the genital tract. Tuttlingen: Endo-Press GmbH; 2016. p. 62–6.
23. Rosen MW, Tasset J, Kobernik EK, et al. Risk factors for endometrial Cancer or hyperplasia in adolescents and women 25 years old or younger. J Pediatr Adolesc Gynecol. 2019:1–4.
24. Chandra V, Kim JJ, Benbrook DM, et al. Therapeutic options for management of endometrial hyperplasia. J Gynecol Oncol. 2016;27(1):e8.
25. Hashim HA, Ghayaty E, Rakhawy ME. Levonorgestrel-releasing intrauterine system vs oral progestins for non-atypicalendometrial hyperplasia: a systematic reviewand metaanalysis of randomized trials. Am J Obstet Gynecol. 2015;213(4):469–78. https://doi.org/10.1016/j.ajog.2015.03.037.
26. Gallos ID, Yap J, Rajkhowa M, et al. Regression, relapse, and live birth rates with fertility-sparing therapy for endometrial cancer and atypical complex endometrial hyperplasia: a systematic review and metaanalysis. Am J Obstet Gynecol. 2012;207:266.
27. Pillay OC, Te Fong LFW, Crow JC, et al. The association between polycystic ovaries and endometrial cancer. Hum Reprod. 2006;21(4):924–9.
28. Shafiee MN, Chapman C, Barrett D, et al. Reviewing the molecular mechanisms which increase endometrial cancer (EC) risk in women with polycystic ovarian syndrome (PCOS): time for paradigm shift? Gynecol Oncol. 2013;131:489–92.

Printed in the United States
by Baker & Taylor Publisher Services